HUMAN PITUITARY HORMONES

II

DEVELOPMENTS IN ENDOCRINOLOGY

VOLUME 1

HUMAN PITUITARY HORMONES

Circadian and episodic variations

A Workshop Symposium held in Brussels, Belgium, November 29-30, 1979.
Sponsored by the Commission of the European Communities, as advised by the
Committee on Medical and Public Health Research

edited by

E. VAN CAUTER, Ph. D.
School of Medicine,
Free University of Brussels,
and Thyroid Study Unit,
The University of Chicago

and

G. COPINSCHI, M.D., Ph. D.
School of Medicine,
Free University of Brussels

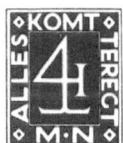

1981

MARTINUS NIJHOFF PUBLISHERS

THE HAGUE / BOSTON / LONDON

for

THE COMMISSION OF THE EUROPEAN COMMUNITIES

IV

Distributors:

for the United States and Canada
Kluwer Boston, Inc.
190 Old Derby Street
Hingham, MA 02043

for all other countries
Kluwer Academic Publishers Group
Distribution Center
P.O. Box 322
3300 AH Dordrecht
The Netherlands

This volume is listed in the Library of Congress Cataloging in Publication Data

ISBN-13:978-94-009-8284-0   e-ISBN-13:978-94-009-8282-6
DOI: 10.1007/978-94-009-8282-6

Publication arranged by :
Commission of the European Communities,
Directorate-General Information Market and Innovation,
Luxembourg

EUR 6857

FOREWORD

During the last decade, circadian and episodic fluctuations
of the plasma levels of pituitary hormones have been demonstrated in man. The interest in the time dependence of the
pituitary secretions partially originates from their close
functional relation with the neuroendocrine mechanisms presumably responsible for the control of the circadian rhythmicity in man.

High frequency blood sampling techniques and specific radioimmunoassays have allowed to describe in detail the variations over the 24-h cycle of the hormonal concentrations in
healthy individuals under basal conditions as well as after
manipulation of external synchronizers such as the sleep-
wake cycle, the dark-light cycle and the feeding schedule.
Alterations in normal hormonal variations have been suggested to play a role in the etiopathogeny of several metabolic and mental diseases, such as obesity or manic-depression.
Important clinical implications regarding treatment and pre-
vention are expected to be developed in the near future.
However, so far, data obtained in different groups are difficult to compare because different hormones were studied
using different protocols and statistical methods. As a
result, unclear or controversial issues are not uncommon.
Also, because of the interdisciplinary nature of biological
rhythm research, studies on 24-h profiles of pituitary hormones have appeared in a wide variety of publications including journals specialized not only in clinical endocrinology and neuroendocrinology but also in psychiatry, chronobiology, sleep or behavioural research and general clinical
investigation. Early in 1977, when this Workshop was proposed to the Committee of Medical Research and Public Health
of the Commission of the European Communities, not a single
reference volume on endocrine rhythms was available. A
unique opportunity to assess the present state of knowledge
and methodology in the field by fostering the discussion
and the exchange of data between leading investigators was
thus provided. The present volume gathers the contributions
of the participants and includes a straightforward trans-
cription of all the discussions. It constitutes an invalua-
ble reference tool for endocrinologists as well as for all
interested in the clinical aspects of biological rhythm
research.

We thank the Committee of Medical Research and Public
Health for evaluation of the Workshop and the Commission of
European Communities for sponsorship. We are grateful to
Mrs. C. Demesmaeker for careful secretarial and editorial
help.

G. COPINSCHI   E. VAN CAUTER

CONTENTS

VIII

QUANTITATIVE METHODS FOR THE ANALYSIS OF
CIRCADIAN AND EPISODIC HORMONE FLUCTUATIONS

Eve Van Cauter

Institut de Recherche Interdisciplinaire, School of Medicine,
The University of Brussels, Belgium and
The Thyroid Study Unit, Department of Medicine, The
University of Chicago, Illinois, USA

INTRODUCTION

The development of sensitive radioimmunoassays and of high
frequency blood sampling techniques has made possible to
measure accurately the variations in plasma levels of pituitary and other hormones over the 24-h cycle. Data generated challenged the concept of hormonal homeostasis and introduced the notion that time of sampling is an important
factor in defining normal and pathological levels. The investigators of hormonal rhythms are faced with the interpretation of data of a new type, namely, time series where at
least two types of temporal variation are present: (1) a
circadian periodicity (low frequency variation); and (2)
short-term, episodic fluctuations (high frequency variation).
Because of the complexity of the data and of their dependence upon time, classical statistical methods currently
used in clinical investigation cannot be generally applied.
The majority of reports on the 24-h profile of blood constituents have therefore been largely descriptive. The
determination of possible correlations between hormonal
variations and sleep stages has also been often based on
visual examination of the data.   The sophistication of
the sampling procedures and of the biochemical determinations in plasma is thus far greater than that of the quantitative

interpretation of the observations. It seems likely that
results well documented by the data could be overlooked or
misinterpreted and that more information could be extracted
from the available data provided suitable quantitative procedures for their interpretation were available.

This paper describes and illustrates methods for the
analysis of 24-h profiles of blood components developed
over the last few years to interpret data collected at the
University of Brussels, Belgium and at the University of
Chicago, USA. Procedures for the analysis of low frequency
(e.g., circadian) components and high frequency (e.g., episodic) components and a preliminary approach to the analysis of correlations between sleep and hormonal variations
will be described separately in the next three sections.

THE CHARACTERIZATION OF THE CIRCADIAN COMPONENT

Several statistical procedures have been combined to derive
a method suitable for the characteristics of 24-h profiles
of hormones and other plasma constituents. The method has
been described in detail elsewhere (1). This presentation
illustrates its potential applications since
its statistical background has been previously discussed (1,
2, 3).

Because 24-h profiles may not present a definite pattern, the first step in the analysis consists of testing
the significance of the observed temporal fluctuations
against the hypothesis of their pure random occurrence.
So-called "white noise" tests are used to determine whether
the profile consists of a random succession of uncorrelated
levels, each data being independent of past and future values, or whether consistent trends, periodicities or ten-
dencies for certain patterns to recur at regular intervals
exist (1).

If the hypothesis of white noise is rejected, a best-
fit pattern describing the low frequency variation of the
profile is built using repeated periodogram calculations.
The periodogram method consists of fitting a sum of sinusoid

functions on the series of data and of selecting those
which contribute significantly to the observed variation.
The estimation of the components found significant with a
minimum probability level of .90 are summed up to build the
best-fit pattern. Such probability levels are standard in
time series analysis (4). Since the method aims at the
description of the circadian or low frequency properties of
the profile, only significant components of periods longer
than 6h00 are retained for inclusion in the best-fit pattern. When bi-circadian (period around 12 h) or tri-circa-
dian (period around 8 h) components are found significant,
the resulting best-fit pattern may exhibit 2 or 3 maxima.
The acrophases and nadirs are, respectively, the times of
occurrence of maxima and minima in the best-fit pattern.
Since a maximum of the best-fit pattern corresponds to consistently elevated values rather than to isolated maximal
levels, acrophases do not necessarily coincide with the
observed maxima. The amplitude of the best-fit pattern is
defined as 50% of the difference between the value at the
acrophase and the value at the nadir and is usually expressed in percent of the overall 24-h mean level. The method
provides confidence intervals for the amplitude, acrophases
and nadirs at a minimal probability level of 90%.

Figure 1A shows a 24-h profile of plasma cortisol in a
healthy male volunteer in whom values were determined at
15-min intervals. The best fit pattern is superimposed and
appears as a continuous smooth line. It described quanti-
tatively the asymmetry of the circadian rhythm of cortisol
with an acrophase at 08:30, declining cortisol levels which
extend over more than 14 hours, a nadir at 00:15, and increasing levels resulting in an early morning maximum lasting no longer than 6 hours. This global circadian pattern
is the result of secretory bursts of variable magnitude and
duration rather than of continuous modulated secretion. In
the case of the profile shown in Figure 1, the 24-h mean of
cortisol is 6.9 μg/dl so that the amplitude expressed in
percent of the 24-h mean is 71%. The confidence interval

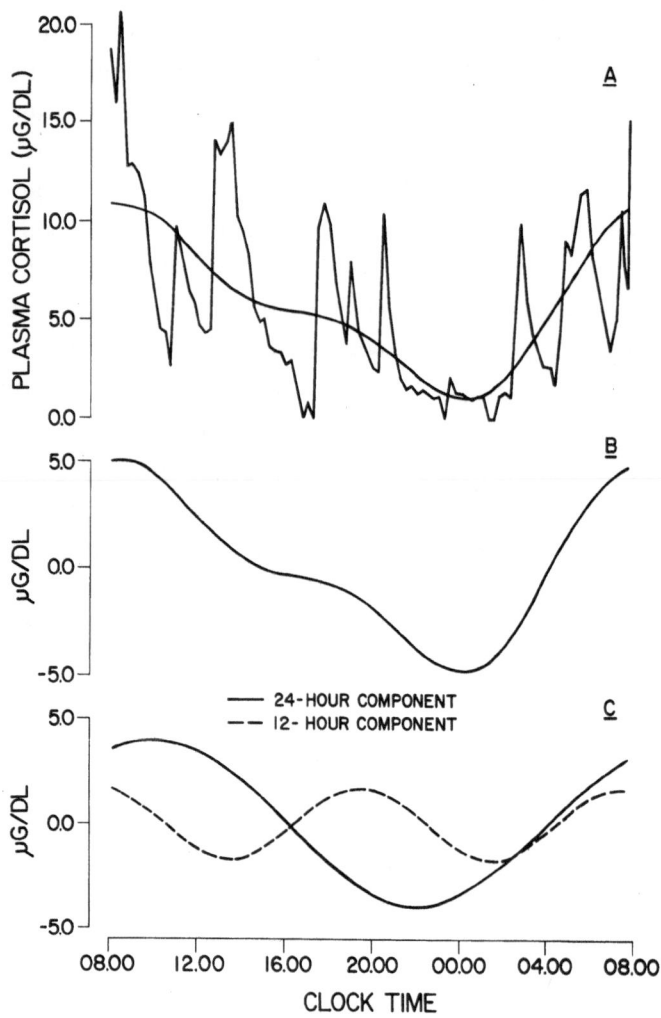

Figure 1: Panel A: Twenty-four hour profile of plasma cortisol
measured at 15-min intervals in a healthy
male. The best-fit pattern is superimposed
as a smooth line.

Panel B: The summing of the two sine waves illustrated in Panel C resulted in this best-fit
pattern which, superimposed to the 24-h mean,
describes the circadian rhythm of cortisol
depicted in Panel A.

Panel C: The 24-h and 12-h sinusoid components found
to contribute significantly to the 24-h
variation of cortisol levels shown in Panel
A by the periodogram method.

for the amplitude is 1.5 µg/dl or 22 % of the mean at a minimum confidence level of 90 %. This means that the probability that the actual amplitude lies between 49 % and 93 % is over 90 %. The best fit pattern, shown separately in Fig. 1B, is the sum of a 24-h and a 12-h sinusoid component, shown in Fig. 1C. The combination of these two sine waves, each fully determined by its amplitude and by its phase, results in the asymmetric pattern fitting the cortisol rhythm. Thus, the best-fit pattern, when described by its amplitude, acrophase and nadir, actually summarizes the information provided by the periodogram method, namely, the periods of the significant components (24-h and 12-h), their amplitudes (4.0 µg/dl and 1.7 µg/dl) and their phases (2h23 and -0h17). While all this information is needed to build the best-fit pattern, the latter provides an objective basis for comparison of 24-h profiles of cortisol recorded under various conditions using only three descriptive parameters of amplitude and of synchronization. The method has withstood the test in the analysis of the effects of jet lag on the pituitary-adrenal periodicity (5).

Fig. 2 shows a 24-h profile of plasma melatonin levels in a control subject determined at 15-min intervals. Details of the protocol and of the melatonin assay appear elsewhere (6). Lights were off from 23:00 to 07:00. In this case, a trimodal best-fit pattern was obtained with acrophases at 10:45, 18:30 and 02:15 and nadirs at 08:00, 14:15 and 21:15. The periods of the underlying components are 23:45, 11:53 and 07:55. The patterns underlines the temporal organization of melatonin levels over the 24-h span in 3 phases, 2 daytime phases corresponding to prolonged secretory episodes in the mid-morning and late afternoon and one large nocturnal increment starting shortly before sleep onset. A "secretory phase" may be defined as the portion of the best-fit pattern comprised between two successive nadirs and characterized by its acrophase, by its value, defined as the value of the best-fit pattern expressed in

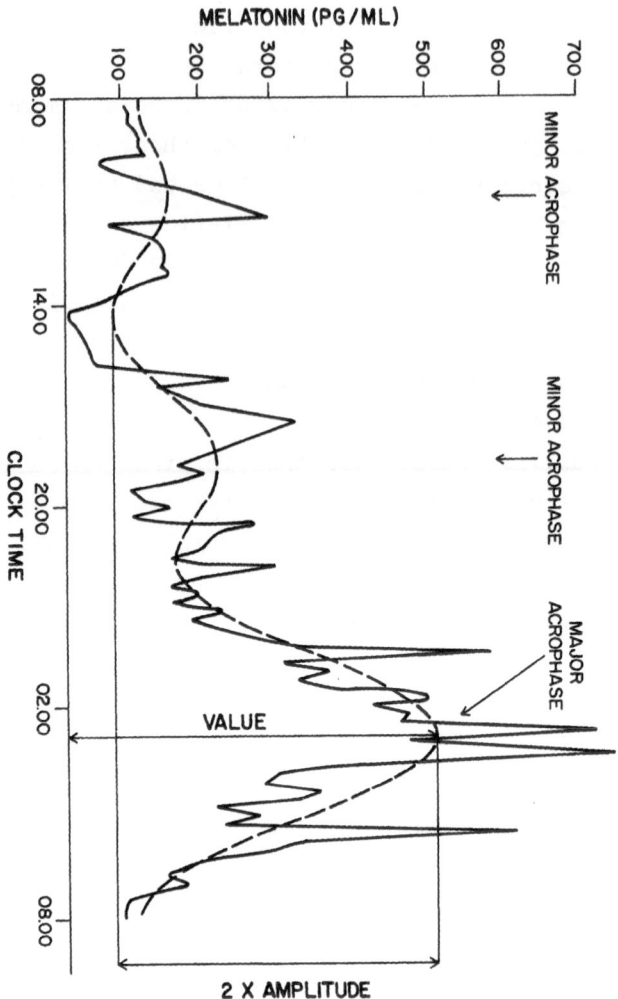

Figure 2 : Twenty-four hour profile of melatonin obtained at 15-min intervals in a healthy male. The best-fit pattern is illustrated in dashed line. The minor and major acrophases are indicated by arrows. The value of the nocturnal acrophase is the value of the best-fit pattern at this acrophase. The amplitude is defined as 50 % of the difference between the maximum and the minimum of the best-fit pattern.

absolute concentration or in percent of the 24-h mean and by its magnitude, which is the difference between the level at the acrophase and the level at the preceding nadir expressed in percent of the level of this nadir. The magnitude of a phase thus describes a relative increase of secretory activity. In the case of the melatonin profile illustrated in Figure 2, the 24-h mean level was 238 pg/ml. The value at the morning acrophase was 170 pg/ml, thus 71% of the 24-h mean and its magnitude was 27% since the value at the preceding nadir (08.00) was 134 pg/ml. The values of the afternoon and nocturnal phases expressed in percent of the 24-h mean were, respectively, 99% and 219% and their magnitudes 133% and 189%. Thus, whereas the value of the nocturnal acrophase is more than twice the value of the largest daytime phase, the relative increase in secretory activity is only 56% higher at night than in the afternoon.

While the nocturnal acrophase of melatonin clearly represents a major secretory event occurring over the 24-h span, whether evaluated in terms of value or in terms of amplitude, in some cases, secretory phases similar on casual examination require the application of objective criteria in order to distinguish "major" and "minor" acrophases. Such criteria are preferably based on comparisons of values rather than magnitudes in order to agree with visual examination. The confidence levels of the best-fit pattern provide such criteria. Indeed, the confidence interval for the amplitude applies as well to the values of the best-fit pattern at the nadirs and acrophases. Those values may be considered to be similar if they do not differ by more than two confidence intervals. Thus, bimodal and trimodal best-fit patterns may have 2 or 3 major acrophases if similar values are observed at these acrophases. In the case of the melatonin profile shown in Figure 2, the confidence interval was 46 pg/ml. The value of the nocturnal acrophase (521 pg/ml) differed from the value at the afternoon acrophase (235 pg/ml) by more than 92 pg/ml so that the profile is indeed characterized by a single major acrophase.

Daytime elevations of plasma melatonin are not uncommon (6, 7). Similar criteria may be applied to nadirs.

The description of the low frequency variation of the profile provided by the best-fit pattern may disclose characteristics overlooked by visual examination. This point is best illustrated by the diurnal phase of PRL secretion. Despite the early observation by Sassin et al. (8) of increased PRL secretion during wakefulness, most subsequent reports on the 24-h profile of PRL suggested that the nocturnal elevation is the sole major secretory event occurring during the 24-h cycle and therefore emphasized the role of sleep in modulating PRL secretion. Figure 3 is drawn from data published by Sassin et al. (8), by Parker et al (9) and by the Brussels group (10) expressed in terms of transverse mean ± SEM. Although as discussed later, this type of data presentation may lead to artefactual interpretations, it was chosen for the sole purpose of comparison. Data were obtained at 1-h intervals in the study by Sassin et al. (panel A), at 20-min intervals in the study by Parker et al. (panel B) and at 15-min intervals in our study (panel C). The number of individual profiles included in the transverse mean is, respectively, 6, 5 and 21. All subjects were healthy young adults. The best-fit patterns for the 24-h transverse profiles are illustrated in dashed lines. Numerical values for the data in panels A and B were estimated from published illustrations. The patterns are strikingly similar with a nadir around noon, a daytime elevation culminating in the late afternoon and a nocturnal rise with an acrophase in the second half of sleep. The concordance between results obtained by the three groups of investigators is amazingly good. Indeed, for panels A, B and C, the values for the daytime acrophase are, respectively 89%, 95% and 90% and for the nocturnal acrophase 166%, 146% and 166%. Whereas, in panel A and C, the magnitude of the nocturnal acrophase corresponds to an increase of more than 100% over the early evening nadir, in panel B, the magnitude of the nocturnal elevation

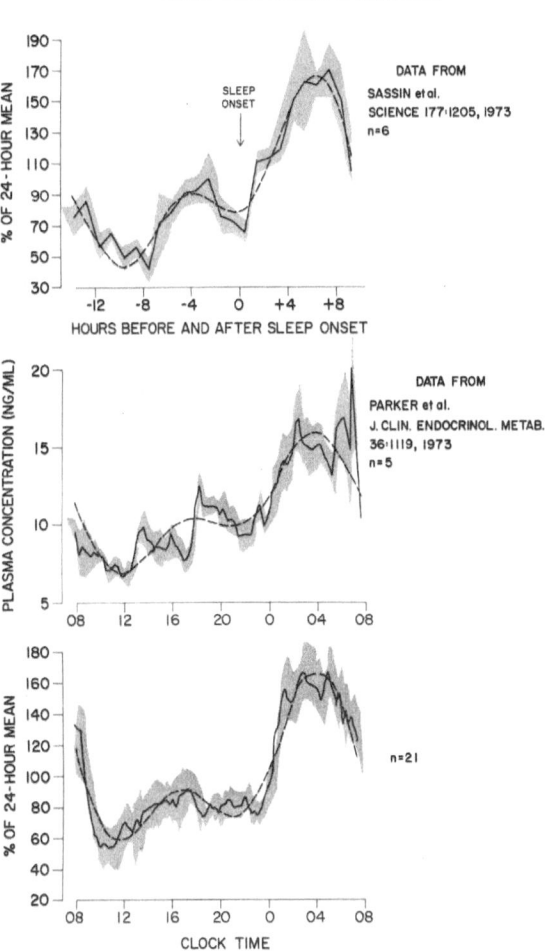

THE 24-HOUR PROFILE OF PROLACTIN

Figure 3: The 24-h profile of prolactin as reported by Sassin et al. (8), Parker et al. (9) and as calculated from a set of 21 individual 24-h profiles obtained in the course of a study by Copinschi et al. (10). Profiles illustrated are transverse mean. The shaded area represents the standard error of the mean above and below the mean. The best-fit patterns are superimposed on the data in dotted lines. Note the bimodality of the patterns and their remarkable similarity.

is only 62%. The calculation of the transverse mean using individual profiles expressed in absolute concentration rather than in percent of the 24-h mean may be responsible for the artefactual smoothness. The relative increases of PRL secretion for the daytime acrophase, as evaluated by the magnitudes, were 49% (panel A), 112% (panel B) and 55% (panel C). When best-fit patterns were calculated for each individual profile included in the transverse mean shown in panel C, a nocturnal acrophase was found significant in all profiles and a daytime acrophase was disclosed in 20 of the 21 profiles. Two profiles were trimodal with 2 acrophases during daytime. Calculating the transverse mean of these 21 individual profiles smoothed the individual variations. Indeed, the average of the individual determinations of the magnitudes was 93% ± 62% for the daytime acrophase and 162% ± 88% for the nocturnal acrophase (mean ± SD).

In fact, the calculation of a transverse mean profile may lead to artefactual interpretation of data on hormonal rhythms. Figure 4 shows hypothetical data to illustrate this point. The results of an imaginary experiment involving the measurement at 2-h intervals of the level of a fictive hormone in 6 volunteers, referred to as A, B, C, D, E and F are presented under the form of individual profiles (left) or under the form of a transverse mean (right). For subjects A, B, C and D, the levels of fictive hormone varied between 90% and 110% of the 24-h mean without any consistent pattern. In contrast, subjects E and F exhibited a sharp increase concomitant with sleep onset. The conclusion of this imaginary experiment is that one-third of the subjects had a sleep-associated elevation of fictive hormone level whereas two-thirds of the subjects had no consistent diurnal variation. However, if the transverse mean of these 6 individual profiles is calculated and illustrated together with the SEM, as is commonly found in the literature, the conclusion that a sharp increase concomitant with sleep onset characterizes the variation of that fictive hormone over the 24-h span might be suggested

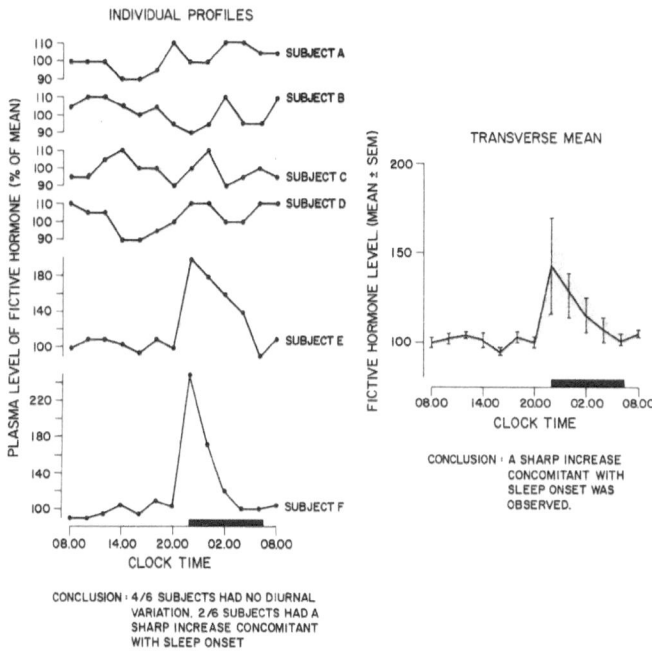

Figure 4: The results of this fictive experiment were simulated in order to illustrate potential artefacts involved in the presentation of the transverse mean profile rather than of individual profiles (see text)

to the casual reader. The example illustrated in Figure 4 constitutes, of course, an extreme case of misuse of the transverse mean. In the case of the 21 PRL profiles included in the transverse mean profile shown in panel C of Figure 3, the calculation of a transverse mean is legitimated by the earlier demonstration of the existence, in each of the individual profiles, or at least, in the case of the daytime secretory phase, in the large majority of them, of the same characteristics as those displayed by the transverse mean. Still, even in this case, the transverse mean partially smoothed the individual variations and provided artefactually lower estimations of the values and magnitudes of the secretory phases. This bias is a consequence of the lack of synchronization among individuals. The choice of an appropriate reference point such as mid-sleep (11) or sleep onset (8) may reduce this bias but is however unlikely to totally eliminate it because of the non-synchronization of episodic secretions. Whereas the calculation of a transverse profile may be a useful way to illustrate the data, the quantitative evaluation of the characteristics of the 24-h pattern under study should be derived from individual profiles.

The best-fit pattern provides means to evaluate objectively the reproducibility of the 24-h variation of a given blood constituent in a set of individuals or in repeated studies of the same individual as well as to demonstrate alterations associated with pathological status or environmental changes. Best-fit patterns may be compared among each other in terms of number and identity of the underlying sinusoidal components. The presence or absence of a given characteristic of a 24-h variation, such as the presence of a daytime acrophase is objectively documented for each profile. Differences in amplitude, acrophases, nadirs and values at the acrophases and nadirs may be considered significant when the corresponding confidence intervals do not overlap. Group statistics may be calculated and compared using standard tests, preferably non-parametric. In particular, the clustering of acrophases or nadirs in a particular portion of the 24-h span may be investigated using the Rao test and other related procedures as described by Batschelet (12).

THE ANALYSIS OF EPISODIC FLUCTUATIONS

A limited number of quantitative characterizations of the "spikes", "peaks", "secretory episodes" or "pulses" observed in 24-h profiles of hormones have been proposed and applied (9, 13-16). No characterization taking into account the variable accuracy of the hormone assay in different ranges of concentration has been proposed so far. This point may be of particular importance since, for several hormones, such as ACTH during certain sections of the 24-h span, the plasma levels are close to the limit of sensitivity of currently available assays. On the other hand, special care has to be taken in evaluating the episodic fluctuations to avoid possible interference with a variation of basal level, such as a circadian rhythm.

Ideally, every "peak", "pulse", "spike" or "secretory episode" observed in a hormonal profile should be first evaluated in terms of its significance with regard to the sensitivity of the assay in the relevant range of concentration. Then, its total duration, duration of its ascending and declining portions and magnitude should be quantified. When relevant, additional parameters such as the corresponding amount of hormone secreted and the apparent "half-life" may be calculated.

The computer program described hereunder has been developed to obtain such a quantitative evaluation of hormonal spikes. The significance of a spike is investigated in terms of relative increments and decrements rather than in terms of absolute concentration. The various steps of the program may be described as follows.

STEP 1 - Input of the Data:
The series of hormonal values is entered together with the limit of sensitivity of the assay and the intra-assay coefficients of variations at different ranges of concentration such as low, medium and high. All samples of a given profile should be measured in the same assay. The possibility of defining sub-sections of the hormonal profile (e.g., sleep and wake periods) in order to characterize separately sub-groups of spikes is offered as an option.

STEP 2 - Preparation of the Data:
Missing data are interpolated linearly. This procedure is limited to isolated data points. Generally, when consecu-

tive data points are missing, the corresponding section of
the hormonal profile should be discarded from the analysis
of episodic variations because of their relatively short
duration as compared to currently used blood sampling intervals. Data below the limit of sensitivity of the assay are
set equal to 50% of this limit. The intra-assay coefficient of variation for a given concentration range actually
represents an average for that range. If the various intra-
assay coefficients of variation were considered as constant
throughout their specific range, abrupt changes in precision of the assay would seem to occur at the limits of the
concentration ranges and so would criteria for significance
of changes in concentration with regard to the precision of
the assay. To avoid this pitfall, a linear interpolation
of the coefficients of variation is performed. An example
of this procedure is illustrated in Figure 5 in the case of
the radioimmunoassay of human melatonin in plasma according
to a modification (17) of the method described by Rollag
and Niswender (18). The limit of sensitivity of the assay
is 20 pg/ml. The coefficients of variation were 17% at 50
pg/ml, 15% at 100 pg/ml and 10% at 500 pg/ml (6). If these
values were considered as representative of a constant average over the ranges 20 - 80 pg/ml, 80 - 200 pg/ml and over
200 pg/ml, quantum jumps in criteria for the significance
of changes in concentration would occur at 80 pg/ml and 200
pg/ml, as illustrated by the horizontal bars shown on
Figure 5. The linear interpolation avoids this pitfall.
In the low concentration range, the linear variation is
extrapolated from 50 pg/ml to 10 pg/ml (50% of the limit of
sensitivity of the assay). If the coefficient of variation
in a specific range of concentration is obtained by averaging several values obtained throughout that range, the same
procedure as illustrated above may be used by ascribing the
average value to the middle of the concentration range.

STEP 3:

A modified profile is obtained by eliminating all non-signi-

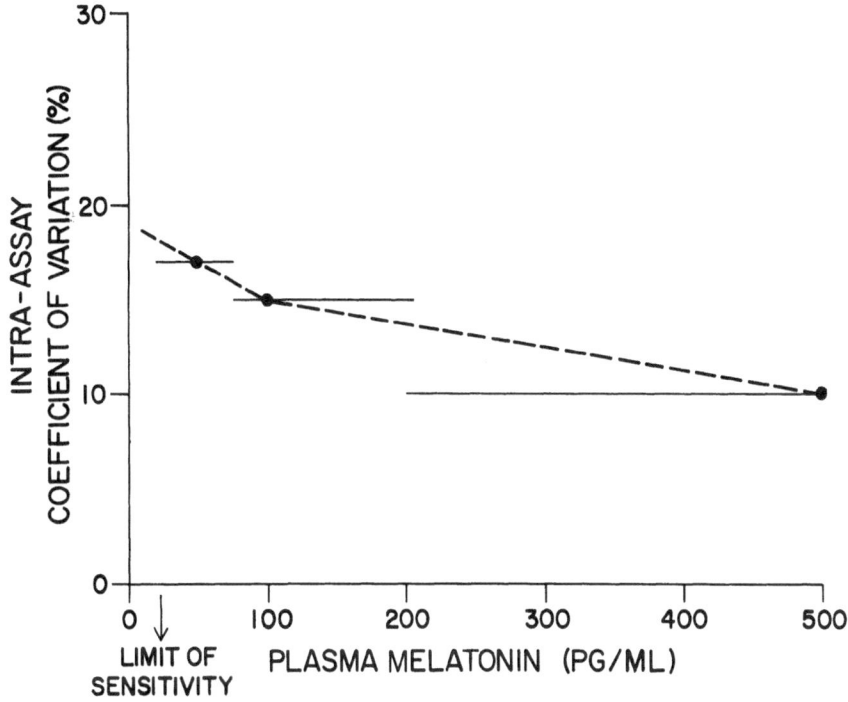

Figure 5: Interpolation of intra-assay coefficient of variation for the radioimmunoassay of human melatonin from specific concentration ranges across the whole physiologic range.

ficant concentration changes. An increase from concentration P_1 to concentration P_2 is considered significant if

$$P_1 \, (1 + CV_{P_1}) \; < \; P_2 \, (1 - CV_{P_2})$$

where CV_{P_1} and CV_{P_2} are, respectively, the coefficients of variation at concentrations P_1 and P_2 obtained from the interpolation described above. Similarly, a decrease from concentration P_1 to concentration P_2 is considered significant if

$$P_1 \, (1 - CV_{P_1}) \; > \; P_2 \, (1 + CV_{P_2})$$

A spike is considered significant if both the increase and the decrease in concentration are significant. If the first significant change in the hormonal profile, starting from the first data point, is a decrease, all preceding data are considered to be part of a "peak" and are set equal to the higher level observed. If the first significant change is an increase, all preceding data are considered to be part of a "trough" and are set equal to the lowest level observed. The program proceeds further by searching for the next significant change and eliminating the non-significant variations by iteration. In the course of a decrease, strings of data amounting to non-significant changes are set equal to the lowest level observed whereas, in the course of an increase, strings of data amounting to non-significant changes are set equal to the highest level. Corrections for consecutive non-significant changes adding up to significant changes are made in a second iteration. The result is a profile where only significant changes of concentration are present.

Figure 6A illustrates a 24-h profile of PRL obtained at 15-min intervals in a healthy volunteer together with the corresponding "smoothed" profile. Plasma PRL was determined by a homologous human radioimmunoassay and expressed in terms of the pituitary PRL research standard n° 71/222 of the Medical Research Council, Great Britain; 1 µU of this standard is equivalent to .045 ng of the standard VLS. The lower limit of sensitivity of the assay is 20 µU/ml. The intra-assay coefficient of variation was 9.8% and found to be approximately constant throughout the physiological range of concentration (19). For computing purposes, the coefficient of variation was rounded to 10%. Every spike present in the smoothed profile (Figure 6B) is significant with respect to the sensitivity of the assay. The total number of significant spikes in this PRL profile was 15. Increases or decreases at the beginning and end of the series of data are not counted as parts of spikes since neither the duration nor the magnitude can be evaluated.

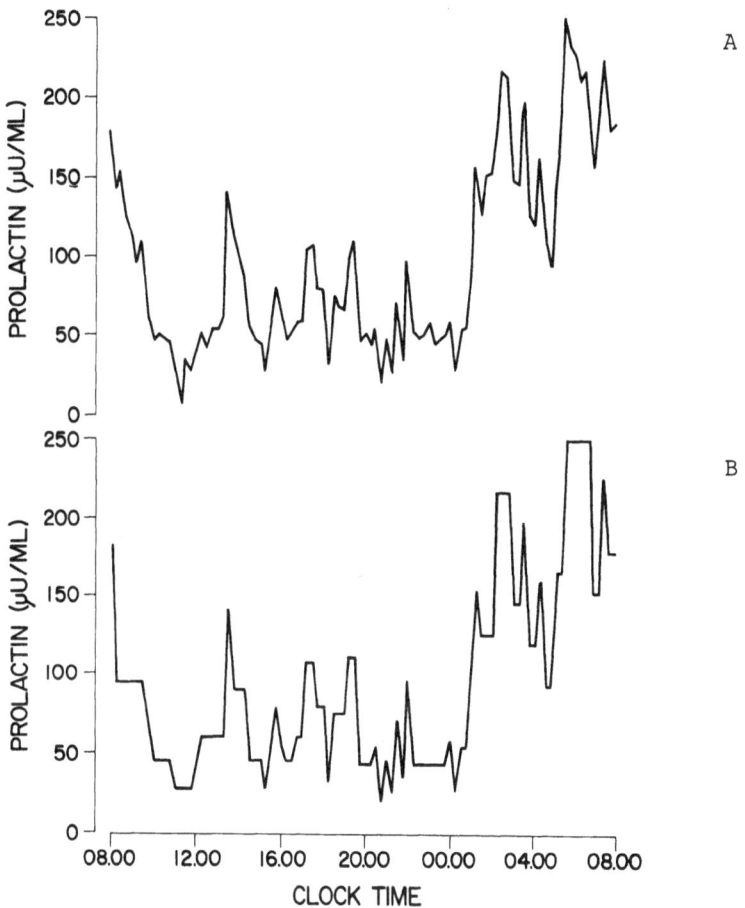

Figure 6:   Twenty-four hour profile of plasma PRL in control
conditions (panel A) and the corresponding smoothed pattern
(panel B) when all changes in concentration non-significant
with regard to the sensitivity of the assay in the relevant
concentration range have been eliminated in order to provide
a straightforward evaluation of the number and magnitude of
secretory peaks.

Though the maximum of several spikes appears in the smoothed profile as plateaus, a record of the times of occurrence
of the observed maximum is kept in memory.

STEP 4:

For each significant·spike, the ascending portion, the declining portion, the total duration, the relative magnitude
and decline and the apparent half-life are calculated according to the following definitions:

Ascending portion: Starts with the first sample after pre-
                      ceding minimum in the smoothed profile
                      and ends with the sample corresponding
                      to the observed maximum. The minimum
                      duration of an ascending portion is
                      thus one sampling interval.

Declining portion: Starts with the first sample after the
                      observed maximum and ends with first
                      sample in the next minimum in the
                      smoothed profile. The minimum dura-
                      tion of a declining portion is thus
                      one sampling interval.

Total duration: Sum of the duration of the ascending
                      and declining portion.

Magnitude: (Value of observed maximum - value of
                      preceding minimum)/value of the preced-
                      ing minimum. The magnitude thus repre-
                      sents an increment of concentration.

Decline: (Value of next minimum - value of ob-
                      served maximum)/value of observed maxi-
                      mum. The decline thus represents a
                      decrement of concentration.

Apparent half-life: A least square regression line in
                      semi-log coordinates is calculated
                      from the observed maximum and the de-
                      clining portion of the spike. The
                      corresponding apparent 1/2 life is de-
                      duced from the slope. This calcula-
                      tion is performed whatever the dura-
                      tion of the declining portion

in order to obtain estimations for
short as well as long spikes.

The values of these parameters for each of the 15 spikes
found significant in the 24-h profile of PRL illustrated in
Figure 6A are listed in Table 2. The observed maximum is
identified in terms of sample number as well as time of
occurrence.

STEP 5:
Statistics for parameters such as total duration, magnitude
and apparent half-life are calculated for the set of significant spikes. In the present example, the average duration of a spike was 64 min $\pm$ 51 min, the average magnitude
153% $\pm$ 133% and the average apparent 1/2 life 36 min $\pm$ 51
min (mean $\pm$ SD). If the option of dividing the 24-h span
in sections of particular interest, such as sleep and wake
periods was chosen in STEP 1, such statistics are also provided for the spikes occurring in these sections only. The
option of storing the values of the parameters constituting
the output of STEP 4 for later evaluation of a larger population of spikes found significant in a set of 24-h profiles recorded using the same protocol in a homogeneous
group of subjects is offered.

SLEEP AND HORMONAL VARIATION

Polygraphic recordings of sleep are generally scored at 20-
sec epochs using standardized criteria (20). Hormonal data
during sleep are commonly collected at time intervals ranging from 5 min to 20 min. Thus, during each time interval
between blood samplings, 15 to 60 sleep data are available.
So far, most studies of possible correlations between hormonal events have been based on visual comparison of a
graphic representation of the succession and duration of
sleep stages Wake, REM, I, II, III and IV with the series
of hormonal data. To make the illustration possible, the
sleep pattern is actually a summary of the scores obtained

TABLE 1: CHARACTERIZATION OF THE SIGNIFICANT PRL SECRETORY SPIKES.

| MAXIMUM | | DURATION (min) | | | MAGNITUDE (Relative increase) | DECLINE (Relative decrease) | APPARENT HALF-LIFE (min) |
TIME	VALUE (μU/ml)	TOTAL	ASCENDING	DECLINING			
13.30	143.00	210	105	105	3.77	0.79	48.6
15.45	83.00	60	30	30	1.77	0.42	38.0
17.30	111.00	105	60	45	1.31	0.70	28.6
19.30	112.00	90	75	15	2.39	0.60	12.6
20.30	56.00	30	15	15	0.24	0.64	10.1
21.00	48.00	30	15	15	1.40	0.42	19.3
21.30	74.00	30	15	15	1.64	0.51	14.4
22.00	99.00	30	15	15	1.75	0.56	16.6
24.00	61.00	30	15	15	0.39	0.56	12.8
1.15	159.00	75	60	15	4.89	0.19	49.7
2.30	218.00	60	30	30	0.69	0.32	56.6
3.30	199.00	30	15	15	0.34	0.39	22.8
4.15	163.00	30	15	15	0.34	0.41	25.3
5.30	250.00	120	45	75	1.60	0.38	136.9
7.15	225.00	30	15	15	0.45	0.20	47.8

at 20-sec epochs. The methodology used to obtain this graphic summary seems to vary from one investigator to another and is usually not specified. We describe here a simple procedure for condensing the sleep record obtained at 20-sec epochs into series of data containing each the same number of points as the corresponding hormonal record and allowing, in a later step, the analysis of cross-correlations using standard statistical methods.

Let Δ be the blood sampling intervals. Sleep data are condensed by calculating for each blood sampling time the percentages of the preceding Δ spent in stages W, REM, I + II, and III + IV (slow wave: SW). A pilot study was conducted in order to determine whether the interval constituted by $\Delta/2$ before blood sampling and $\Delta/2$ after blood sampling should be considered rather than one Δ preceding blood sampling. The results were very similar with both methods. Using the Δ preceding blood sampling is probably preferable because it seems more likely that hormonal events would follow neural events rather than the opposite.

Figure 7 illustrates sleep and PRL data obtained at 15-min intervals in a control subject after 16 nights of adjustment to sleep recording and blood sampling conditions. Sleep was scored at 20-sec epochs and is illustrated in Figure 7A summarized over 1-min intervals. The excellent quality of sleep of the subject is noteworthy. No awakenings occurred during the sleep period and the record has all the characteristics of textbook descriptions; namely the known alternance of REM - non REM stages with decreasing amounts of slow wave sleep and increasing amount of REM as sleep progresses towards morning awakening. Panel B, C and D of Figure 7 show, respectively, the evolution of SW, I + II and REM stages. At each time of blood sampling, the corresponding value shown on panels B, C and D represents the percentage of the preceding 15-min intervals spent, respectively, in SW, I + II and REM stages. An excellent visualization of the REM - non REM cycles is provided by the evolution of the percent of REM stage illustrated in panel D.

22

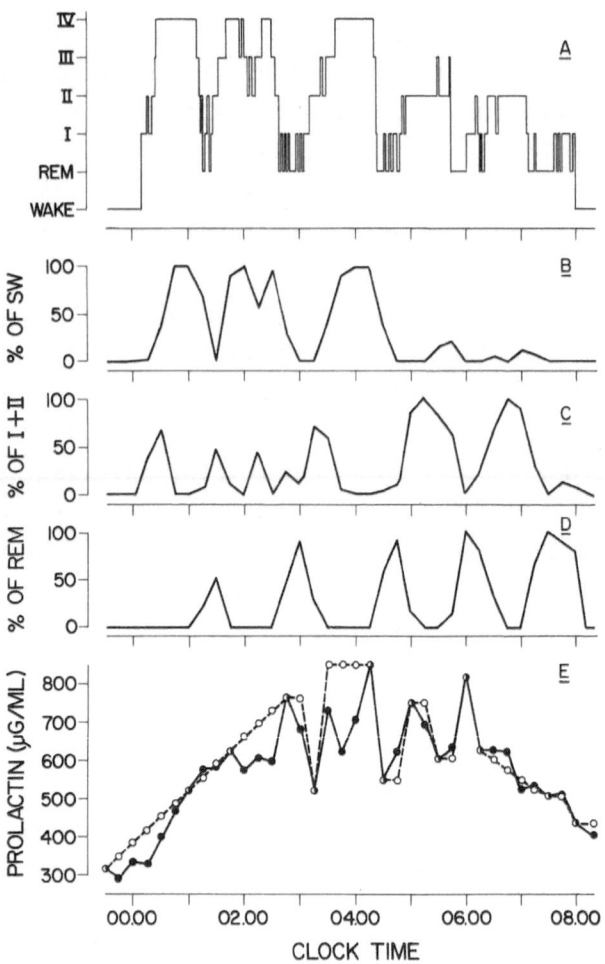

Figure 7: Sleep and PRL levels sampled at 15-min intervals in a normal subject after 16 nights of adjustment to recording conditions. A standard sleep pattern is shown on panel A, whereas panels B, C and D illustrate respectively, the percentages of the 15-min interval preceding hormone sampling spent in stages III + IV (slow wave), I + II and REM. The PRL determinations (●) are shown together with the smoothed profile (o) obtained after elimination of all concentration changes non-significant with respect to the sensitivity of the assay.

The plasma levels of PRL are plotted in Figure 7E, together
with the smoothed profile obtained after eliminating all
non-significant changes in concentration according to the
procedure described in the preceding section. Four significant PRL spikes and five REM - non REM cycles occurred
during sleep. The first PRL spike corresponded to the increment associated with sleep onset and extended over two
REM - non REM cycles with dominant SW sleep. The second
PRL spike was concomitant with an episode of stage II sleep.
The third spike occurred in parallel with a REM episode and
the fourth appeared associated with a predominance of
stages I + II. Cross correlation coefficients between PRL
levels across sleep and percent of SW, I + II and REM in
the 15-min interval preceding the hormonal determination
were respectively .15, .06, and .08.

CONCLUSIONS

The methods described here aim at a quantitative, rather
than qualitative, description of the circadian and episodic
hormone fluctuations in plasma and of their relationship
with sleep. It is expected that such procedures will help
defining the patterns of spontaneous hormonal changes in
basal conditions, provide reference values for their characteristics and contribute to the understanding of their
control mechanisms. Then, alterations in pathological
states or after environmental changes may be objectively
detected and quantified. Methods for the detailed analysis
of interrelations between fluctuations of various hormones
in plasma and correlation with neurological events are presently being developed.

ACKNOWLEDGEMENTS

We thank Dr. S. Refetoff for advice and criticism, Dr. D.F.
Kripke for stimulating discussions and Mrs. Y.W. Richmond
for secretarial help. This work was performed on a PDP 11/
34 computer made available by Dr. L.J. DeGroot at the University of Chicago and was partially supported by APMO Foundation, Brussels.

REFERENCES

1. Van Cauter, E, Method for the characterization of 24-hour temporal variations of blood components. Am J Physiol 6:E255, 1979

2. Van Cauter, E, S Huyberechts, Problems in the statistical analysis of biological time series: The cosinor test and the periodogram. J Interdiscipl Cycle Res 4:41, 1973

3. Van Cauter, E, Methods for the analysis of multifrequential biological time series. J Interdiscipl Cycle Res 5:131, 1974

4. Jenkins, GM, and DG Watts, Spectral Analysis and Its Applications. San Francisco, Holden Day, 1968

5. Desir, D, E Van Cauter, J Golstein, VS Fang, E Martino, C Jadot, JP Spire, P Noël, S Refetoff, and G Copinschi, Effets of jet lag on hormonal patterns. I. Procedures, variations in total plasma proteins and disruption of ACTH-cortisol periodicity. J Clin Endocrinol Metab in press, 1981

6. Fevre-Montange, M, E Van Cauter, S Refetoff, D Desir, J Tourniaire, and G Copinschi, Effects of jet lag on hormonal patterns. II. Adaptation of melatonin circadian periodicity. J Clin Endocrinol Metab in press, 1981

7. Weinberg, U, RD D'Eletto, ED Weitzman, S Erlich, and CS Hollander, Circulating melatonin in man: Episodic secretion throughout the light-dark cycle. J Clin Endocrinol Metab 48:114, 1979

8. Sassin, JF, AG Frantz, ED Weitzman, and S Kapen, Human prolactin: 24-hour pattern with increased release during sleep. Science 177:1205, 1972

9. Parker, DC, LG Rossman, and EF Vanderlaan, Sleep-related, nyctohemeral and briefly episodic variation in human plasma prolactin concentration. J Clin Endocrinol Metab 36:1119, 1973

10. Copinschi, G., R Leclercq, J Golstein, C Robyn, D Desir,, MH Delaet, E Virasoro, L Vanhaelst, M L'Hermite, and E Van Cauter, Seasonal modifications of circadian and ultradian variations of ACTH, cortisol, β-MSH, hPRL and TSH in normal man. Chronobiologia 4:A106, 1977 (Abstract)

11. Krieger, DT, and J Aschoff, Endocrine and other biological rhythms, In: Endocrinology, DeGroot, LJ (ed.), Vol. II, New York, Grüne and Stratton, p. 2079, 1979

12. Batschelet, E, Recent statistical methods for orienta-
    tion data, In: Animal Orientation and Navigation,
    Galler, SR et al (eds.), NASA Symposium, 1970, U.S.
    Government Printing Office, 1972

13. Weitzman, ED, D Fukushima, C Nogeire, H Roffwarg,
    TF Gallagher and L Hellman, Twenty-four pattern of
    the episodic secretion of cortisol in normal sub-
    jects. J Clin Endocrinol Metab 33:14, 1971

14. Santen, RJ and CW Bardin, Episodic luteinizing hormone
    secretion in man. J Clin Invest 52:2617, 1973

15. Krieger, DT, W Allen, F Rizzo and HP Krieger, Charac-
    terization of the normal temporal pattern of plasma
    corticosteroid levels. J Clin Endocrinol Metab 32:
    266, 1971

16. Christian, LE, DO Everson and SL Davis, A statistical
    method for detection of hormone secretory spikes.
    J Animal Sci 46:699, 1978

17. Fevre, M, T Segel, JF Marks and RM Boyar, LH and mela-
    tonin secretion patterns in pubertal boys. J Clin
    Endocrinol Metab 47:1383, 1978

18. Rollag, MD and GD Niswender, Radioimmunoassay of serum
    concentrations of melatonin in sheep exposed to
    different lighting regimens. Endocrinology 98:482,
    1976

19. Badawi, M, S Bila, M L'Hermite, FR Perez-Lopez and
    C Robyn, Comparative evaluation of radioimmunoassay
    methods for human prolactin using anti-ovine and
    anti-human prolactin sera, In: Radioimmunoassay and
    Related Procedures in Medicine, International Atomie
    Energy Agency, Wien, Vol. I, p. 411, 1974

20. Rechtstaffen, A and A Kales, A manual of standardized
    terminology, techniques and scoring system for sleep
    stages of human subjects. Public Health Service,
    Government Printing Office, Washington, D.C., 1968

DISCUSSION

WEITZMAN: Your methods are elegant and begin to approach the problems that all of us face in dealing with the variability of the data and their reproducibility among and within indiviudals. How do you deal with a change in waveshape which is not dramatic? It is easy to detect the change in cortisol rhythm between normal subjects and patients with Cushing's syndrome even on a qualitative basis. However, if in the same individual, the components of the circadian waveshape change to some extent though not greatly but would nevertheless show an error term after fitting sine functions, how can one detect and quantify such changes?

VAN CAUTER: To quantify changes in waveshape, a high frequency of sampling is required. The sampling interval should be not longer than 30 minutes, and preferably shorter. Then, the best-fit pattern will provide an accurate quantitative representation of the shape of the profile and thus offer a precise visualization of possible changes in shape. To quantify such changes, one may then define parameters directly deduced from the best-fit pattern. For instance, we showed that the symmetry of the cortisol rhythm was modified after jet lag by defining a period of minimal secretion and measuring its length, which was scattered over a longer time span after jet lag, but returned to normal later. Thus, after having obtained a best-fit pattern, it is still necessary to find out which parameters should be defined in order to obtain an adequate quantification of a change in waveshape. However, this work is facilitated by the very good visualization, excluding sporadic fluctuations, provided by the best-fit pattern.

ASCHOFF: Dr. Weitzman is certainly referring to the dramatic changes of shape between synchronized and free-running rhythms. The change is then from a right skewed curve to a left skewed curve with a completely different acrophase. Such changes in acrophases can be adequately quantified. The real problem is then "what is the meaning of this acrophase?"

ROSSMAN: Why do you use a 90% confidence interval in the Fisher test? Also, in your 24-hour pattern of PRL, the diurnal peak is much larger than what we observed in our individual profiles. Even though in your fitting of our data, an afternoon acrophase is apparent, the diurnal secretion was very minimal in our profiles and we chose not to describe it.

VAN CAUTER: Regarding the significance level, whereas a .05 probability level is commonly used in standard statistics, in time series analysis, probability levels of 10% and 20% are more frequently used because of the complexity of the testing procedures. Regarding the PRL pattern, you were able to see that the best-fit pattern calculated using your published transverse mean profile of 17 individuals showed a highly significant diurnal acrophase. In order to obtain such a diurnal phase representing roughly a 100% increase in PRL level, using the transverse mean profile, some of the individual profiles and probably the majority of them, must have had a significant afternoon elevation.

ROSSMAN: I agree. However, this afternoon elevation is not large enough to be considered a significant contribution to the circadian waveform.

VAN CAUTER: The diurnal phase of PRL corresponds to an elevation of PRL level over late morning values of approximately 100%. It is a very reproducible characteristic of the 24-hour profile of PRL which was first recognized by Dr. Sassin. The transverse profiles obtained by Dr. Sassin's laboratory and by Dr. Parker's laboratory can practically be superimposed and could also be superimposed to our data, if we would calculate a transverse mean. Exceptionally, there are some individual profiles which do not exhibit a diurnal elevation. In our studies, it happened in two out of twenty profiles.

ROSSMAN: I think the methodology is needed to evidence this diurnal phase.

ASCHOFF: In your study on the cortisol rhythm in Cushing's disease, you interpreted the average group acrophase of 10.0 $\pm$ 6.4 hours as a "lack of synchronization". I disagree with this interpretation since each individual could be beautifully synchronized but with a different acrophase.

VAN CAUTER: I meant "inter-individual" synchronization.

ASCHOFF: OK. The inter-individual variability in phasing of some of these rhythms is presently one of the most interesting problems and relatively little is known. In certain diseases, the entrainment power of social zeitgebers, if such zeitgebers exist, may be weakened resulting in a larger dispersion of acrophases among such individuals. Would you agree with that?

VAN CAUTER: Yes.

ASCHOFF: On some of the profiles, you showed the best-fit pattern had two acrophases, one major and one minor. It seemed to me, however, that on certain profiles, a third acrophase could have been present. How do you determine the number of acrophases to be included in your best-fit pattern?

VAN CAUTER: A maximum of 3 acrophases can be included since we want to describe only the low frequency properties of the profile. The number of acrophases included is related to the percentage of variance of the profile accounted for.

THE SLEEP-WAKE PATTERN OF CORTISOL AND GROWTH HORMONE SECRETION DURING NON-ENTRAINED (FREE-RUNNING) CONDITIONS IN MAN

Elliot D. Weitzman, Charles A. Czeisler, Janet C. Zimmerman
and Joseph M. Ronda

Laboratory of Human Chronophysiology, Department of Neurology,
Montefiore Hospital and Albert Einstein College of Medicine
Bronx, New York.

INTRODUCTION

It is now well established that all the peptide hormones secreted from the pituitary in man are related to the daily sleep-wake cycle. In addition to a temporal pattern of episodic secretion, the timing of the daily rhythm has been shown to be closely associated with sleep stages (1-6). The field of biological rhythm research has demonstrated that biological organisms have endogenous oscillations and that when these rhythms are no longer entrained to specific daily time cues (zeitgebers) they will develop free-running rhythms with period lengths greater than or less than 24 hours (circadian) (7-15).

In order to study the nature and timing of the physiological controls which determine the inter-relationship among these correlative measured periodic events such as sleep, sleep stages, body temperature and hormones, we have established a comprehensive multi-variable study of the chronophysiology of man living in a time-free environment with a non scheduled daily pattern of living (16-19). We have instituted a Laboratory of Human Chronophysiology where subjects can be studied in temporal isolation. We have provided social communication which has the major advantage of allowing us to make certain biological and psychological measurements. We therefore have applied previously developed methods to obtain frequent plasma samples to normal human subjects who live for weeks to months in our "time free" environment to describe the relationships between hormonal blood concentrations, sleep and sleep stages. We present here a summary of the timing of the secretion of cortisol and growth hormone in relation to the sleep-wake cycle during entrained (scheduled) and free-running (non-scheduled) conditions.

METHODS

We have carried out detailed and prolonged measurements of sleep-waking function in human subjects for time periods ranging from 25 to 105 calendar days. We measured polygraphic sleep-stage characteristics, minute by minute body temperatures and frequent (approx. 20 minutes) blood sampling for cortisol and growth hormone in normal adult men living in an environment free of all time cues, under entrained, free-running and re-entrained conditions.

A special environment was established where the individual subjects lived for many weeks (16,17). A three room apartment (study, bedroom and bathroom) was arranged without windows, the walls sound attenuated and a double door entrance constructed as a temporal isolation facility (TIF). A closed circuit TV system and voice intercom monitored the subject's activities.

Ten male subjects were individually studied. The first group (3 subjects, (AA, AB and AC) was studied for 15 calendar days and the second group (6 subjects, (AD-H and AJ) for 25 calendar days. No subject had significant psychopathology, medical illness, nor were any on drugs. Each subject kept a written daily diary of sleep times for at least 2 weeks and maintained a regular scheduled sleep-wake schedule in accord with their usual habits. After entry in the TIF, an entrained condition of 3 or 4 scheduled 24 hour sleep-wake periods preceded the non-scheduled "free-running" portion of the study. The entrained clock times were determined by the subject's recorded habitual lights off-lights on time at home. The subject was told that his sleep time would be scheduled for certain portions of the study but was not advised of the clock times nor the duration. Following the entrained portion, each subject was told that he could choose to go to sleep and awaken at any time he wished. He was asked not to "nap" although he was permitted to go to sleep whenever he wished. A decision to go to sleep, therefore, represented bedrest for that biologic "day." Food was available to the subject on demand as breakfast, lunch, dinner and a "snack." The subject could request any meal type at any time. A set of buttons were available which when pushed was coded on a paper punch tape and indicated the behavior the subject was about to initiate and the elapsed time from the beginning of the study. These behaviors included bedrest onset, activity onset, urination, defecation, shower, blood sample times, exercise and mealtimes.

The subject was totally isolated from contact with all non-laboratory persons but communicated by intercom and direct discussion with selected laboratory staff. The supervising staff members were scheduled on a random basis as to time of day and duration of work-shift to prevent the subject from obtaining a time cue.

The following measurements were made for each subject.

(1) Polygraphic-Sleep Recording -The interval between the subject's decision to sleep and lights-out with full electrode application was less than 15 minutes. All polygraphic records were scored by standard methods (20).

(2) Rectal Temperature - A rectal thermistor probe was maintained by each subject throughout the entire study except for brief daily periods of defecation. The temperature was automatically recorded every minute on the punch paper tape and a print-out.

(3) Plasma Cortisol and Growth Hormone - Blood samples were obtained at approx. 20 minute intervals using an indwelling specially designed catheter system (2,16). This venous catheter was changed at 2-5 day intervals using alternating arm veins without interrupting the sampling. Plasma cortisol assays were performed using the competitive protein binding technique (21). The samples were assayed in duplicate using $25\mu l$ aliquot for each assay. HGH was assayed in duplicate from each plasma sample by radioimmunoassay using $20\mu l$ of plasma for each assay.

(4) Special Mathematical Techniques and Computer Algorithms -In addition to the usual statistical method of analysis and computer plotting and display routines, several mathematical techniques were created to assist in the analysis of the data (16,17). These include a) estimate of period length using a minimum variance fit, b) waveform eduction and c) averaged timed event relationship. The minimum variance technique consists of finding the minimum value of repetitive estimates of variance (standard deviation) of all data points for a specified range of period lengths. This least variance value determines the period length used to obtain the educed wave form. The educed wave form is the mean curve derived from the sequential data points, summed across a specified number of cycles (e.g. biological days). The averaged time event relationship consists of obtaining a mean value of each individual time point before and after a specific defined event, for the parameter selected, (e.g. 720 minute values of body temperature before and after sleep onset during the entire "free-running" experimental segment for a subject).

RESULTS

During the entrained condition all subjects had the normal episodic patterns of secretion of cortisol with very low values just prior to and during the first 3 hours of sleep, followed by a series of secretory episodes during the latter half of the night. An intermittent episodic secretory pattern was present during the waking day (Figs 1,2). The educed waveform pattern at the calculated period length during the entrained condition clearly demonstrated the circadian phase relation to the timing of the sleep episode (Figs 3,4). During the free running condition however a change in both the timing and wave-shape of the cortisol curve was evident. There was a phase advance of the nadir by 100 to 105 degrees. Since the mathematical process of waveform eduction produces a mean curve at a defined period length, the technique will obscure, because of the averaging process, specific timed related events which might be present.

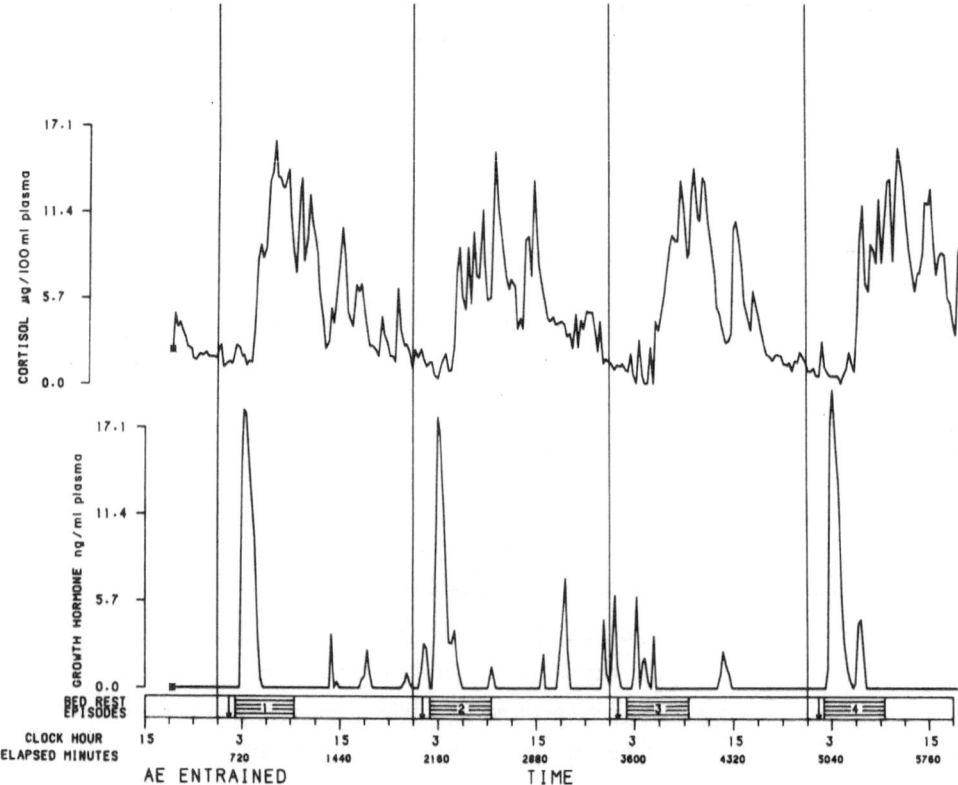

Figure 1.   Secretory pattern of growth hormone and cortisol in one subject (AE) during 4 days of entrainment.

Examination of the individual cortisol plasma concentration time series revealed that on many non-scheduled (free-running) biological days, cortisol was secreted just prior to sleep onset and then would stop being secreted for several hours after sleep onset; a pattern not seen during entrainment (Figs 1,2). In order to define this pattern we developed the technique of "evoking" an averaged Timed Event Relationship (TER) of the hormonal concentration in regard to any chosen recurring event (Figs 5,6).

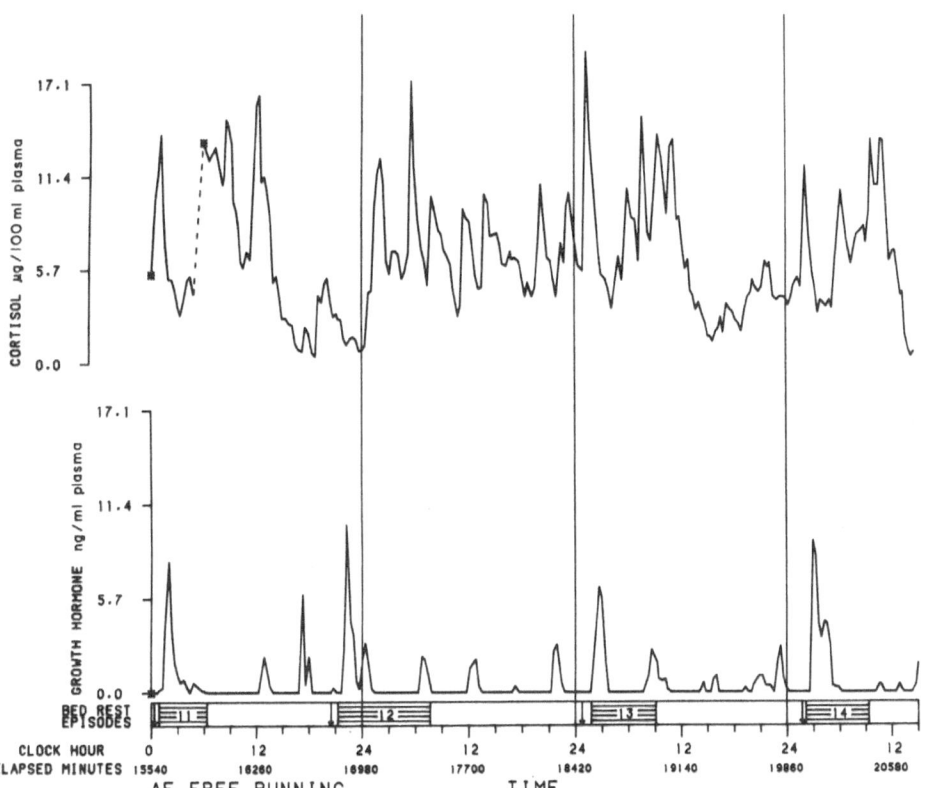

Figure 2.   Secretory pattern of growth hormone and cortisol in one subject (AE) during 5 days of non-entrainment.

The results of obtaining a TER "time-locked" to sleep onset clearly demonstrated that all subjects had an inhibition of cortisol secretion during the 1 to 3 hours after sleep onset during the free-running condition (Fig. 6).

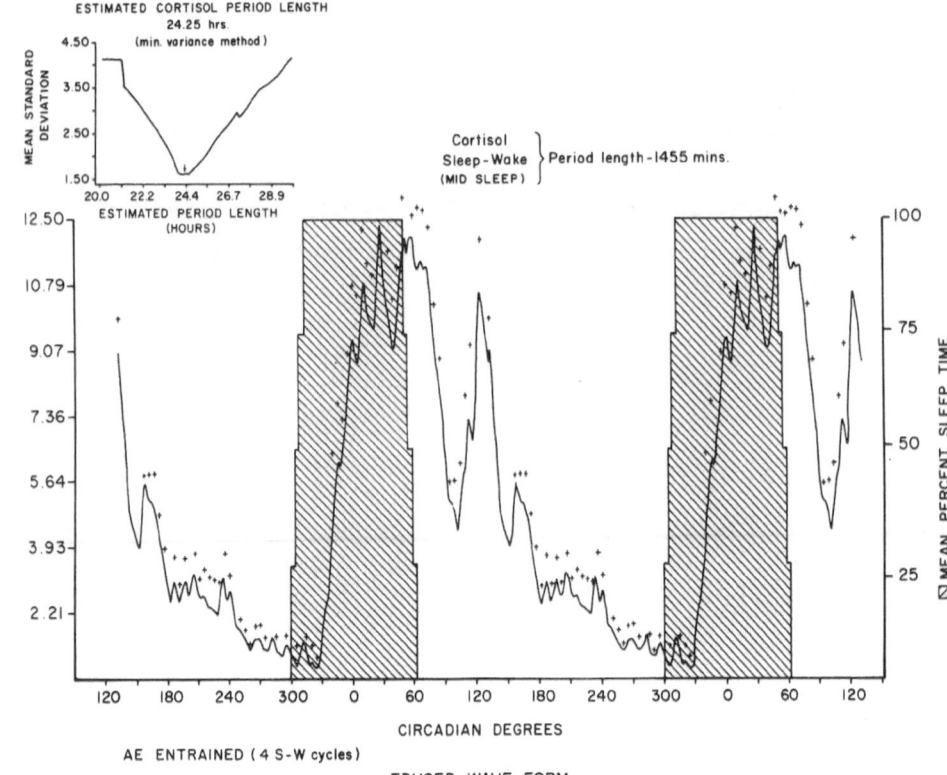

Figure 3.   Educed wave-form and period length estimate of cortisol
and sleep-wake pattern during entrainment (subject AE),
(4 biological days). The sleep pattern educed wave-form
was obtained at the same period length as cortisol and is
derived by averaging the percentage of time asleep at each
defined data point across the same sequence of circadian
cycles.

Therefore during the free-running condition a phase advance of
cortisol occurred in relation to the sleep episode, the overall wave shape
was changed and a specific sleep related inhibition of cortisol secretion
was apparent. During the re-entrainment condition, a similar pattern was
evident since the phase relationship between the cortisol rhythm and sleep
had not yet returned to normal. Evidence that this sleep related inhibition
may well be operative even in subjects habitually living on a 24 hour
routine may be deduced from the data obtained during the transition from
the entrained to the free-running condition on those nights when a phase
delay of sleep onset on a single night exceeded 2-3 hours. On those
occasions, the hormone was released just before sleep and then
immediately inhibited after sleep onset.

It thus appears that the episodic pattern of cortisol secretion is influenced both by an endogenous rhythmic component, not directly related to the behavioral sleep-wake cycle and a specific sleep (or lights out in bed) related component. Whether other daily behavioral events such as meal times, etc. are also determinants of the episodic pattern will require further detailed analysis of the extensive data we have obtained in these studies.

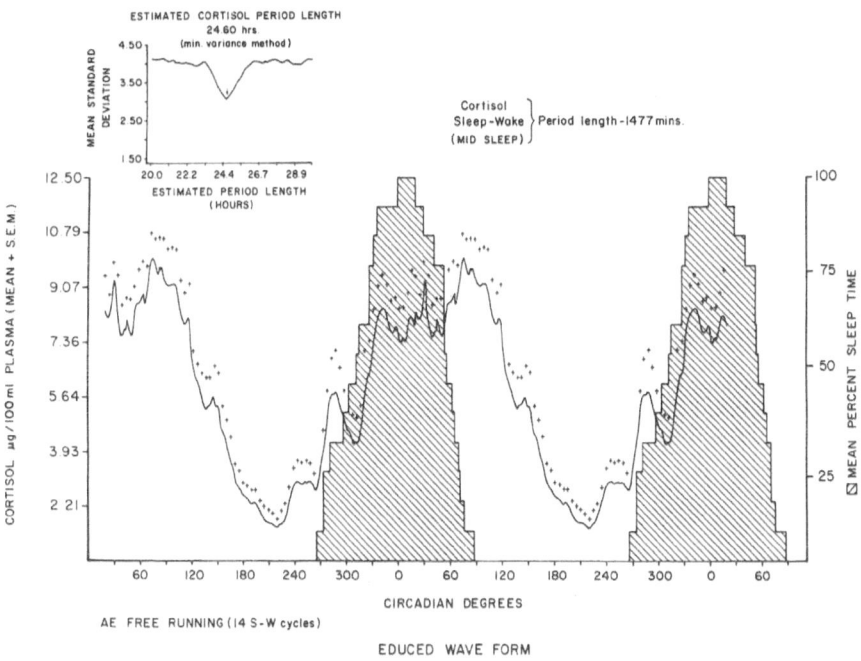

Figure 4. Educed wave-form and period length estimate of cortisol and sleep-wake pattern during non-entrainment (subject AE - 14 biological days).

Growth Hormone Patterns

HGH was found to be secreted in an episodic normal manner in all subjects with the typical pattern of brief episodes of secretion (1-2 hours) followed by long inter-episode intervals (6-12 hours) with no HGH detectable (4,22) (Figs 1,2). The hormonal concentration was less than the overall average (1 ng/ml) 80% of the time. A striking highly consistent relationship between sleep onset and an episode of HGH secretion was found for all 3 experimental conditions for all subjects (5,22,23) (Figs 5,6). A clear secretory episode followed sleep onset approx. 90% of the time. Thus far no independent rhythm of HGH could be detected but further analysis for an ultradian, or specific behavioral related event will be searched for.

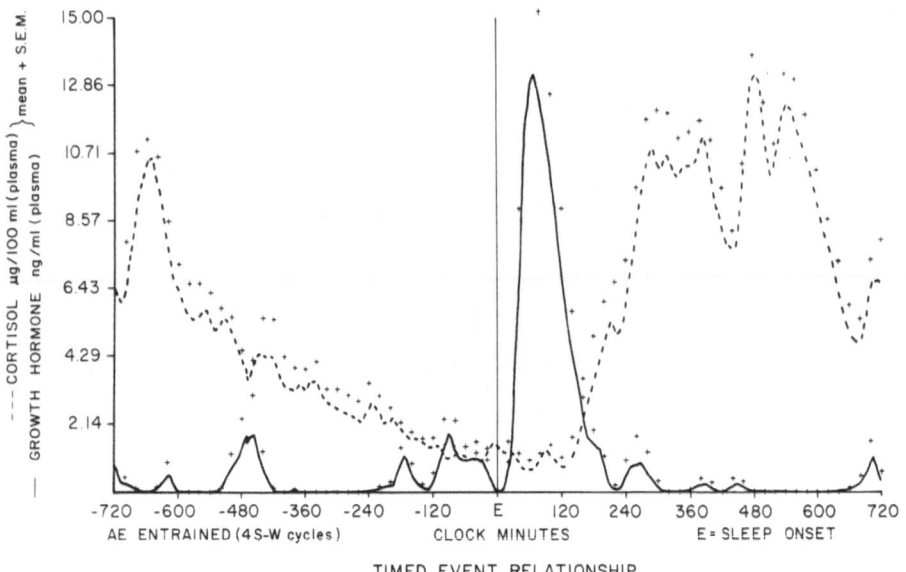

Figure 5.   Timed event relationship between sleep onset, cortisol and growth hormone in subject AE during the entrained (4 days) condition.

We also analyzed the temporal pattern of the change of cortisol and GH at the time of waking for both entrained and free-running conditions for all sleep episodes (Figs 7,8). All subjects had a sharp but brief elevation of cortisol, associated with an inhibition of GH at awakening when entrained. This waking response was also present during free-running.

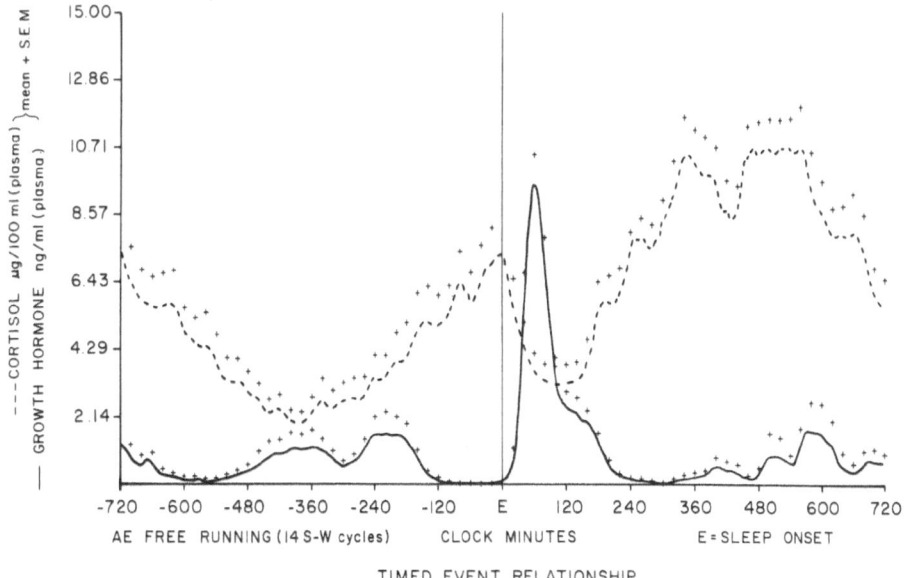

Figure 6. Timed event relationship between sleep onset, cortisol and
growth hormone in subject AE during non-entrained conditions
(14 biological days).

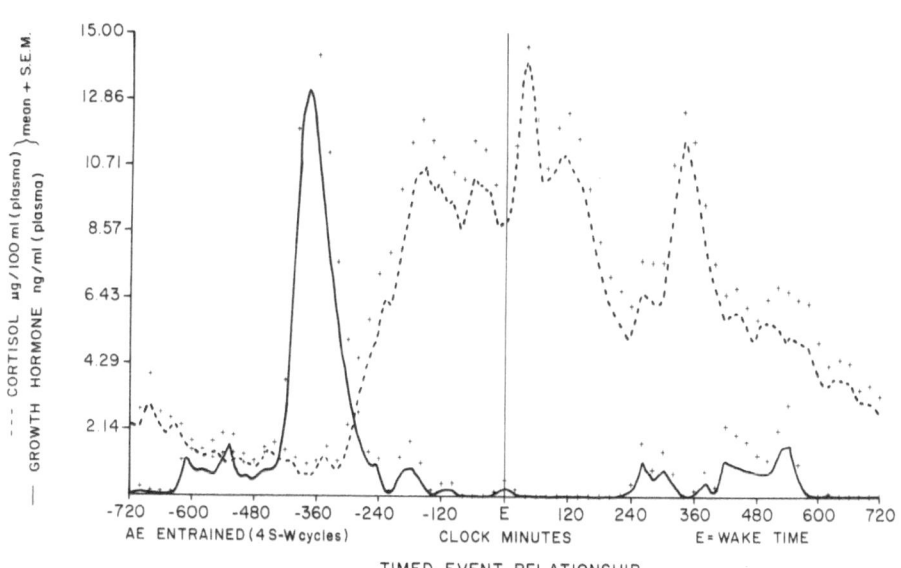

Figure 7. Timed event relationship between wake time, cortisol and
growth hormone in subject AE during the entrained conditions
(4 days).

The timing of the peak value of cortisol after awakening (lights on) was similar for all subjects and conditions, namely at 30-40 minutes (Figs 7,8). The opposite pattern was found for GH. Just prior to awakening there was a variable concentration of GH. When the mean concentration of GH was elevated just prior to awakening, such as occurred during prolonged sleep periods, there was a sharp decrease of GH concentration within minutes of the wake time (lights on) to undetectable values; this period of inhibition lasting for approximately 4 hours after the daily sleep episode was terminated. When the GH concentration was at very low values just prior to awakening they also remained at undetectable levels for the 4 hours after lights on.

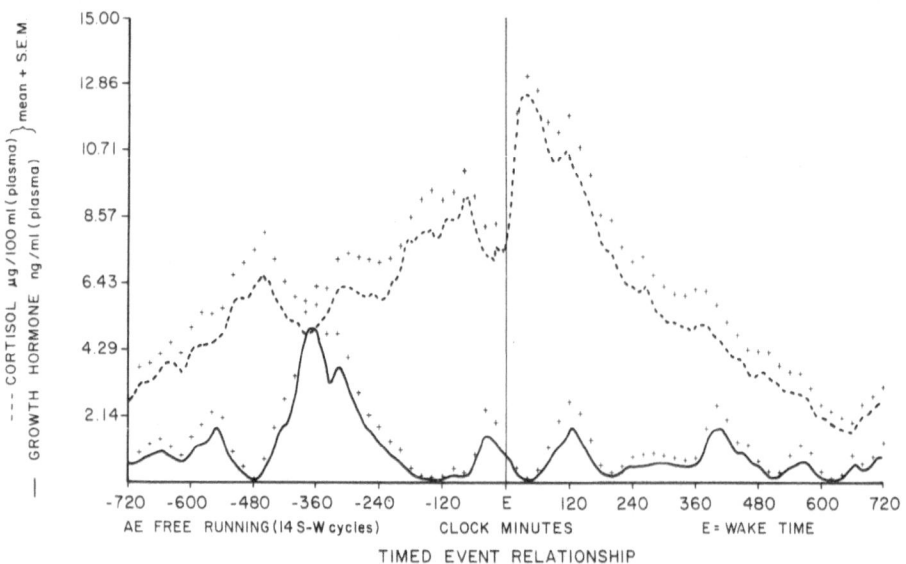

Figure 8. Timed event relationship between wake time, cortisol and growth hormone in subject AE during non-entrained conditions (14 biological days).

CONCLUSIONS

Measurements of plasma cortisol throughout each study demonstrated two components of the circadian cortisol curve during free-running as compared to the entrained condition. One component has a phase advance (6-8 hours) relative to sleep onset whereas a second component clearly follows sleep onset. This second component appears to be a sharp inhibition of cortisol secretion during the first 2-3 hours of sleep interrupting a rising phase of the hormonal curve. Growth hormone secretion, on the other hand, was intimately related to the first 2 hours after sleep onset. A sharp episode of hormonal secretion occurs just after sleep onset for almost all sleep periods. No other independent circadian rhythm of GH has been detected thus far. There appear to be brain mechanisms which simultaneously control the yoked release of ACTH-Cortisol and inhibit GH, as well as the simultaneous inhibition of cortisol and release of GH. When there is "activation" (waking-REM sleep) there is inhibition of GH and secretion of cortisol and when stages 3+4 sleep occurs there is inhibition of ACTH-cortisol and secretion of GH.

These and previous reported studies emphasize the lawfulness of neuroendocrine biological rhythm functions in man and demonstrate the importance of the methodology using temporal isolation and the analysis of "free-running" rhythms to unravel these chronobiological processes.

REFERENCES

1. Weitzman, ED, H Schaumburg, and W Fishbein, Plasma 17-Hydroxycorticosteroid levels during sleep in man. Journal of Clinical Endocrinology 26:121-127, 1966

2. Weitzman, ED, D Fukushima, C Nogeire, H Roffwarg, TF Gallagher, and L Hellman, Effects of a prolonged 3-hour sleep-wake cycle on sleep stages, plasma cortisol, growth hormone and body temperature in man. Journal of Clinical Endocrinology 33:14-22, 1971

3. Hellman, L, F Nakada, J Curti, ED Weitzman, J Kream, H Roffwarg, S Ellman, DK Fukushima, and TF Gallagher, Cortisol is secreted episodically in Cushing's syndrome, Journal of Clinical Endocrinology 30:411-422, 1970

4. Weitzman, ED and L Hellman, Temporal organization of the 24 hour pattern of the hypothalamic-pituitary axis, Biorhythms and Human Reproduction, M. Ferin, T. Halberg, R. Richart, and R. VandeWiele (eds), New York, John Wiley 23:371, 1973

5. Weitzman, ED, RM Boyar, S Kapen, and L Hellman, The relationship of sleep and sleep stages to neuroendocrine secretion and biological rhythms in man, In Recent Progress in Hormone Research, R. Greep (ed.), New York, Academic Press 31:399-446, 1975

6. Weitzman, ED, Circadian rhythms and episodic hormone secretion in man, Annual Review of Medicine 27:225-243, 1976

7. Pittendrigh, CS and S Daan, The stability and lability of spontaneous frequency, Journal of Comparative Physiology 106:223-252, 1976

8. Pittendrigh, CS and S Daan, A functional analysis of circadian pacemakers in nocturnal rodents. IV. Entrainment: Pacemaker as clock. 106:291-331, 1976

9. Pittendrigh, CS and S Daan, Circadian oscillations in rodents: A systematic increase of their frequency with age. Science 186:548-550, 1974

10. Pittendrigh, CS, Circadian rhythms and the circadian organization of living systems. Journal of Comparative Physiology, Cold Spring Harbor Symposium on Quantitative Biology 25:159-184, 1961

11. Aschoff, J and R Wever, Spontanperiodik des Menschen bei Ausschluss aller Zeitgeber. Die Naturwissenschaften 49:337-342, 1962

12. Aschoff, J, Physiological and Behavior Temperature Regulation, J.D. Hardy, A.P. Gagg and J.A. Stolwijk (eds), Springfield, Charles C. Thomas, 905-919, 1970

13. Aschoff, J, U Gerecke, A Kureck, H Pohl, P Reiger, U V.Saint Paul, and R Wever, Interdependent parameters of circadian activity rhythms in birds and man. Biochronometry, M. Menaker (ed), Washington, D.C.: National Academy of Science, p.3, 1971

14. Daan, S and CS Pittendrigh, A functional analysis of circadian pacemakers in nocturnal rodents: II. The variability of phase response curves. Journal of Comparative Physiology 106:253-266, 1976

15. Wever, R, The Circadian System of Man, New York, Springer Verlag, 1979

16. Weitzman, ED, CA Czeisler, and MD Moore-Ede, Sleep-wake neuroendocrine and body temperature circadian rhythms under entrained and non-entrained (free-running conditions in man). Biological Rhythms and Their Central Mechanism, M. Suda, O. Hayaishi and H. Nakagawa, (eds), Elsevier/North Holland Biomedical Press, 1979

17. Czeisler, CA, Human circadian physiology: Internal organization of temperature, sleep-wake and neuroendocrine function in an environment free of time cues. Ph.D. Dissertation, Stanford University, 346, 1978

18. Weitzman, ED, CA Czeisler, JC Zimmerman, and J Ronda, Timing of REM and stages 3 + 4 sleep during temporal isolation in man, Sleep 2, Raven Press, New York (In Press), 1980

19. Czeisler, CA, JC Zimmerman, J Ronda, MC Moore-Ede, and ED Weitzman, Timing of REM sleep is coupled to the circadian rhythm of body temperature in man. Sleep, (In Press), 1980

20. Rechtschaffen, A and A Kales, (eds), A Manual of Standardized Terminology, Techniques and Scoring System for Sleep Stages of Human Subjects, University of California at Los Angeles, Brain Information Service/Brain Research Institute, 1968

21. Murphy, BP, W Engelberg, and CJ Pattee, Simple method for determination of plasma corticords. Journal of Clinical Endocrinology 23:293, 1963

22. Takahashi, Y, DM Kipnis, and WH Daughaday, Growth hormone secretion during sleep. Journal of Clinical Investigation 47:2079-2090, 1968

23. Sassin, JF, DC Parker, JW Mace, RW Gotlin, LC Johnson, and LG Rossman, Human growth hormone release: Relation to slow-wave sleep and sleep-waking cycles. Science 165:513-515, 1969

Due to a technical problem, the discussion following Dr. Weitzman's presentation could not be tape recorded.

SEARCH FOR A PRIMATE MODEL OF HUMAN
SLEEP-RELATED HORMONE SECRETION

H.-J. Quabbe[*]

Department of Internal Medicine, Section of Endocrinology,
Klinikum Steglitz, Freie Universität Berlin. Hindenburgdamm
30, D-1000 Berlin 45, FRG.

INTRODUCTION

In man, an influence of the sleep/wake cycle on the secretory pattern of certain hormones is well documented. The secretion of growth hormone (GH), prolactin (PRL) - and luteotropin (LH) during puberty - is stimulated by the occurrence of sleep, while thyrotropin (TSH) (and possibly LH during the early follicular phase in adult women) may be inhibited (1). Sleep-deprivation and sleep-reversal experiments have been used to prove that sleep itself affects hormone secretion in these cases irrespective of the time of the day. These studies have revealed that different hormones have different links to sleep. Thus, a major GH secretory episode occurs regularly during the first slow-wave-sleep (SWS) phase of nocturnal sleep and only little or no GH is secreted during the remaining sleep (2, 3, 4). In contrast, PRL secretion increases with the onset of sleep, then the plasma concentration remains elevated and highest values are often reached towards the end of sleep. TSH plasma concentrations attain highest levels in the evening before the onset of sleep, and this seems to be the result of an endogenous circadian rhythm. Sleep onset is then accompanied by a decrease of TSH, which suggests an inhibitory influence of sleep on TSH secretion. However, other authors have described different patterns of TSH secretion (9, 10, 11, 12, 13).

[*]Original studies of the author were supported by Deutsche Forschungsgemeinschaft.

A link not only to the sleep/wake cycle but also to the non-REM/REM (REM = rapid eye movement) sleep-phase cycle has been suggested for nocturnal PRL secretory episodes. However, this has not been generally confirmed (5, 6, 7, 8). During daytime, the secretion of GH and of PRL is probably augmented by the occurrence of napping (5, 6, 14, 15). Thus, there is a link of the secretory mechanism of these hormones not only to the sleep/wake and the sleep-phase cycle but also the the rest/activity cycle during daytime.

Very little is known on the mechanism of the sleep-hormone link. At the present time - apart from a few clinical observations - no convincing experimental information is available. Theoretically, the following possibilities may be discussed :

1. The link is established via neuronal pathways connecting sleep/wake-regulating structures of the thalamus, the anterior and posterior hypothalamus and the ponto-mesencephalic brain stem with the hypothalamic (mediobasal) hypophysiotropic area. The main neurotransmitters which are involved in the regulation of the sleep/wake cycle (serotonin, norepinephrine) are known also to be important for the modulation of pituitary hormone release. However, the evidence for a role of these neurotransmitters in the link between sleep and pituitary hormone secretion is meager. In addition, while sleep disorders (e.g. narcolepsy) have been shown to be accompanied by a disturbance of the sleep-hormone link (16, 17), there is no proof that this disturbance is due to anatomical damage of a neuronal circuit or to dysfunction of its related neurotransmitter mechanisms.

2. A humoral transmission of the sleep/wake influence on the endocrine hypothalamus has not yet been considered but offers an alternative possibility. The mediobasal hypothalamus is adjacent to the third ventricle, and substances transported in the cerebrospinal fluid (CSF) probably have direct or indirect access to its neurons. The pineal gland or other circumventricular organs may secrete substances into the CSF which could either relay information on the arousal state of the brain to the hypophysiotropic area or

could concomitantly modulate the activity of sleep-regulating and hormone-regulating structures. The so-called "sleep-factors" (18, 19, 20) would also be hypothetical candidates for a CSF-transported influence on both sleep and hormone modulation.

3. Finally - as a more remote possibility - information arriving via the blood stream could have a concomitant influence on the sleep/wake cycle and the hypothalamo-pituitary system. Thus, the plasma concentration of certain amino acids, especially tryptophane, may be important for CNS neurotransmitter metabolism (21) and may also influence pituitary hormone secretion (22). Other factors - related to food intake and absorption - may have similar modulatory influences. For instance, intestinal distension is a stimulus for a sedating effect relayed via the vagus and the nucleus of the solitary tract to the noradrenergic locus coeruleus and by implication to the sleep/wake-regulating system (23). At the same time, food intake stimulates cholecystokinin-secretion, and this substance seems to have a direct sedating effect at the CNS (24). On the other hand, food-intake modulates pituitary GH secretion (25).

The sleep-endocrine link is not only of interest to the students of physiological mechanisms in endocrinology or sleep research. Disturbances of the 24-h hormonal secretory pattern and its link to the sleep/wake cycle have been described in a number of clinical conditions, especially in psychiatric and psychosomatic diseases. Thus, in the syndrome of psychosocial dwarfism, nocturnal sleep-related GH secretion is absent, and this may be a causal factor in the growth arrest which occurs during the periods of maternal deprivation (26). LH secretion offers another example. It becomes linked to the sleep/wake cycle with the beginning of puberty and loses this link when adulthood has been reached. However, in the psychosomatic disease anorexia nervosa - which is characterized by a return to an immature personality - the LH secretory pattern as well reverts to the immature stage of the pubertal sleep-linked secretion (27). The mechanism by which the CNS severs or reestablishes such a link during a disease is unknown.

While there is a fairly complete picture of the influence of
the sleep/wake and the rest/activity cycle on the secretory pattern of at least some hormones, investigations into
its mechanism have been hampered by the lack of an animal
model. GH is probably the hormone with the strongest link
to sleep in man. Attempts to find a sleep-hormone link in
animals have therefore mainly been centered on this hormone.
Unfortunately, neither in the rat nor in some other animals,
has an influence of sleep on the secretion of GH been found.
The dog as well does not exhibit a sleep-GH link under physiological conditions (28, 29, 30). Two studies in primates have not yet yielded conclusive results (31, 32). We
have therefore investigated the rhesus monkey for the existence of a link between the sleep/wake and the rest/activi-
ty cycle on the one hand and the secretion of GH, PRL and
TSH on the other.

The rhesus monkey offers several advantages for the study of
such a link. First , their phylogenetic closeness to man
makes non-human primates the best candidates for the existence of such a link. Secondly, their hormone regulation is
very similar to that of man, while other animals (e.g. the
rat) sometimes have dissimilar responses in certain test
conditions, especially for GH (33). Thirdly, the sleep
pattern of the rhesus monkey resembles closely that of man,
including its EEG expression (34). Its sleep-phase cycle of
approximately 45-50 min is long enough for the detection of
a link between sleep-phases and hormone secretory episodes
if compared to the plasma half-time of pituitary hormones
(e.g. the plasma half-time of GH in man is approximately 20
min). Finally, the blood volume of the rhesus monkey is
large enough to allow frequent sampling (e.g. every 15 min)
of blood for the determination of several hormones over extended periods of time (e.g. 24-h or longer). The size of
its brain allows more selective neurophysiological experiments (e.g. section of nerve bundles or coagulation of
nuclei) than that of smaller animals.

EXPERIMENTAL APPROACH

12 male adolescent (n = 7) or adult (n = 5) rhesus monkeys

were used. They lived in fully climatized animal quarters
which were noise-isolated against the exterior. All experiments were performed with the animals remaining in their
usual social surrounding. Special care was taken to assure
stress- and disturbance-free conditions. Therefore, the
animals were adapted to chronic chair living and then fitted
with chronic right atrial catheters and electrodes for chronic electroencephalogram (EEG), electro-oculogram (EOG) and
electromyogram (EMG) recording. Catheter and electrodes
were connected by a swivel mechanism to lines passing
through the wall into the adjacent room. The light changed
slowly over ten minutes from light to dark at 20.00 h and
from dark to light at 6.00 h. Light intensity was approximately 300 lux at daytime and less than 1 lux at night-time.
This illumination allowed TV closed-circuit observation of
the animals during waking and sleeping. The animals were
fed at 8.30 h and 16.00 h, while water was available ad li-
bitum.

Hormone profiles were obtained by sampling blood every 15
min under the following conditions :
1. no disturbance with blood sampling either separately
    during lights-on or lights-off or for 24-h or 96-h un-
    interruptedly,
2. nap-deprivation during daytime from 8.00 to 13.00 h, with
    further sampling until 16.00 h,
3. sleep-deprivation during night-time from 20.00 to 1.00 h,
    with further sampling until 4.00 h,
4. selective SWS or REM-sleep deprivation during the entire
    night from 20.00 to 6.00 h.

During daytime, the activity of the animals was rated as active, quiet or napping by observation on the TV screen
every 5 min, and, during the night, a continuous EEG/EOG/EMG
was obtained, which allowed sleep-stage determination according to criteria established for human sleep-staging (40).
Nap- and sleep-deprivation was achieved by the presence of a
person in the animal quarter who - when necessary - aroused
the attention of the animals by non-stressful procedures
(walking, speaking, etc.). SWS- and REM-sleep deprivation

was achieved by activation of a white-noise generator whenever the respective sleep-stage appeared on the EEG-tracing.

Rhesus monkey hormones were determined by heterologous
radioimmunoassays with antibodies directed against human
hormones. These assays were validated against rhesus-mon-
key hormone standards.[1] GH was determined in the experiments (n = 112) of all animals, while PRL was determined in
85 experiments in 8 animals and TSH in 57 experiments in 5
animals.

RESULTS AND DISCUSSION

Validation of experimental conditions

Many pituitary hormones respond to stress with large and
sudden secretory bursts. Hence, the study of the physiological pattern of hormone secretion and of its possible relation to the sleep/wake cycle makes it necessary to assure
stress-free experimental conditions. The following evidence suggests that our animals were not under the influence of
acute or chronic stress.

The first 2-3 weeks of chair adaptation are usually accompanied by weight loss due to reduced intake of water and
food. Thereafter, the animals regain their previous weight,
eat and drink normally, and young animals continue to grow
and to mature sexually. Subjectively the animals show no
signs of abnormal behavior. Their sleep pattern is composed
of a regular alternation of N-REM and REM sleep phases with
the expected temporal distribution : preponderance of SWS
during the first part of the night and of REM sleep during
the second half (Fig. 1). Total sleep time and relative
distribution of the different sleep phases in the group of
animals are in reasonable agreement with other published
data on rhesus monkey sleep (35, 36, 37) (Table 1). These
observations suggest that the animals were fully adapted to
chronic chair living and were not chronically stressed.

[1]Rhesus monkey hormone standard preparations were kindly do-
nated by Dr. W.D. Peckham, Pittsburgh, USA.

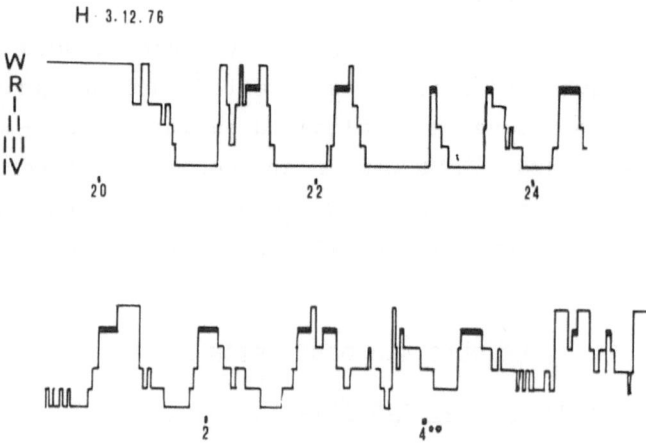

Figure 1 : Sleep pattern of a chronically chaired rhesus monkey. No
blood samples were taken during this night. W : waking; R : REM sleep;
I/II/III/IV : sleep stages 1-4 of non-REM sleep.

Table 1. Comparison of sleep data from our own animals with data
published in the literature. For easier comparison, the original data
from other publications were partly transformed into the mean percent
values presented in this table.

Total sleep time (% of dark time)	N-REM	REM (% of sleep time)	SWS	
80	85	15		Ref. 35
		11.1	13.6	Ref. 36
81.4		12.2		Ref. 37
80.6	83.4	12.7	16.6	present series

On experimental days, frequent blood sampling was an additional factor which might have disturbed the animals. Did
this constitute an acute stress ? When blood samples were
taken during the day and during the night, the animals often became aware of the procedure. During the day, light

napping was often disturbed by the sampling, but, during
more profound naps, the taking of a blood sample would often go unnoticed by the animal. During the night, a short
EEG-arousal reaction often followed the flushing of the catheter after a blood sample had been taken. During sleep
stage-1, a short awakening was sometimes observed. During
deeper N-REM sleep, sometimes a short change to a lighter
sleep stage occurred, but, during N-REM stage-4 and during
REM sleep, usually no change in sleep-stage could be detected. The mean time awake during the night as well as the
percent of sleep-time spent in stage REM and in stage SWS
respectively were not significantly different between nights
without and with blood sampling (19.4, 13.4, and 10.2 % vs
19.4, 12.1 and 12.0 %).

The animal's core temperature reacted very sensitively with
sudden increases to changes in the environment, e.g. the
entrance of unfamiliar persons into the animal quarters.
However, no influence of the blood sampling procedure was
detected when temperature curves from experimental days
were compared with those from non-experimental days. These
curves were obtained in some animals for extended periods
of time (several weeks or months) by continuous telemetric
recording of the abdominal core temperature from previously
implanted temperature-radioprobes.[1]

The existence of a circadian rhythm of cortisol secretion
as well as the absolute plasma concentration of cortisol
were assumed to be additional evidence for the absence or
presence of acute or chronic stress. Cortisol was therefore determined in each blood sample by radioimmunoassay. A
circadian rhythm of the plasma cortisol concentration was
present. Values were high in the morning and low in the
afternoon and the first part of the night. During the latter time, often periods of apparent secretory quiescence
existed. When a stress was clearly present (e.g. catheter
trouble which necessitated manipulation at the animal head),

[1] Studies done by Dr. J. Georgiev, Institut für Versuchstier-
kunde und Versuchstierkrankheiten, Freie Universität Berlin.

a sudden cortisol response usually disrupted the circadian
pattern, and much higher cortisol plasma concentrations
were measured. We therefore interpret the presence of a
smooth circadian pattern of plasma cortisol and the absence
of excessive secretory spikes during most experiments as
evidence for a non-stressful experimental condition.

Thus, several parameters -including a normal sleep-phase
pattern- indicate that our experimental conditions allow the
determination of the physiological pattern of pituitary hormone secretion as much as this is possible under laboratory
conditions (which always imply severe restrictions of mobi-
lity of the animals). We have preliminary evidence that the
hormone patterns described below are similar in animals living chronically in primate chairs and other animals living
in cages and connected to the electrocannular feedthrough
swivel by a protected cable. It should therefore be possible to detect any existing sleep-hormone link in these animals.

Hormone secretory patterns

GH in these animals is secreted episodically. However,
while in humans, there is characteristically a major GH secretory episode linked to the occurrence of the first nocturnal SWS-phase (38), this is not the case in the rhesus
monkey. Secretory episodes occur throughout the 24-h day
(Fig. 2). On many occasions there is a secretory episode
at the time of the dark/light change in the morning, which
is followed by several hours of little or no secretion.
Then secretory episodes occur fairly but not absolutely regularly with a tendency to higher maximal GH plasma concentrations towards the evening. The episodes occur with less
regularity during the night, and lower absolute concentrations are often found during the early morning hours (still
in darkness). In individual animals there is a certain reproducibility of the pattern from day to day, but sometimes,
and without any apparent reason, a quite dissimilar pattern
may be found as to frequency and height of the secretory
spikes.

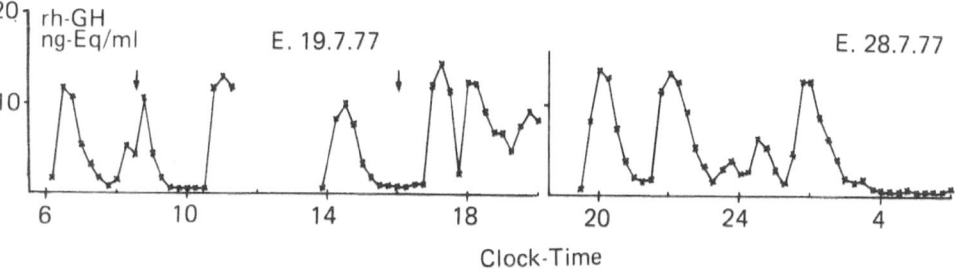

Figure 2 : GH secretory pattern during undisturbed conditions. Separate daytime and night-time curves of monkey E. are shown. Interruption between 11.30 and 13.45 h was due to technical difficulties. Arrows indicate feeding times.

The different deprivation procedures have failed to produce any evidence for an influence of the sleep/wake cycle, the rest/activity cycle during daytime or the sleep-phase cycle during the night on this secretory pattern of GH. Prominent GH secretory episodes occur during nap-deprivation (Fig. 3) as well as during sleep deprivation (Fig. 4). Selective SWS-deprivation has no inhibitory effect on GH secretion during the night, and GH secretion does not increase signi-ficantly during nights with selective REM sleep deprivation (Fig. 5). Thus, in contrast to the findings in humans, GH secretion in the rhesus monkey is not linked to the sleep/wake and the sleep-phase cycle. This is similar to the situation in the rat which also shows no correlation of GH secretion with sleep (28). It confirms results obtained

52

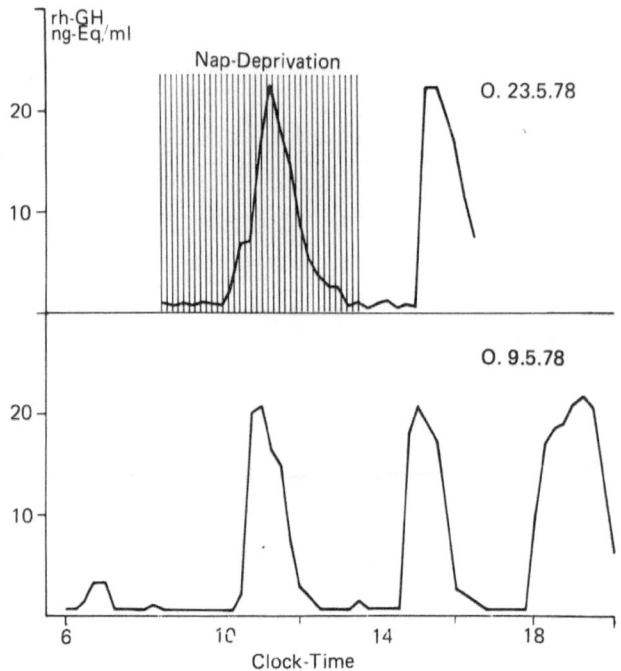

Figure 3 : *Daytime GH secretory pattern in monkey O during undisturbed conditions (lower part) and during nap deprivation. Deprivation is indicated by the shaded area. Note similar secretory episode during undisturbed conditions and during nap deprivation.*

under less strictly controlled conditions in the rhesus monkey (32). In view of the phylogenetic closeness between the rhesus monkey and the baboon, it seems likely that a suggestive relation of GH secretion to SWS in the latter species - seen in a pilot study (31) - was due to a chance relationship in a restricted number of observations.

PRL secretion in man occurs episodically during the 24-h day. There is an increase of the PRL plasma concentration during the night, and this is sleep-dependent. Highest concentrations are often reached towards the end of the night (5, 39). In our rhesus monkeys as well, PRL is often secreted in bursts. However, during long periods of time, there are only low-amplitude oscillations of the plasma PRL concentration which are within the limits of accuracy of

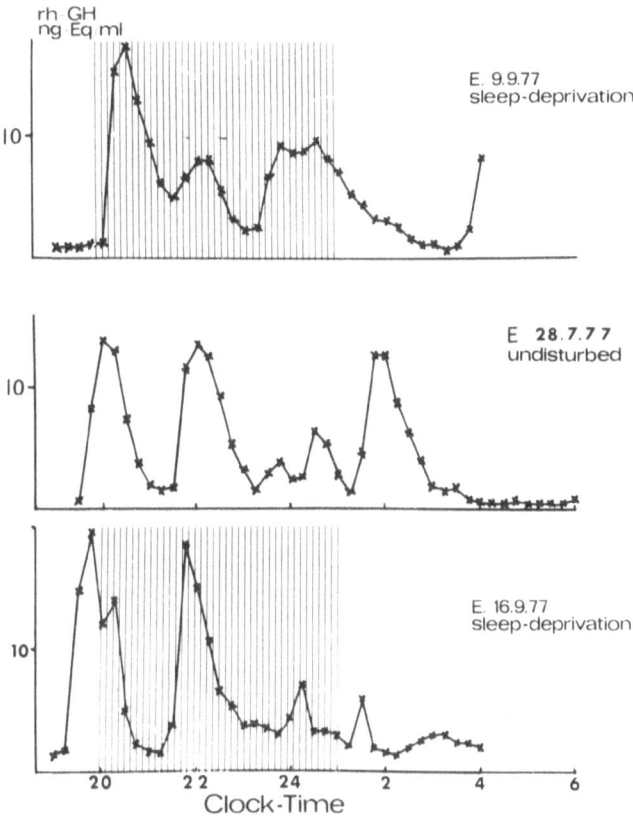

Figure 4 : Night-time GH secretory pattern of monkey E during undisturbed conditions (middle) and during sleep deprivation (upper and lower).

the assay and thus cannot with certainty be ascribed to episodic secretion (Fig. 6). The mean PRL plasma concentration is significantly higher during the night than during the day when complete 24-h observations are analyzed. In most 24-h profiles, two or three periods of elevated PRL plasma concentrations are visible : in the morning, in the late afternoon and during the night. However, the exact timing and the amplitude of these increases are somewhat variable in individual animals from day to day and also bet-

54

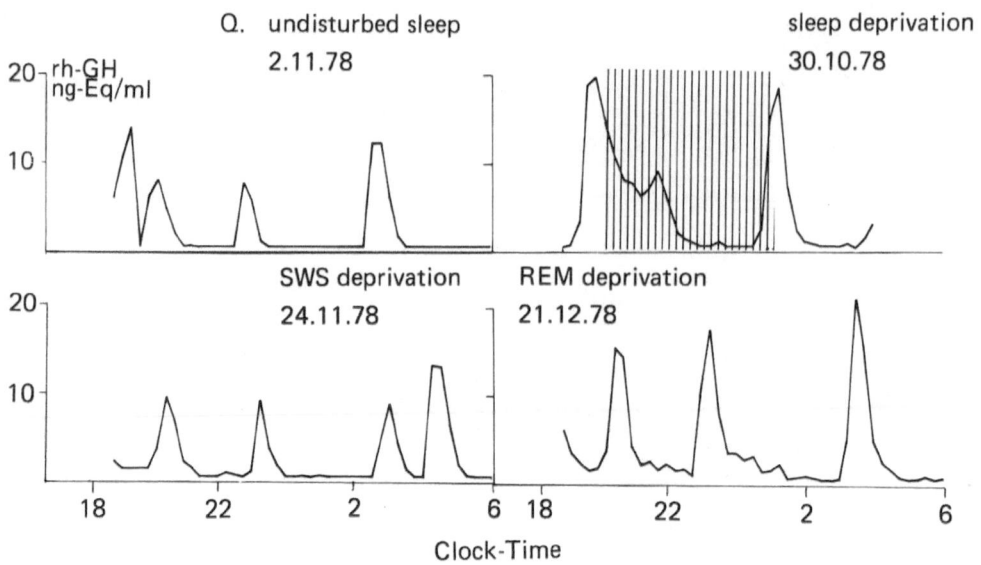

Figure 5 : Night-time GH secretory pattern in monkey Q during undisturbed sleep, during total sleep deprivation (shaded area) and during selective SWS and REM sleep deprivation. Note basic similarity of the secretory pattern irrespective of experimental conditions. The last secretory peak on 30.10.78 clearly begins before termination of the sleep deprivation.

ween animals. During nap deprivation at daytime and during sleep deprivation at night-time, PRL increases are absent (Fig. 6). However, during selective SWS or REM sleep deprivation, they do occur.

The interpretation of these results is difficult. The PRL maxima during daytime occurred shortly after the feeding times. However, in individual animals, the increases also began before feeding. During nap deprivation, the increases did not occur, although the animals were fed at the normal time. This does not support feeding as a cause of PRL elevation in the morning and the afternoon. Stress is a stimulus to PRL secretion in man. However, in our animals, PRL stress responses were clearly distinguishable by their

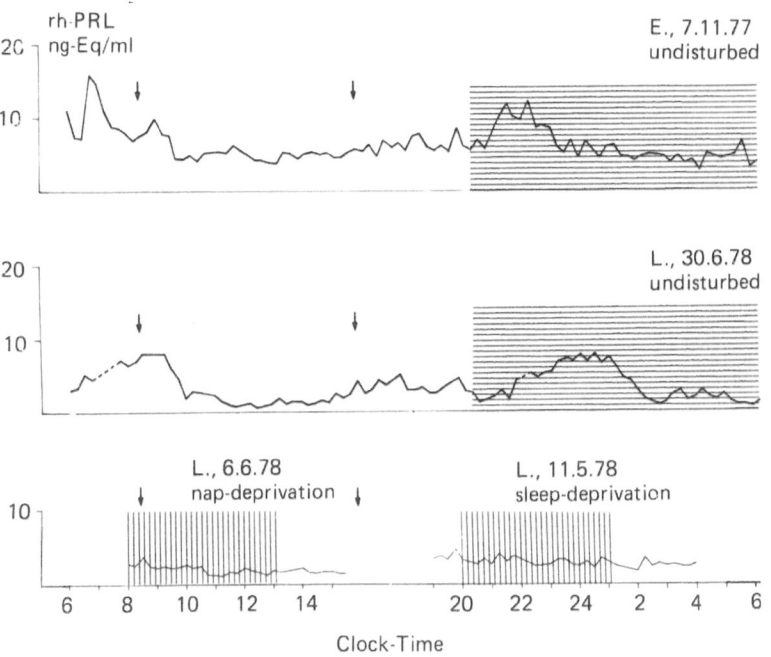

Figure 6 : PRL secretory pattern (24-h) during undisturbed conditions in 2 monkeys (E. and L.) and during nap and sleep deprivation respectively. Horizontal shading indicates lights-off. Vertical shading indicates deprivation time. Arrows : feeding times.

untimely, sudden, high-amplitude appearance in contrast to the usual slow and low-amplitude increases in the morning, the afternoon and the night. Nevertheless, it cannot be ruled out at the present time that environmental changes (cleaning, presence of personnel in the animal quarter, etc) contributed to the PRL increases during daytime.

The PRL elevation during the night was absent during total sleep deprivation, but not during selective sleep-phase deprivation. This is compatible with facilitation of noc-turnal PRL secretion by sleep in the rhesus monkey, compara-ble to the situation in man. However, during nocturnal sleep deprivation, lights were kept on until the deprivation ended at 1.00 h. Therefore, a facilitatory influence of darkness on nocturnal PRL secretion must also be considered. On the other hand, the onset of darkness and of sleep after the termination of sleep deprivation did not result in an increase of the PRL plasma concentration. This does not support a direct influence of either factor on nocturnal PRL secretion. Therefore, at the present time, the pattern of PRL secretion in the male rhesus monkey seems to be best explainable by the existence of an endogenous periodicity of relatively weak expression (in view of the high degree of variation in the pattern). A direct link of nocturnal PRL secretion to the sleep/wake cycle seems unlikely on the basis of the available information. However, a facilitatory role of sleep in the nocturnal PRL elevation may exist although distinction between the influence of light and that of sleep requires further experiments.

The results from studies on the 24-h secretory pattern of TSH in the human are somewhat controversial. While there is agreement that TSH is secreted episodically, higher plasma concentrations during the night as well as a suppressive effect of sleep on plasma TSH have been reported (9-14). In our animals, the TSH secretory pattern was surprisingly variable. In particular, the excursions of the plasma concentration during secretory episodes varied greatly in individual animals from day to day and between animals. This complicates the interpretation of the results.

Slightly higher nocturnal TSH plasma concentrations were seen when the group means of daytime and night-time concentrations were compared, although the difference fell short of being significant. However, in individual animals, there was often no clear day/night or wake/sleep difference (Fig. 7). Unexplained sudden large increases of TSH sometimes occurred during the day as well as during the night. Nap deprivation and total sleep deprivation failed to induce consistent changes of the TSH secretory pattern.

The 24-h pattern of the TSH plasma concentration in the male rhesus monkey is thus comparable with that in male human subjects, as described by some authors (10, 12). The increase of the plasma TSH concentration in the evening and the suppressive effect of sleep reported by others (9) has not been found in our animals. The cause of the high varia-

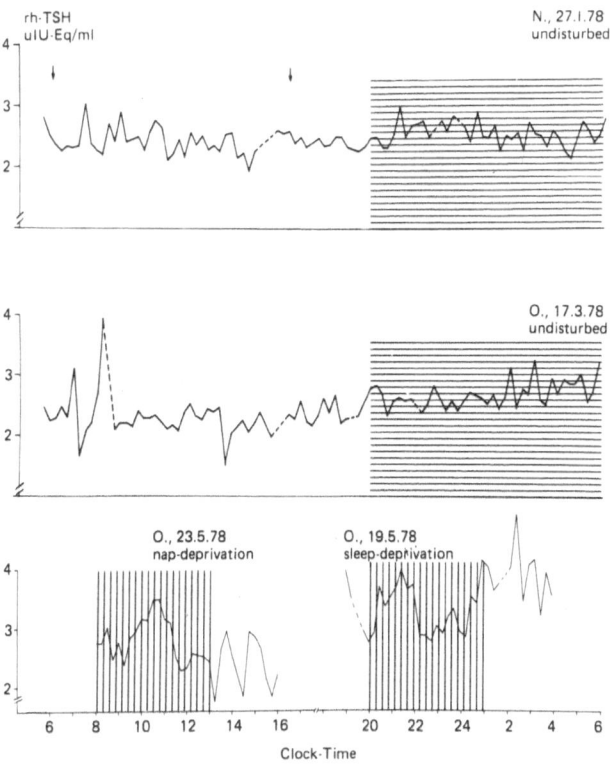

Figure 7 : *TSH secretory pattern (24-h) during undisturbed conditions in 2 monkeys (N. and O.) and during nap and sleep deprivation respectively. Symbols as in Fig. 6. Dotted lines indicate missing samples. Note absence of depressive effect of sleep onset on TSH plasma concentration during undisturbed conditions and following sleep deprivation (the episodic excursions of plasma TSH are higher in monkey O. on the days of nap and sleep deprivation than during undisturbed conditions). However, similar excursions were present on other occasions during undisturbed conditions and also on 17.3.78 during the early morning hours.*

bility of the TSH secretory pattern remains unexplained at the present time. Evaluation of the data showed no consistent influence of the time of the year (although the number of experiments in each season is too small for the application of statistical tests of significance). The strict control of the environment rules out changes of room temperature or humidity as causal factors.

Conclusions

Taken together, the results of our studies on the 24-h pattern of pituitary hormone secretion in the male rhesus monkey have revealed some differences between this primate
species and man. Most importantly, the strong link of GH
secretion with the sleep/wake cycle - regularly found in the
human - does not exist in the rhesus monkey. An influence
of sleep on the secretion of PRL has not been entirely ruled
out but does not seem to have the same importance as in man.
For TSH a comparison with man is not yet feasible, since
different reports on the human TSH secretory pattern are
not entirely concordant. It seems, however, that the rhesus monkey cannot be used as a model for human sleep related hormone secretion, at least for GH, PRL and TSH. This
makes it unlikely that other animals - phylogenetically
more remote from man - will be useful for such studies.

REFERENCES

1. Weitzman, ED, RM Boyar, S Kapen and L Hellman, The relationship of sleep and sleep stages to neuroendocrine secretion and biological rhythms in man. In : <u>Recent Progress in Hormone Research</u>, Greep, R (ed.), New York Academic Press, vol. 31, 399-446, 1975

2. Takahashi, Y, DM Kipnis and WH Daughaday, Growth hormone secretion during sleep. J Clin Invest 47:2079-2090, 1968

3. Honda, Y, K Takahashi, S Takahashi, K Azumi, M Irie, M Sakuma, T Tsushima and K Shizume, Growth hormone secretion during nocturnal sleep in normal subjects. J Clin Endocrinol Metab 29:20-29, 1969

4. Parker, DC, JF Sassin, JW Mace, RW Gotlin and LG Rossman, Human growth hormone release during sleep : Electroencephalographic correlation. J Clin Endocrinol Metab 29:871-874, 1969

5. Parker, DC, LG Rossman and EF Vanderlaan, Sleep-related nyctohemeral and briefly episodic variation in human plasma prolactin concentrations. J Clin Endocrinol Metab 26:1119-1124, 1973

6. Parker, DC, LG Rossman and EF Vanderlaan, Relation of sleep-entrained human prolactin release to REM-Non REM cycles. J Clin Endocrinol Metab 38:646-651, 1974

7. Sassin, JF, AG Frantz, ED Weitzman and S Kapen, Human prolactin : 24-hour pattern with increased release during sleep. Science 177:1205-1207, 1972

8. Mendelson, WB, LS Jacobs, JD Reichman, E Othmer, PE Cryer, B Trivedi and WH Daughaday, Methysergide. Suppression of sleep-related prolactin secretion and enhancement of sleep-related growth hormone secretion. J Clin Invest 56:690-697, 1975

9. Parker, DC, AE Pekary and JM Hershman, Effect of normal and reversed sleep-wake cycles upon nyctohemeral rhythmicity of plasma thyrotropin : Evidence suggestive of an inhibitory influence in sleep. J Clin Endocrinol Metab 43:318-329, 1976

10. Vanhaelst, L, E Van Cauter, JP Degaute, and J Golstein, Circadian varitions of serum thyrotropin

levels in man. J Clin Endocrinol Metab 35:479-482, 1972

11. Patel, YC, FP Alford and HG Burger, The 24-hour plasma thyrotrophin profile. Clin Sci 43:71-77, 1972

12. Weeke, J and HJG Gundersen, Circadian and 30 minutes variations in serum TSH and thyroid hormones in normal subjects. Acta Endocrinol (Kbh) 89:659-672, 1978

13. Copinschi, G, M L'Hermite, J Golstein, R Leclercq, D Desir, L Vanhaelst, E Virasoro, C Robyn and E Van Cauter, Interrelations between circadian and ultradian variations of PRL, ACTH, cortisol, βMSH and TSH in normal man, In: Progress in Prolactin Physiology and Pathology, Robyn, C, and M Harter (eds.),Amsterdam, Elsevier, 165-172, 1978

14. Alford, FP, HWG Baker, HG Burger, DM de Kretser, B Hudson, MW Johns, JP Masterton, YC Patel and GC Rennie, Temporal patterns of integrated plasma hormone levels during sleep and wakefulness. I. Thyroid stimulating hormone, growth hormone and cortisol. J Clin Endocrinol Metab 37:841-847, 1973

15. Othmer, E, WB Mendelson, WR Levine, WB Malarkey and WH Daughaday, Sleep-related growth hormone secretion and morning naps. Steroids Lipids Res 5:380-386, 1974

16. Besset, A, A Bonardet, M Billiard, H Descomps, A Craste de Paulet and P Passouant, Circadian patterns of growth hormone and cortisol secretions in narcoleptic patients. Chronobiologia 6:19-31, 1979

17. Takahashi, Y, K Takahashi, T Riguchi, Y Niimi, A Miyasita and Y Ishii, Pituitary hormone secretions and narcolepsy. In : Advances in Sleep Research, vol 3, Narcolepsy, Guilleminault, C, WC Dement and P Passouant (eds.), New York, Spectrum Publications, 543-563, 1976

18. Pappenheimer, JR, TB Miller and CA Goodrich, Sleep-promoting effects of cerebrospinal fluid from sleep-deprived goats. Proc Natl Acad Sci (USA) 58:513-517, 1967

19. Monnier, M, L Dudler, R Gächter and CA Schoenenberger,
     Transport of the synthetic peptide DSIP through the
     blood-brain-barrier in rabbit. Experientia 33:1609-
     1610, 1977

20. Nagasaki, H, M Iriki, S Inoué and K Uchizono, The
     presence of a sleep-promoting material in the brain
     of sleep-deprived rats. Proc Japan Acad 50:241-246,
     1974

21. Wurtman, RJ and JD Fernstrom, Control of brain neuro-
     transmitter synthesis by precursor availability and
     nutritional state. Biochem Pharmacol 25:1691-1696,
     1976

22. Knopf, RF, JW Conn, SS Fajans, JC Floyd, EM Guntsche
     and JA Rull, Plasma growth hormone response to
     intravenous administration of amino acids. J Clin
     Endocrinol Metab 25:1140-1144, 1965

23. Kukorelli, T and G Juhasz, Sleep induced by intesti-
     nal stimulation in cats. Physiol Behav 19:355-358,
     1977

24. Rubinstein, EH and RR Sonnenchein, Sleep cycles and
     feeding behaviour in the cat : role of gastrointes-
     tinal hormones. Acta Cient Venez 22:125-128, 1971

25. Roth, J, SM Glick, RS Yalow and SA Berson, Secretion
     of human growth hormone : physiological and experi-
     mental modification. Metabolism 12:577-579, 1963

26. Wolff, G and J Money, Relationship between sleep and
     growth in patients with reversible somatotropin
     deficiency (psychosocial dwarfism). Psychological
     Med 3:18-27, 1973

27. Boyar, RM, J Katz, JW Finkelstein, S Kapen, H Weiner,
     ED Weitzman and L Hellman, Anorexia nervosa : im-
     maturity of the 24-hour luteinizing hormone secre-
     tory pattern. New Engl J Med 291:861-865, 1974

28. Willoughby, JO, JB Martin, LP Renaud and P Brazeau,
     Pulsatile growth hormone release in the rat :
     failure to demonstrate a correlation with sleep
     phases. Endocrinology 98:991-996, 1976

29. Quabbe, H-J, Chronobiology of growth hormone secretion. Chronobiologia 4:217-246, 1977

30. Takahashi, K, Y Takahashi, S Takahashi and Y Honda, Growth hormone and cortisol secretion during nocturnal sleep in narcoleptics and in dogs. In : Psychoneuroendocrinology, Hatotani, N, Tsu and Mieken (eds.). Basel, Karger, 67-76, 1974

31. Parker, DC, M Morishima, DJ Koerker, CC Gale and CJ Goodner, Pilot study of growth hormone release in sleep of the chair-adapted baboon : potential as a model of human sleep release. Endocrinology 91: 1462-1467, 1972

32. Jacoby, JH, JF Sassin, M Greenstein and ED Weitzman, Patterns of spontaneous cortisol and growth hormone secretion in rhesus monkeys during the sleep-waking cycle. Neuroendocrinology 14:165-173, 1974

33. Martin, JB, Brain regulation of growth hormone secretion. In : Frontiers in neuroendocrinology, Martin, L and WF Ganong (eds.). New York, Raven Press, 4: 129-168, 1976

34. Weitzman, ED, DF Kripke, C Pollak and J Dominguez, Cyclic activity in sleep of macaca mulatta. Arch Neurol 12:463-467, 1965

35. Kripke, DF, ML Reite, GV Pegram, LM Stephens and OF Lewis, Nocturnal sleep in rhesus monkeys. EEG clin Neurophysiol 24:582-586, 1968

36. Reite, ML, JM Rhodes, E Kavan and WR Adey, Normal sleep patterns in macaque monkey. Arch Neurol 12: 133-144, 1965

37. Weitzman, ED, MM Rapport, P McGregor and J Jacoby, Sleep patterns of the monkey and brain serotonin concentration : effect of p-chlorophenylalanine. Science 160:1361-1363, 1968

38. Sassin, JF, DC Parker, JW Mace, RW Gotlin, LC Johnson and LG Rossman, Human growth release : relation to slow-wave sleep and sleep-waking cycle. Science 165:513-515, 1969

39. Sassin, JF, AG Frantz, S Kapen and ED Weitzman, The nocturnal rise of human prolactin is dependent on

sleep. J Clin Endocrinol Metab 37:436-440, 1973

40. Rechtschaffen, A, A Kales (eds.), RJ Berger, WC
    Dement, A Jacobson, LC Johnson, M Jouvet, LJ
    Monroe, I Oswald, HP Roffwarg, B Roth and RD Walter,
    A manual of standardized terminology, techniques and
    scoring system for sleep stages of human subjects.
    Public Health Service, US Government Printing Office,
    Washington, DC, 1968

ACKNOWLEDGMENTS

The experiments in monkeys were done in cooperation with
Drs. M. Gregor, D. Gianella-Neto and C. Bumke-Vogt.
Technical assistance was given by Ms. M. Rösick and B.
Henning. The manuscript was typed by Ms. J. Weirowski.

DISCUSSION

ASCHOFF: You mention that the variability in TSH pattern could probably not be due to seasonal effects because the animals were kept in standardized conditions. Did I understand correctly?

QUABBE: We have compared the patterns during different seasons and were unable to show consistent seasonal changes. However, the number of experiments performed in each season is too small to allow statistical evaluation.

ASCHOFF: Apart from a possible physiological endogenous seasonal rhythm present in those animals, there is now increasing evidence, coming not only from Hanover but also from Canada, that even under rigorously controlled 12:12 light-dark conditions, and controlled temperatures all over the year, some factors producing seasonal effects may still be present in such chambers.

VAN CAUTER: You show that the differences in GH patterns between man and monkey consist of a larger number of secretory spikes during wakefulness in the monkey. However, the human GH patterns published in the literature are mostly, if not exclusively, obtained in males. Our preliminary data suggest that, in females, it seems that the number of secretory spikes during wakefulness is much larger than in males. Were your monkeys males or females? Can you comment on sex differences in the 24-h pattern of GH?

QUABBE: All our monkeys were males. I cannot comment on sex differences in GH patterns. I agree, and this may be very important, that in man one can have almost the same GH pattern as in monkeys or in the rat under certain conditions, such as prolonged fasting and diabetes, which may be viewed as a type of prolonged intracellular fasting. Even in humans, there is probably a pulsing mechanism in the hypothalamus which tends to produce fairly regular, every 3 to 5 hours, episodic secretion of GH which is suppressed during certain times of the day and released during sleep, especially slow wave sleep.

VAN CAUTER: I would like to comment on the distribution of GH secretory spikes during wakefulness in the monkey. These spikes last about 2 hours and are distributed over a 12 to 14 hour period. There is only a limited number of ways to distribute 2-h peaks over a 12-h period and therefore one should be very cautious in concluding that peaks have a tendency to recur at specific times.

QUABBE: More precisely, there is a tendency for a GH peak to occur always at the time of the dark-light change in the morning at 06.00. (We had a 10:14 sleep-wake cycle.) Then, there is a period of 3 to 4 hours with almost no secretion until the next burst and so on. This distribution is more apparent on the mean curve. With advancement in the 24-h day, there is a tendency to disruption of this synchronized regulation. It is our impression that there may be group synchronization by the dark-light change in the morning which breaks down as the day progresses. But although there is a certain regularity, the reproducibility within and among individuals from day to day is not always good.

HANSEN: I would like to comment on your very beautiful GH results. Patterns similar to yours were also observed in the rat. Are there other animals in which similar GH secretory patterns have been reported?

QUABBE: The rat and the monkey are the only two animals which show a fairly regular pattern of GH spiking. No comparable studies exist in other species. It seems that the rat is more regular than the monkey in the periodicity of the peaks. The mean period is about 3 - 4 hours in the rat. In some of our studies in which we extended the sampling over 36 hours, we performed a frequency analysis and we detected significant periodicities of 24 hours and 4 - 5 hours. Thus, it seems that the period of spike recurrence is a little longer in the monkey than in the rat, but the variability is certainly much larger in the monkey that in the rat.

WEITZMAN: In patients with narcolepsy, who have multiple sleep episodes during the day, we found a similar increase of GH secretion with a decreased period length between episodes. Thus, patterns similar to the ones observed in monkey may occur in man. Regarding your sleep deprivation studies, were the animals deprived all day or only during segments of the day?

QUABBE: Sleep deprivation was only during the night from 20.00 to 01.00. The observation was then continued until 04.00. Thus, the animals were deprived of the first five hours of sleep. Our intention was not to perform a sleep-reversal study but to investigate whether the early GH increase associated with sleep onset is suppressed when the animal is deprived of sleep and whether it appears again later when the animal is allowed to sleep.

WEITZMAN: Was there nap deprivation all day?

QUABBE: The nap deprivation was from 08.00 to 13.00 and then the animals were allowed to nap from 13.00 to 16.00.

WEITZMAN: If you had kept the animals awake from 07.00 to 22.00, you could have developed a consolidated sleep period at night very similar to human sleep with stages III - IV at the beginning of sleep and a recurrent REM - non-REM cycle with much fewer awakenings. Thus, the human sleep - wake cycle can be mimicked in monkeys by preventing day time sleep, which is usually absent in man. Regarding the 3-hour GH cyclicity your data seem to show, I wonder if these monkeys were free running since they had their own sleep - wake cycle. Under free running conditions, the rhythm of GH secre-

tion and the sleep - wake cycle may have different periods.
If a synchronized sleep - wake cycle was enforced, a relationship between GH secretion and sleep onset might appear.

QUABBE: The nap deprivation and sleep deprivation
were always performed on separate days. The animals developed very good sleep cycles with a slow-wave phase in the
beginning of sleep. Actually, analyzing the sleep data on
days with and without blood sampling, we found on the average no differences between the two conditions. Our first
results seemed to indicate that there was, in our monkeys,
a relationship between sleep onset and GH spiking. However, this was mere chance as we found out when the number
of experiments was increased.

Regarding your second question, these animals were
under strict sleep - wake and dark - light controlled
conditions and it is our impression that this 4 to 5 hour
periodicity breaks up during day time and is re-established
the next morning. It is especially apparent in the mean
curve of approximately forty-five 24-h profiles that there
is always a peak in the morning between 06.00 and 07.00,
after lights on, and then no peak for several hours and
then comes the next peak. The nadirs on the mean curve
disappear until the next morning as a result of inter-
individual desynchronization since the individuals continue to spike. We are currently performing experiments
with lights-on delays and awakening delays to further
investigate these phenomena.

ADAPTATION OF 24-HOUR HORMONAL PATTERNS AND SLEEP TO JET LAG

Eve Van Cauter[1,6], Samuel Refetoff[6], Daniel Desir[2], Claude
Jadot[3], Michelle Fevre-Montange[9], Victor S. Fang[7],
Jacqueline Golstein[1], Marc L'Hermite[4], Claude Robyn[4], Pierre
Noel[5], Jean-Paul Spire[8] and Georges Copinschi[2]

[1]Institute of Interdisciplinary Research (LMN), [2]Laboratory
of Experimental Medicine, [3]Department of Psychiatry,
[4]Department of Gynecology and Obstetrics, [5]Department of
Pediatric Neurology, School of Medicine, Free University of
Brussels, Belgium and [6]Thyroid Study Unit, [7]Endocrinology
Laboratory, [8]Laboratory of Clinical Neurophysiology, The
University of Chicago, Illinois, USA and [9]Laboratory of
Endocrinology, Hôpital de l'Antiquaille, University of Lyon,
France.

INTRODUCTION

Effects of rapid transmeridian time shifts on behavioral
and biological parameters such as vigilance, heart rate,
and urinary excretion of electrolytes and corticosteroids
have been demonstrated (1, 2, 3). Because of the key role
played by hormones in the adaptation to the environment,
disruptions in the temporal organization of hormonal secretion might be involved in the production of the jet lag
syndrome. The current availability of sensitive hormone
assays has made it possible to test this hypothesis. Moreover, assessment of jet lag induced changes of the 24-h
hormonal profiles and their pattern of adaptation is expected to bring further insight into the control of the
various hormonal rhythms, the identity of their zeitgebers
and their possible interrelationships.

In the present investigation, healthy males were submitted to seven 24-h studies over a total period of 10
weeks while they underwent a westward and an eastward 7-h
time shift by jet. During each 24-h session, blood was

sampled at 15-min intervals and sleep and psychological indexes of anxiety and depression were recorded. The protocol of the study and the adaptation of the pituitary-adrenal periodicity and of the melatonin rhythm have been described in detail elsewhere (4, 5). We present here an overview of these results as well as preliminary data on the 24-h profiles of prolactin (PRL) and compare the adaptation of sleep and of the various hormonal patterns to the subjective evaluation of adaptation provided by the anxiety and depression scores.

SUBJECTS AND METHODS

Subjects

Five healthy male volunteers, aged 21 - 29, were studied. Their selection involved an interview, a physical examination and a psychiatric evaluation. Normality of their physical condition was further assessed by a battery of biological tests including a thorough endocrine evaluation, and by electroencephalographic and electrocardiographic recordings (4). Positive factors for selection included emotional stability, adherance to regular social, professional, feeding and sleep schedules and absence of personal or family history of endocrine and psychiatric disturbances. All volunteers gave a written consent after full explanation of the aims and means of the study.

Protocol of the Investigation

The study rooms in Brussels, Belgium and in Chicago, USA, were of similar design. The time zone difference between these locations was 7 hours. The investigation spanned from October 17th to January 1st. Climatic conditions were detailed elsewhere (4).

Except during travel, throughout the investigation, the subjects adhered to a 16:8 light-dark cycle (lights off from 23:00 to 07:00, local time) and to regular meals at 08:00, 12:30 and 19:00, local time (LT). During travel,

they were exposed to the usual airport and aircraft conditions and sleep was prevented. Owing to the airline schedule, on the westward trip, the duration of daylight and
the exposure to light (natural or artificial) were prolonged from, respectively, 10 and 16 hours to 16 and 23
hours. Sleep deprivation also lasted 23 hours. On the
eastward trip, exposure to light and sleep deprivation were
prolonged to 33 hours. However, the duration of natural
darkness was shortened from approximately 15 hours to an
average of 9 hours with unchanged preceding and following
periods of daylight. Study 1 was performed in Brussels
after four nights of adjustment to the blood sampling and
sleep recording conditions. Studies 2, 3 and 4 begun ~1
(25 h), 11 and 21 days after arrival in Chicago. All subjects remained in Chicago for 30 days. Studies 5, 6 and 7
corresponded to ~1 (33 h), 11 and 21 days after return to
Brussels. A day of readjustment to the study unit preceded
each 25-h blood sampling session. Details of the blood
sampling procedure were given elsewhere (4).

Measurement in Plasma Samples

Blood samples were immediately centrifuged at 4°C. Total
plasma proteins (TPP) were then measured in order to detect
possible plasma dilutions resulting from the sampling procedure. Thirty-six of the 3264 samples were found to be
significantly diluted and were discarded (4). Plasma ACTH,
cortisol, melatonin and PRL were measured on each sample.
Technical details for ACTH, cortisol and melatonin assays
were given elsewhere (4,5). Plasma PRL was measured by a
radioimmunoassay and results expressed in μU of the pituitary research standard n° 71/222 of the Medical Research
Council, Great Britain (6). One μU of this standard is
equivalent to .045 ng of the VLS standard. Samples from a
single subject were always analyzed in the same assay. For
statistical purposes, values below the limit assay sensitivity were set equal to 50% of this limit and missing data
were linearly interpolated.

Sleep Analysis

The polygraphic recordings of sleep were scored at 20-sec intervals using a standardized procedure (7). The total sleep period was defined as the period between sleep onset and final morning awakening. During the total sleep period, interrupted time segments of wakefulness, stage REM, stage I and II, stages III and IV and stage IV only were summed up. The actual duration of sleep was defined as the total sleep period minus the duration of wakefulness interrupting the sleep. The amounts of stage REM and stage IV were expressed in percent of the actual duration of sleep. The distribution of REM and of stage IV sleep was evaluated by comparing the percentage of time spent in each of these stages in the first (REM_1, IV_1) and second (REM_2, IV_2) halves of the total sleep period, and by calculating the ratios ($REM_2 - REM_1$)/total REM and ($IV_2 - IV_1$)/total IV (5).

Psychological Evaluation

Psychopathological evaluation using the Hamilton scales for anxiety and depression (8, 9) was carried out with each study by the same investigator (C.J.).

Statistical Analysis

The low frequency (e.g., circadian) components of each individual profile of TPP, ACTH, cortisol, melatonin and PRL were evaluated using a method based on the building of a best-fit pattern described in detail elsewhere (10). The amplitude of the rhythm, its acrophases and nadirs, its major acrophases and the confidence intervals were defined and calculated (4). Mean TPP levels during ambulation and recumbency were compared for each individual profile by a t test with a minimal probability level of 0.05. To characterize the period during which serum cortisol levels are low, the "period of minimal secretion" (PMS) was defined as starting when concentrations lower than 50% of the 24-h mean level were observed for more than two consecutive samples, and ending when concentrations higher than 50% of the 24-h mean level were obtained for more than

two consecutive samples. To quantify fragmentation of the
PMS occurring in the course of adaptation to jet lag, the
duration of the longest uninterrupted portion of the PMS or
the major PMS (MPMS) was calculated and expressed in percent of the PMS. For PRL profiles, the acrophases were
classified as "wakefulness acrophase" or "sleep acrophase"
depending upon their time of occurrence. Unless otherwise
specified, all group data are given as mean $\pm$ SD. Times
are expressed in hours and minutes of the local 24-h clock
time.

RESULTS

The four top panels of Figure 1 illustrate the 24-h profiles of TPP, cortisol, melatonin and PRL obtained in one
representative subject in study 1, before leaving Brussels.
In the unperturbed state, TPP levels were higher during
ambulation (A) than during recumbency (R). This presumably
posture-dependent variation resulted in a significant circadian rhythm (4). The 24-h profiles of ACTH and cortisol
were essentially concordant (4). They exhibited the classical characteristics of the pituitary-adrenal periodicity
with maximal levels around 07:30 LT, decreasing concentrations throughout the daytime, a period of minimal secretion
lasting approximately 4 hours around midnight followed by a
sharp early morning rise (4). The 24-h rhythm of plasma
melatonin consisted of a well-defined increase in secretory
activity starting in the evening and culminating approximately 2 hours after lights were turned off and one hour
after the onset of sleep. During daytime, melatonin levels
were generally low although diurnal acrophases were sometimes observed (5). In agreement with previous findings
(12), PRL followed a bimodal pattern with minimum levels
around noon, a late afternoon phase of increased secretory
activity and a subsequent major nocturnal elevation culminating around mid-sleep. Episodic fluctuations of cortisol,
ACTH, melatonin and PRL occurred throughout the 24-h span.

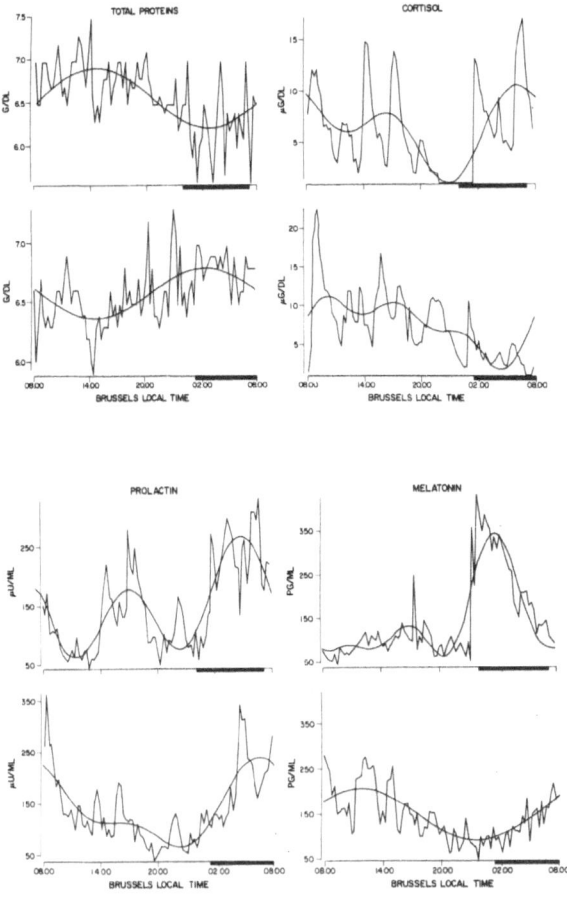

Figure 1: Twenty-four hour profiles of total plasma proteins
(TPP), cortisol, melatonin and prolactin (PRL) of one representative subject in study 1, before travel (top panels) and in study
5, one day after eastward shift (lower panels). Black bars indicate the sleep periods. The best-fit pattern is superimposed on
the data.

Criteria for Evaluation of Adaptation

In an attempt to obtain a quantitative analysis of the process of adaptation to jet lag, criteria for deviations from
normalcy were defined for each parameter recorded using the

results of study 1 as reference. Differences in the 24-h
mean levels or amplitudes of the circadian rhythm specifically associated with a jet lag effect were not significant
at the group level (4, 5). Therefore, the criteria for
adaptation takes mainly into consideration the synchronization of each profile to the local time and its conformity
with the shape of the reference profile. The circadian
amplitudes of the profiles will be compared and their evolution throughout the investigation analyzed in a separate
section. The terms "synchronization", "partial synchronization" and "desynchronization", as defined below, refer
to the time of occurrence of an acrophase or nadir with respect to the reference acrophase or nadir. The criteria
for "adaptation", "partial adaptation" or "no adaptation"
take into account not only the synchronization but also,
when relevant, the conformity with the shape of the reference pattern.

Conditions for synchronization of an acrophase (or
nadir) to the LT are illustrated in Figure 2. The reference acrophase was defined as the average acrophase of
study 1 for the group of subjects. The average confidence
interval for acrophases (or nadirs) of hormonal patterns
was roughly one hour (4). Since differences may be considered significant when the corresponding confidence intervals do not overlap (10), acrophases (or nadirs) were considered to be "synchronized" to LT if they occurred within $\pm$
2 hours of the reference acrophase (or nadir) expressed in
LT. Because the time zone difference between Brussels and
Chicago was of 7 hours, an acrophase (or nadir) was considered to be "partially synchronized" if it occurred between
2 and 5 hours from the reference acrophase (expressed in LT)
in the direction opposite to the preceding time shift. An
acrophase (or nadir) was considered to be "desynchronized"
when it was neither synchronized nor partially synchronized.
Desynchronization thus includes cases where the acrophase
(or nadir) remained synchronized on Brussels time when the
subject was in Chicago and vice-versa, as well as cases

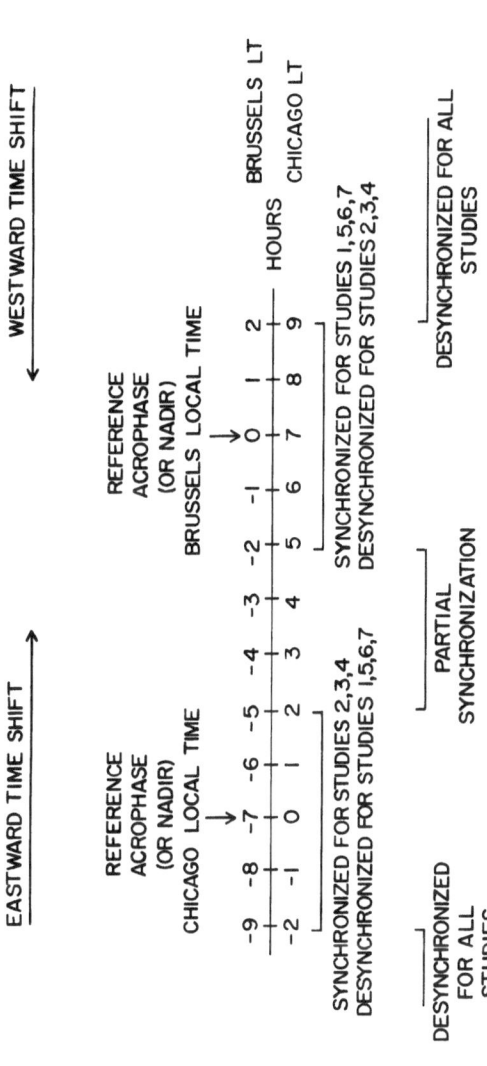

Figure 2: Criteria for synchronization, partial synchronization or desynchronization of an acrophase (or a nadir) according to its time of occurrence in relation to the time shift. The reference acrophase (or nadir) is the average acrophase (or nadir) in study 1. Chicago LT lags 7 hours behind Brussels LT. Westward shift implies a 7-hour delay and eastward shift a 7-hour advance.

where the rhythm was totally disrupted with an acrophase (or nadir) occurring outside of the ranges for synchronization or for partial synchronization on any of the two local times. For example, if the reference acrophase is 08.00 LT, acrophases observed in subsequent studies will be considered as "synchronized" if they occur between 06.00 and 10.00 LT, as "partially synchronized" if they occur after 03.00 but before 06.00 in Chicago LT after eastward shift or before 13.00 but after 10.00 in Brussels LT after westward shift, and as "desynchronized" if they occur outside the range 06.00 - 13.00 in Brussels or outside the range 03.00 - 10.00 in Chicago.

Using these criteria for synchronization, the 24-h profiles of blood constituents, the sleep records and the psychological evaluations were scored "0" for "adapted", "50" for "partially adapted" and "100" for "not adapted" as follows:

24-h profile of ACTH and cortisol: Since ACTH and cortisol profiles were largely concordant throughout the investigation, the process of adaptation was evaluated using the cortisol profiles which provide a more accurate estimation for the circadian components because episodic fluctuations are of lesser magnitude (4). Detailed analysis of the results showed that the major acrophase and the period of minimal secretion (PMS) adapt at a different rate (4). Separate criteria were defined to describe these differences. Whereas, under basal conditions, the cortisol pattern had one major acrophase and one major nadir, two major acrophases and/or nadirs occurred in the course of adaptation and were interpreted as reflecting a splitting of the rhythm as is commonly observed when environmental zeitgebers of a biological rhythm are manipulated (12). In the criteria hereafter, the terms "acrophase" and "nadir" refer to the major acrophase and nadir.

    a. Criteria for time of maximal secretion:
        reference: one acrophase at 07.26 (LT).

"adapted": one acrophase synchronized on LT.

"partially adapted": one acrophase partially synchronized OR two acrophases, one of which
sychronized or partially synchronized on LT.

"not adapted": one desynchronized acrophase OR two
desynchronized acrophases

b. Criteria for time of minimal secretion:

reference: one nadir at 00.00 (LT). The average
MPMS for the group in study 1 is 93% $\pm$ 8%
(mean $\pm$ SD).

"adapted": One nadir synchronized on LT. The
MPMS $\geqslant$ 85% (mean - 1SD).

"partially adapted": one nadir partially synchronized on LT OR two nadirs, one of which synchronized or partially synchronized on LT OR
77% (mean - 2SD) $\ll$ MPMS $<$ 85% (mean - 1SD).

"not adapted": one desynchronized nadir OR two
desynchronized nadirs OR MPMS $<$ 77% (mean -
2SD).

24-h profile of melatonin: Criteria are based only on
the synchronization of the major nocturnal acrophase since
low melatonin levels occurred for periods of time too long
to define nadirs or PMS (5). Splitting did not seem to be
associated with adaptation (5).

reference: one acrophase at 01.15 (LT).

"adapted": one acrophase synchronized on LT.

"partially adapted": one acrophase partially synchronized on LT.

"not adapted": all major acrophases are synchronized.

24-h profile of PRL: The adaptation of the sleep and
wakefulness acrophases was evaluated separately as they appeared differently influenced by the time shifts. Whereas,
under basal conditions, the PRL pattern had one sleep and
one wakefulness acrophase, splitting of the wakefulness
acrophase occurred in the course of adaptation to jet lag.

a. Criteria for sleep acrophase:

reference: one acrophase at 04.18 (LT).

"adapted": one sleep acrophase synchronized on LT.

> "partially adapted": one sleep acrophase parti-
>   ally synchronized on LT.
> "not adapted": the sleep acrophase is desynchro-
>   nized.
> b. Criteria for wakefulness acrophase:
> reference: one wakefulness acrophase at 17.27
>   (LT).
> "adapted": one wakefulness acrophase synchronized
>   on LT.
> "partially adapted": one wakefulness acrophase
>   partially synchronized on LT OR two wakeful-
>   ness acrophases with one synchronized or par-
>   tially synchronized on LT.
> "not adapted": no wakefulness acrophase OR one
>   desynchronized wakefulness acrophase.

24-h profile of TPP: The difference between mean TPP
levels during ambulation and recumbency (A-R) was used to
quantify disruptions. In study 1, 4 of 5 subjects had a
significant positive A-R (4).

> "adapted": A-R significantly positive.
> "partially adapted": A-R non-significant
> "not adapted": A-R significantly negative.

Sleep records: Examination of the sleep records indicated that patterns obtained in study 1 should not be used
as reference since an abnormal amount of awakenings occurred despite 4 nights of adjustment to the sleep recording
conditions. Patterns obtained in studies 6 and 7 were
similar to textbook descriptions and were used as reference
to evaluate disruptions in other studies. Disturbances of
sleep observed in the course of the investigation included
increased percent of wakefulness, decreased percent of REM
stage, increased percent of stage IV and abnormal distribution of REM stages across sleep (4). In studies 6 and 7,
on the average, the percentage of wakefulness was 6% $\pm$ 5%,
the percentage of REM 27% $\pm$ 7%, the percentage of stage IV
20% $\pm$ 7% and the ratio $(REM_2 - REM_1)$/total REM was positive
in all records.

"adapted": % of wakefulness $<$ 11% (mean + 1SD)

% of REM $>$ 20% (mean - 1SD)

% of IV $<$ 27% (mean + 1SD)

Positive ratio $(REM_2 - REM_1)$/total REM

"partially adapted": One of the following occurs:

% of wake $>$ 11%

% of REM $<$ 20%

% of IV $>$ 27%

negative ratio $(REM_2 - REM_1)$/total REM

"not adapted": two or more of the conditions listed above are present.

Psychological status: Because of the larger interindividual variability commonly encountered in psychological scoring, the results from studies 1 and 7 were used as reference in order to increase the number of individual determinations. The reference score for depression was 2 ± 2 and the reference score for anxiety was 3 ± 2 (4).

"adapted": depression score $<$ 4 (mean $\pm$ 1SD)

anxiety score $<$ 5 (mean + 1SD)

"partially adapted": 4 $<$ depression score $<$ 6 (mean + 2SD)

5 $<$ anxiety score $<$ 7 (mean + 2SD)

"not adapted": depression score $>$ 6

anxiety score $>$ 7

Occurrence of Disruptions in the Course of Adaptation

The lower panels of Figure 1 show the TPP and hormonal profiles obtained one day after the eastward flight, Chicago-Brussels. Disruptions are evident. The TPP levels were higher during recumbency than during ambulation rather than the opposite. The acrophase of the cortisol rhythm was partially synchronized on the new clock time but the PMS remained centered on Chicago time and was fragmented in 3 portions with an MPMS of 38%. The melatonin rhythm was totally disrupted with the major acrophase occurring in the middle of the daytime period rather than at night. Finally,

despite immediate adaptation of the nocturnal PRL elevation
to the time shift, alterations of the organization of PRL
secretion during wakefulness are obvious.

Figure 3 illustrates the evolution of the cortisol,
melatonin and PRL major acrophases in the same subject
throughout the investigation, together with the corresponding sleep-wake and natural and artificial dark-light cycles.
Under basal conditions (study 1), the melatonin acrophase
occurred first, approximately one hour after sleep onset,
was then followed by the PRL acrophase and finally by the
early morning cortisol acrophase. This temporal succession
was maintained in all studies except for study 5, one day
after eastward shift. In study 2, the 3 acrophases shifted
almost in parallel but were not fully synchronized on the
new clock time. Full synchronization occurred in study 3.
In study 5, the PRL acrophase immediately synchronized with
the displacement of sleep but melatonin and cortisol secretions were totally disorganized, with melatonin acrophase
during the middle of the daytime period and split cortisol
acrophases, one on Chicago LT and the other partially synchronized to Brussels LT.

The criteria for adaptation defined above will also
detect disruptions in 24-h profiles of blood constituents,
sleep records or psychological status which are not related
to transmeridian time shift. In studies 1 or 7, possible
individual discrepancies from the reference characteristics
cannot be associated with adaptation to jet lag. Nevertheless, they will be detected by the criteria for adaptation
and included in the average score for the group in these
studies.

For each parameter and for each study, the average disruption score at the group level is shown on Figure 4. Fig.
4G illustrates the evolution of the global disruption score,
averaged across all parameters and all subjects. The period
of minimal pituitary-adrenal secretion, as quantified by
the cortisol nadirs, PMS and MPMS, stands out as an exception since its disruptions were more severe one day after

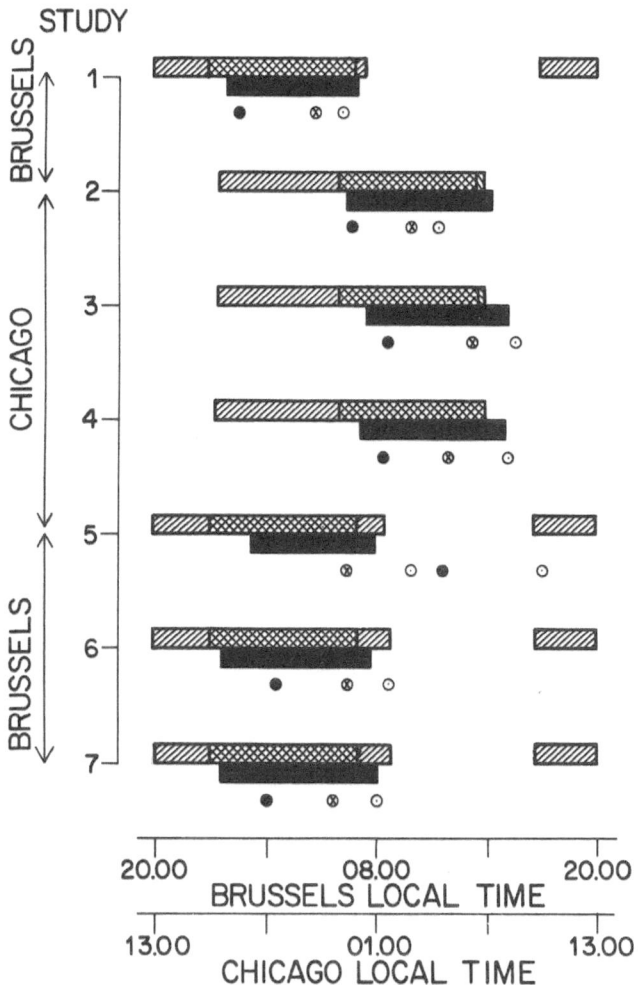

Figure 3: Evolution of the major acrophase for melatonin (●),
PRL (θ) and cortisol (θ) throughout the investigation for one
representative subject. Black bars indicate the sleep periods.
Right-hatched bars show the period of natural darkness, left-
hatched bars the period with lights off and cross-hatched bars
the period of superimposed natural darkness and lights off.

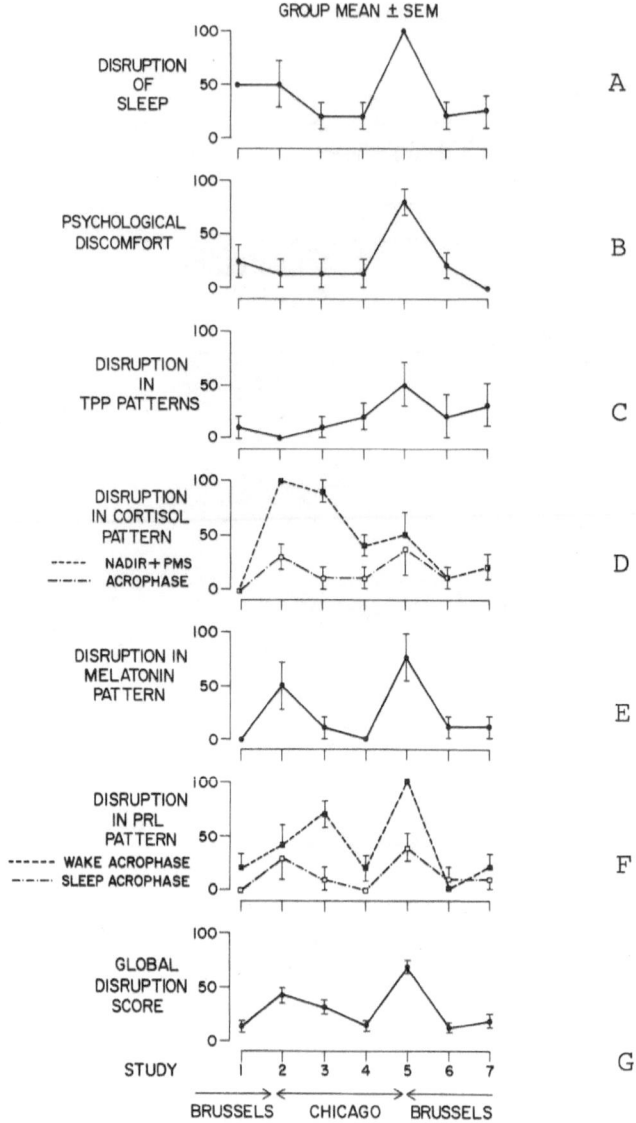

Figure 4: Evolution of the average disruption score for the various parameters recorded (panels A through F) and of the global disruption score (panel G) throughout the investigation. Note that the average global score is lower in study 2 (one day after westward travel) than in study 5 (one day after eastward travel) but higher in study 3 (after 11 days in Chicago) than in study 5 (after 11 days in Brussels).

westward (study 2) rather than eastward travel and persisted for more than 11 days in Chicago (study 4) (Fig. 4D).
For all the other parameters so far examined, low disruption scores were obtained in studies 1 (before travel), 4
(after 21 days in Chicago), 6 (after 11 days in Brussels),
and 7 (after 21 days in Brussels) and disruptions were more
severe after the eastward flight than after the westward
flight. Persistent temporal disorganization was observed
in study 3 (after 11 days in Chicago), not only for the
minimal cortisol secretion but also for the PRL acrophase
during wakefulness. However, both parameters were fully
adapted to local time 11 days after return to Brussels. No
indexes of psychological discomfort were significant in
study 2, one day after westward flight, despite partial
disruptions in sleep, pituitary-adrenal periodicity and
melatonin and PRL rhythms.

Evolution of Relative Circadian Amplitudes

Figure 5 illustrates the group average of the relative circadian amplitude of the TPP, ACTH, cortisol, melatonin and
PRL patterns. In studies 1, 4, 6 and 7, when jet lag effects were presumably absent, the average amplitude, expressed in percent of the 24-h mean, was 5% $\pm$ 3% for TPP,
80% $\pm$ 37% for ACTH, 94% $\pm$ 17% for cortisol and 66% $\pm$ 17%
for PRL. The dispersion of individual values, as determined by the SD, is wider for ACTH than for cortisol, probably because of the larger number and greater magnitude of
the secretory episodes (4). For melatonin, a significant
decrease in amplitude, apparently unrelated to time shifts,
was observed as the investigation progressed from October
to January (5). The average melatonin amplitude was 89% $\pm$
27% for studies 1 and 4 and 55% $\pm$ 21% for studies 6 and 7.

Statistical analysis of matched pairs before travel
and one day after arrival (studies 1-2 and 4-5) failed so
far to demonstrate changes in relative circadian amplitude,
significant at the group level, for any of the hormones
studied. However, in the case of the pituitary-adrenal

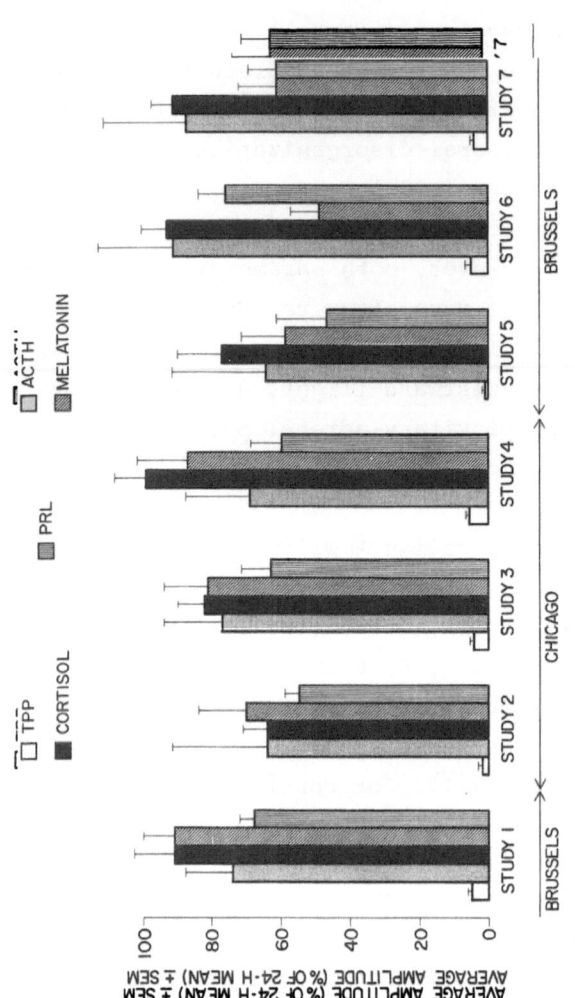

Figure 5: Average circadian amplitudes of TPP, ACTH, cortisol, melatonin and PRL throughout the investigation. Note the decrease in melatonin amplitude in studies 6 and 7 as compared to studies 1 and 4 and the apparent overall reduction in amplitude immediately after travel for TPP, pituitary-adrenal periodicity and PRL.

periodicity, this negative result may well be related to the small number of subjects since 7 of the 9 individual transmeridian transitions were accompanied by a reduction of the circadian amplitude of the cortisol rhythm. For PRL, a decrease in amplitude occurred in 4 of the 5 subjects after westward shift but only in one subject after eastward shift. As shown in Figure 5, the average circadian amplitude for TPP, ACTH, cortisol and PRL were lower in studies 2 and 5, when compared to all other studies. However, they did not reach a level of statistical significance.

CONCLUSIONS

After both westward and eastward shift, disruptions in sleep and temporal organization of hormonal secretion were observed. Eleven days after travel in both directions, sleep and the major acrophase for cortisol, melatonin and PRL were adapted to local time. Disruptions in these "fast-adapting" parameters were, on the average, more severe after eastward than after westward transportation. In contrast, the rate of adaptation of the quiescent period of the pituitary-adrenal rhythm and the daytime PRL acrophase was slower after westward trip, with disturbances persisting for 11 days, and in some individuals for 21 days, after arrival in Chicago. Since the circadian rhythm of TPP has been shown to be posture-dependent (13), the partial disruption in the 24-h profile of TPP, observed only after the eastward shift, was probably caused by the longer period spent without recumbency. Psychological indexes of discomfort were observed after eastward shift only, concomitantly with greater disturbances of sleep and melatonin and PRL secretion. The objective disruptions in biological and neurological parameters observed after westward jet lag were not associated with any subjective discomfort one day after travel. To conclude that alterations in sleep and hormonal secretion are responsible for the jet lag syndrome and that they modulate the associated psychological manifestations will require further correlation analysis and inclusion of data on other hormones collected during this investigation.

ACKNOWLEDGEMENTS
Thanks are due to Dr. J. E. Dumont for continual support, to Dr. L. J. DeGroot for use of his PDP 11/34 computer and to Mrs. Yolanda W. Richmond for secretarial help.

REFERENCES

1. Klein, KE, HM Wegmann, and BI Hunt, Desynchronization of body temperature and performance circadian rhythm as a result of outgoing and homegoing transmeridian flights. Aerospace Med 43:119, 1972

2. Lafontaine, E, J Lavernhe, J Courillon, M Medvedeff, and J Ghata, Influence of air travel east-west and vice-versa on circadian rhythms of urinary elimination of potassium and 17-hydroxycorticoids. Aerospace Med 38:944, 1967

3. Nicholson, AN, Duty hours and sleep patterns in air crew operating world-wide routes. Aerospace Med 43:138, 1972

4. Desir, D, E Van Cauter, J Golstein, VS Fang, E Martino, C Jadot, JP Spire, P Noël, S Refetoff, and G Copinschi, Effects of jet lag on hormonal patterns. I. Procedures, variations in total plasma proteins and disruption of ACTH-cortisol periodicity. J Clin Endocrinol Metab in press, 1981

5. Fevre-Montange, M, E Van Cauter, S Refetoff, D Desir, J Tourniaire, and G Copinschi, Effects of jet lag on hormonal patterns. II. Adaptation of melatonin circadian periodicity. J Clin Endocrinol Metab in press, 1981

6. Badawi, M, S Bila, M L'Hermite, FR Perez-Lopez, and C Robyn, Comparative evaluation of radioimmunoassay methods for human prolactin using anti-ovine and anti-human prolactin sera, In: Radioimmunoassay and Related Procedures in Medicine, International Atomic Energy Agency, Wien, vol. 1, 411-422, 1974

7. Rechtschaffen, A, and A Kales, A manual of standardized terminology, techniques and scoring system for sleep stages of human subjects. Publich Health Service, Government Printing Office, Washington, D.C., 1968

8. Hamilton, M, A rating scale for depression. J Neurol Neurosurg Psychiat 23:56-62, 1960

9. Hamilton, M, The assessment of anxiety states by rating. Brit J Med Psych 32:50-55, 1959

10. Van Cauter, E, Method for the characterization of 24-hour temporal variations of blood components. Am J Physiol 6:E255-E264, 1979

11. Sassin, JF, AG Frantz, S Kapen, and ED Weitzman, The nocturnal rise of human prolactin is dependent on sleep. J Clin Endocrinol Metab 37:436, 1973

12. Krieger, DT and J Aschoff, Endocrine and other Biological rhythms, In: Endocrinology, DeGroot LJ (ed.), New York, Grune and Stratton, vol. ii, p. 2079, 1979

13. DeCostre, P, U Buhler, LJ DeGroot, and S Refetoff, Diurnal rhythm in total serum thyroxine levels. Metabolism 20:782-791, 1971.

DISCUSSION

Questions from the audience were answered by Drs. Copinschi, Desir, Fevre and Van Cauter.

WEITZMAN: Regarding the concept of east-west and west-east differences, Dr. Klein and co-workers, in Germany, showed rather convincingly that it does not make any difference whether you are going home or away from home. The only thing that matters is whether you fly east (less than 180° phase shift), which is a phase advance or whether you fly west, which is a phase delay. The evidence that there is an asymmetry of the phase-response curve supports this concept.

Regarding the issue of the relationship of PRL and REM - non-REM cycles, did I understand correctly you used the end of the REM period in your analysis?

DESIR: Yes.

WEITZMAN: REM periods vary in length. One could use the beginning or the mid-point of the REM periods or even the mid-point of a short REM - non-REM cycle. Just looking at the end of the REM cycle may not be the best way to search for a possible relationship between PRL and REM - non-REM cycles. Did you look at other aspects of sleep?

DESIR: Other aspects of the analysis of the sleep data are still under progress. We first tried to reproduce the results of Parker and co-workers published in 1974 using an identical methodology and we failed to reproduce these results. I am not aware of other reports investigating a possible relationship between PRL episodic secretion and REM - non-REM cycles using other criteria.

VAN CAUTER: We made another type of analysis in order to investigate the relationship between PRL peaks and sleep stages. Using a computer program specifically designed for that purpose, data points which are, respectively, in the increasing and in the declining portion of the secretory episodes were defined. Then, the proportion of "increasing data" in non-REM stages and the proportion of "declining data" in REM stages was calculated and normalized for the respective duration of REM and non-REM stages. So far, using only the profiles obtained in Brussels before travel and 21 days after return from Chicago, we could not find any correlation between PRL peaks and REM - non-REM cycles.

WEITZMAN: One of the dramatic aspects of the PRL 24-h profiles is the very sharp fall upon awakening. Did you find that consistently in this study?

DESIR: In our profiles, the most dramatic event was the increase with the sleep onset. The maximum PRL level did not occur always at the beginning of the sleep or at the end of sleep. In some cases, the fall is not dramatic but consists instead of a slow decrease during the second part of the sleep period. We observed this not only in the basal study performed in Brussels before travel but also after transmeridian flights.

QUABBE: It seems that, in your data, the rise of PRL started before sleep onset.

DESIR: Indeed, in a certain number of profiles, the rise starts 30 minutes or one hour before the time of lights-off.

ASCHOFF: You emphasized that there were no effects of jet lag on the amplitude of the pituitary-adrenal periodicity. There was some depression but the results were not significant. Maybe this should be analyzed further because it seems that the amplitude is a very important parameter of adaptation processes. With body temperature, it becomes clear that there are striking eastward-westward differences in the depression of the amplitude of the rhythm, the amplitude being dramatically decreased after eastward flight and practically unchanged after westward flight. Moreover, there seems to be a correlation between the amount of depression of the amplitude and the speed of re-entrainment.

KRIEGER: Your last slide showed the percent of correlation and non-correlation between ACTH peaks and cortisol peaks. Is there any difference in amplitude between the peaks that are correlated and the ones that are not?

COPINSCHI: This is an important question. The analysis is still under progress.

WEITZMAN: I wonder if non-correlated peaks occur more frequently when the basal concentration of ACTH is already relatively high because, in such a condition, the adrenal cortex is already strongly stimulated.

VIGNERI: Don't you think that when a lack of correlation between ACTH and cortisol peaks is observed, it mainly results from the fact that these two hormones have very different metabolic clearance rates and distribution volumes so that the changes in secretion rate may be blunted?

COPINSCHI: It is a possibility. Our analysis is too preliminary to answer this question.

VAN CAUTER: The reason why the analysis was somewhat delayed is that our analysis was initially based on the use of the Weitzman criteria for the definition of a peak. However, these criteria are based on the consideration of an increment in hormone level expressed in absolute concentration units. After examining the results, it became obvious that we had to perform another analysis taking into account the specific coefficients of variation of the assays in the different concentration ranges, low, medium, and high. Indeed, in certain profiles, we would find an ACTH peak concomitant with a cortisol peak but the ACTH peak would not be significant using the Weitzman criteria whereas it obviously was significant since the physiological response was present. We had some instances where a cortisol peak corresponding to an increment of 50 - 60% was present when no ACTH peak was detected. On the other hand, ACTH peaks are generally more frequent and of larger magnitude than cortisol peaks as was reported by Gallagher and others.

WEITZMAN: When you give increasing amounts of multiple injections of ACTH, the adrenal cortex responds by increasing the duration of its rate of secretion of cortisol, not by increasing the amplitude beyond a certain point.

VAN CAUTER: Data look as if there was some inertia of the adrenal which could not respond fast enough to repeated stimulations so that two peaks of ACTH may result only in one peak of cortisol.

COPINSCHI: What Dr. Weitzman just referred to is true for pharmacological doses of ACTH. To my knowledge, with physiological doses, there is still an increase of the cortisol response when there is an increase in the magnitude of the ACTH increment.

CERESA: One must consider that the response of the adrenal glands to ACTH stimulation is biphasic with a rapid discharge within the first 3 - 4 minutes and then a very slow rise in secretion. Maybe the first phase corresponds to discharge of cortisol already present or in the last step of steroidogenesis.

WEITZMAN: I am surprised that you did not find a change in amplitude in the course of the phase shift. You in fact show that after time shift in one direction, the cortisol levels of the subject are below 50% of the 24-h mean for a longer period than under basal conditions. One would expect that, in those days, the total quantity of cortisol secreted and the mean amplitude would be decreased.

COPINSCHI: In our study, neither the absolute amplitude nor the relative amplitude (expressed in percent of the 24-hour mean) were significantly affected at the group level.

WEITZMAN: Did you measure urinary corticosteroids?

COPINSCHI: No.

WEITZMAN: The issue of association or dissociation of melatonin secretion and sleep stages is presently an important one because in the animals, melatonin secretion is so powerfully tied to the light-dark cycle. I brought a slide showing a study of the urinary concentration of melatonin in a human subject in the course of a free-running experiment. As you can see, as the subject free ran, there was a clear dissociation between the timing of melatonin output in the urine and sleep. Even though there was a very powerful relationship during the baseline study, the melatonin output preceded sleep in free running conditions. There is some additional evidence that one can dissociate sleep and lights out from the time of melatonin output. I wonder whether the drop of melatonin after the flight to Chicago might be related to a shorter total sleep time. The subjects may have been awake in the dark when they were in bed in Chicago and you must know that since you did all the recordings of sleep. If the total sleep was reduced, that would probably decrease the amount of melatonin secreted if there is a relationship between sleep and melatonin secretion.

FEVRE: We observed this dramatic drop only after eastward shift, not after westward shift.

VAN CAUTER: The volunteers were investigated in Chicago two days after the flight. At that time, they had a little more wakefulness periods than in the basal study but considerably less than in the study after return to Brussels. On the other hand, when you fly to the U.S., you prolong your day so that the exposure to daylight is about double what it would be in the normal day. This is especially true at the time when the flight occurred, at the end of October.

WEITZMAN: Yes, except that we have also artificial light. Do you think that daylight is different from artificial light?

VAN CAUTER: Yes. Madame Fevre's data show that the amplitude of the melatonin rhythm decreased significantly as the investigation progressed from October to December. It may be that we observed simultaneously two effects: synchronization of the circadian rhythm with the sleep-wake or dark-light cycle and an effect of the decreasing natural daylight.

ROBYN: Did you investigate whether there was any time relationship between the secretory episodes of melatonin and of prolactin during daytime?

FEVRE: This analysis is under progress.

MINORS: Are you aware of the data of Dr. Arendt showing bi-annual rhythms of melatonin in humans?

FEVRE: Yes, but the frequency of sampling was much lower than in this study.

MINORS: It is true but they did show seasonal effects. In fact, there seems to be a 6-month period so that the 3-month period you cover in your study might be going from a peak to a trough.

WEITZMAN: In San Diego, Dr. Lewis from N.I.H. presented a study in human subjects where he turned on the light in the middle of the night and observed a dramatic decrease of plasma melatonin, as measured by an assay involving mass spectrometry. Thus, it is possible that, in man, if the lights are strong enough, you can inhibit the melatonin secretion.

ASCHOFF: All the data presented here indicate a shift
of rhythms in the direction of the flight, advance shift
after eastward flight and delay shift after westward flight.
If you measure only at day one and ten days later, you cannot be sure whether there has not been internal desynchronization of the subjects, that means that not all rhythmic
functions moved in the same direction. There may be a parti-
tioning of the circadian system which can only be observed
if you measure the functions day after day. The data presented here don't indicate that this happened but one has
to be very careful not to overlook such a possibility.

WEITZMAN: If you look at jet lag as a resetting of
the clock in some direction, you make the assumption that
the system moves in that direction. However, from 180°
shift studies, there is evidence that the system may change
by a phase of the day. It is a problem of data analysis.

EFFECT OF AN IMPOSED 21 HOUR SLEEP-WAKE CYCLE UPON THE RHYTHMICITY OF HUMAN PLASMA THYROTROPIN.

Supported by the Medical Research Service of the Veterans Administration

L.G. Rossman[*], D.C. Parker[*], A.E. Pekary[+], and J.M. Hershman[+]

[*]San Diego Veterans Administration Medical Center, La Jolla, California
[+]Wadsworth Veterans Administration Medical Center, Los Angeles, California

INTRODUCTION

Though nycthohemeral variation in the plasma concentration of human thyrotropin (TSH) initially proved difficult to demonstrate (1-6), its occurrence now appears to be fairly well established (7-14). However, an unusual degree of variation in the clocktime of occurrence of these daily maxima across the night exists in these reports in which peaks were found in the 2100-0000 hr (10, 11, 14); 0000-0400 hr (7, 8, 10); or 0300-0700 (9, 12, 13) intervals. In earlier work (15), we presented evidence confirming the existence of nychtohemeral variation in plasma TSH concentrations, and showed that it was rhythmically repetitive over several nights. Our results further indicated that nycthohemeral maxima most consistently occurred prior to the onset of sleep in the 2100-0100 hr interval across usual normal sleep-wake cycles that were well maintained. We could find no convincing evidence in support of any sleep-related enhancement in TSH release (8-10, 14). Instead, a unique occurrence amongst nightly patterns of release of human anterior pituitary hormones was seen in which diminished TSH release characterized the course of undisrupted sleep of normally maintained sleep-wake cycles. Shifts in the time of entering polygraphic sleep were associated with alteration in the concentration and timing of resultant TSH maxima in a way that suggested the presence of an inhibitory influence in sleep upon a circadian mechanism for TSH release. In addition, during study of acute reversal of sleep-wake cycle (15), a sharp dampening in TSH amplitude that made phase unrecognizable at its expected locus followed within 12 hr of the shift of sleep into the 1100-1830 interval. A similar result followed within 24 hr after 1200-2100 hr sleep in a study of 30 hr sleep-wake cycles. Thus an important additional effect upon phase of the TSH rhythm seemed to be occurring after sleep was delayed by 180° from its usual locus. To further evaluate the effect of sleep itself upon the rhythmicity of anterior pituitary release of TSH here we have studied several subjects in whom a 21 hr sleep-wake schedule was imposed upon its imputed circadian oscillator. We hoped that this study of rhythmic period and phase and of inhibitory state effects would give us further insight into the mechanisms basic to rhythmic TSH release and help to clarify some of the uncertainty regarding the locus of basal TSH maxima.

MATERIALS AND METHODS

Four healthy young men, between the ages of 23 and 27 participated in this study. One subject was withdrawn from the study during the accommodation period because of a low normal hematocrit basally. All three remaining subjects were euthyroid and presented no endocrinological abnormalities. Each subject was well accommodated to the sleep study environment and techniques by participation in previous studies as well as by time spent in an initial 24 hr period of accommodation in this study. Then a 21 hour sleep-wake cycle was imposed upon the subjects over the next 12 days. Here they were allowed 6 hr and 20 min of bedtime followed by 14 hr and 40 min of carefully monitored wakefulness serially across 21 hr intervals.

Subjects' sleep periods were monitored polygraphically and scored by standardized techniques (16). Subjects were not allowed to lie in bed or sleep during the wakeful periods. The artificial illuminative cycle, which was of low intensity light at its peak, conformed to the imposed 21 hr sleep-wake cycle. Exposure to the natural light:dark cycle was unimpeded during wakefulness and bedroom windows were not darkened in any significant way during sleep. During wakefulness subjects remained aware of the 24 hr temporal cues of clocks, radios, and television scheduling and that of hospital routines going on about them so that exposure to social cues of 24 hr periodicity was maintained across the 12 days. During the wakeful segment of the 21 hr sleep-wake cycle, the subjects were fed 6 identical feedings containing 23 g protein, 42 g carbohydrates and 13 g fat every 2 hours commencing 40 minutes after awakening. This diet yielded the equivalent of 2584 calories/24 hr.

Blood samples of 2 ml were drawn through a 10 ft. extension line of blood pressure monitor tubing attached to a small bore indwelling catheter that had been emplaced and secured in an antecubital vein. Between samples this line was maintained with a heparin lock system containing 5 U/ml of normal saline. Plasma was immediately separated in a 4 ml heparinized vacutainer tube and promptly frozen at $-20^{\circ}C$

until hormone assay. We thought our usual consecutive sampling at
20 min intervals would result in withdrawal of too much blood (nearly
2 liters) from a subject. So the study was designed to have over-
lapping blood sampling amongst subject pairs along with catheter
and sampling "vacation days" for the subject pairs in order that the
entire study could be evaluated hormonally while still avoiding this
pitfall of excess blood sampling. However, the withdrawal of one
subject left us with occasional sectors where only one subject
contributed data to the study. All subjects have 24 hr periods of
1/2 hr sampling occurring at overlap points on Day 1-2, 5, 8, and 12.
All other periods of sampling were at hourly intervals. Subjects 301
and 305 had an identical sampling schedule: 18-21 hr sampling
vacations occurred within D_{2-3}, D_{5-6} and D_{9-10}. Subject 316's
vacations from sampling were within D_4, D_{7-8} and D_{10-11} (c.f. figures
1-3).

The plasma TSH concentrations were measured by a highly sensitive
RIA technique (17). The minimum detectable dose was 0.02 µU/tube and
50% suppression of I^{125} labeled TSH occurred with 0.33 µU of TSH per
tube. One hundred µl of each plasma sample was measured in duplicate.
The intra-assay coefficient of variation was 4.3% at 5.7 µU/ml. Each
subject's entire study was assayed in the same assay. Results were
expressed as % of his trans-study mean in order to minimize inter-sub-
ject differences. Fortran IV programs compiled and utilized on an
HP 2100 A computer aided in the analysis of this data. The significance of the least squares fitting of cosine curves to the data was
estimated using Halberg's cosinor methodology (18). The use of the
autocorrelation function and its Fourier transform, the variance
spectrum has been previously described (19, 20, 21).

RESULTS AND DISCUSSION

The time series of plasma TSH concentrations across the 12 day study
period during which a 21 hr sleep-wake schedule (S 6-1/3 h:W 14-2/3 h)
was imposed are shown in actigraphic format in figures 1-3. Each
figure is of the TSH data of a single normal young man who was allowed
full access to the natural L:D cycle and other 24 hr sociotemporal
cues in his hospital environment during wakefulness each day. The
first important point seen was that all 3 figures exhibit essentially
similar patterns in all 3 men's TSH variation across the study. This

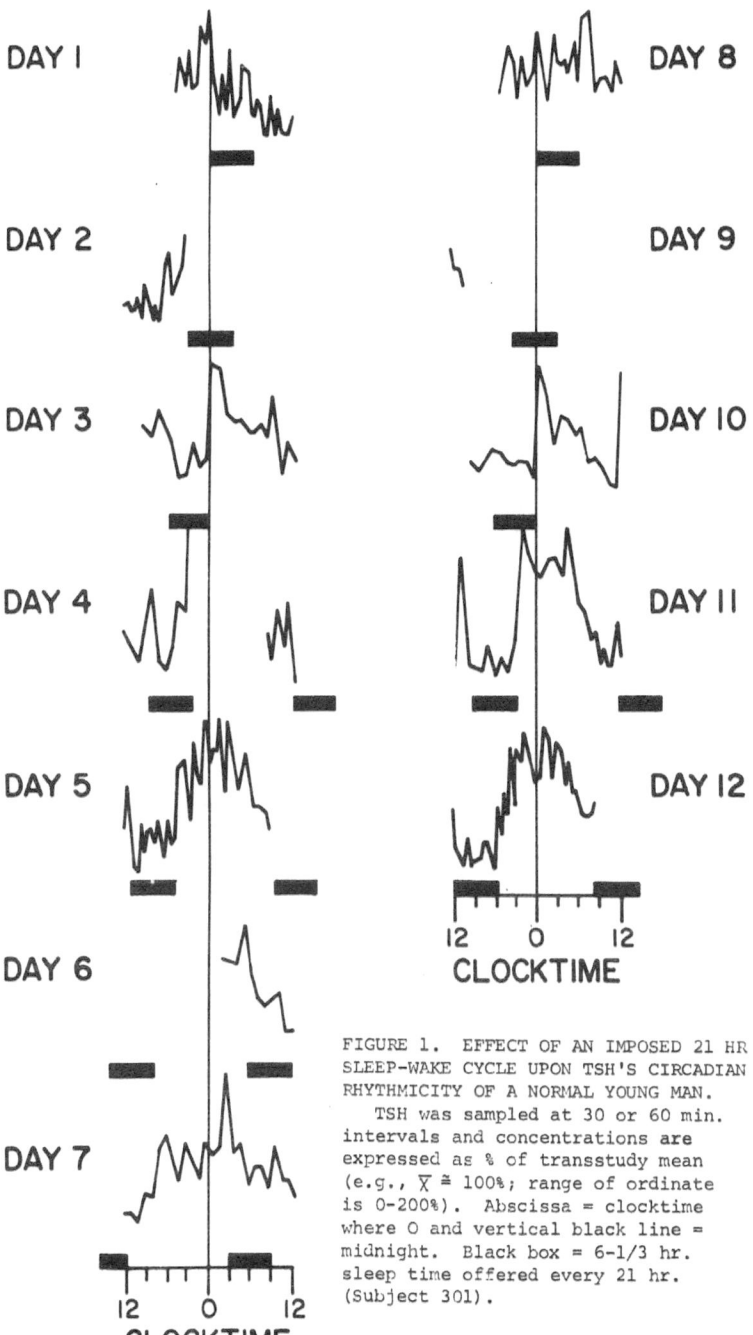

FIGURE 1. EFFECT OF AN IMPOSED 21 HR SLEEP-WAKE CYCLE UPON TSH'S CIRCADIAN RHYTHMICITY OF A NORMAL YOUNG MAN.

TSH was sampled at 30 or 60 min. intervals and concentrations are expressed as % of transstudy mean (e.g., $\overline{X} \cong 100\%$; range of ordinate is 0-200%). Abscissa = clocktime where 0 and vertical black line = midnight. Black box = 6-1/3 hr. sleep time offered every 21 hr. (Subject 301).

100

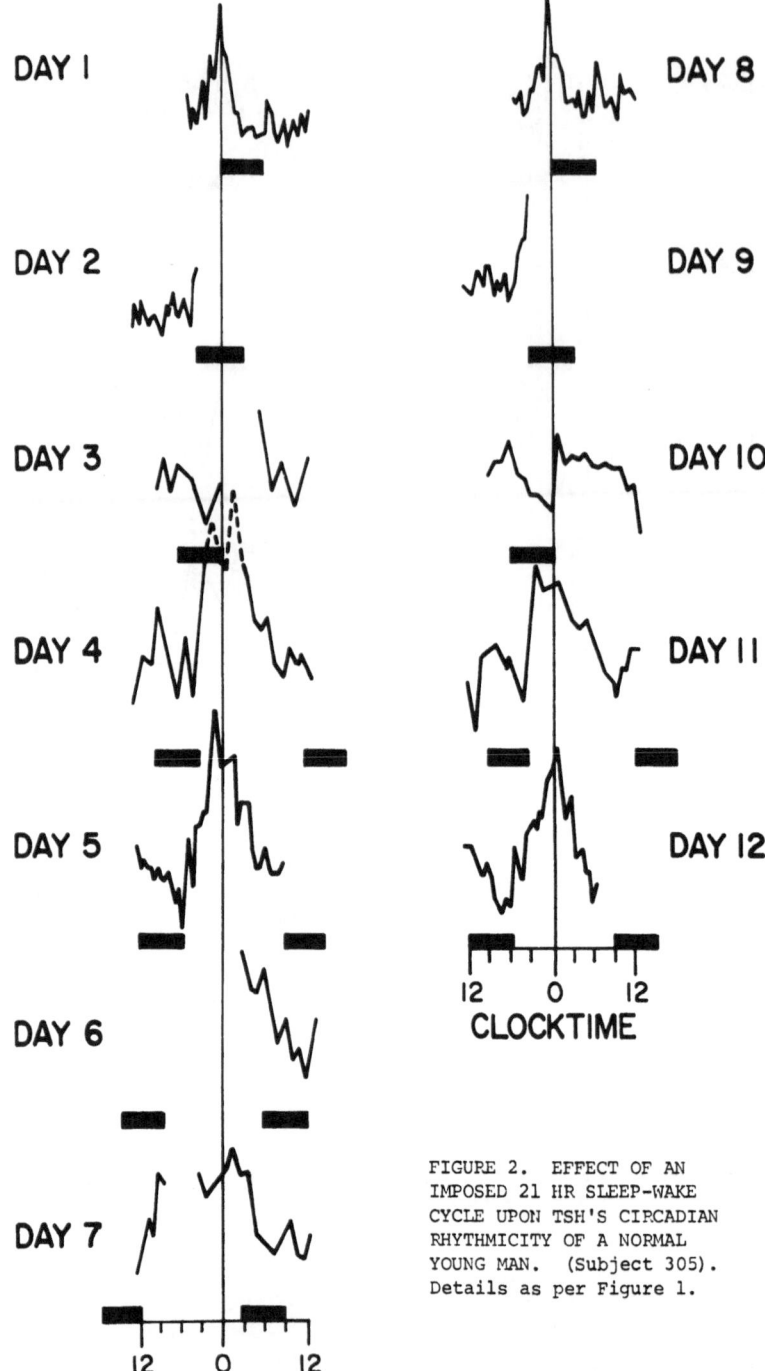

DAY 1

DAY 2

DAY 3

DAY 4

DAY 5

DAY 6

DAY 7

DAY 8

DAY 9

DAY 10

DAY 11

DAY 12

12   0   12
CLOCKTIME

12   0   12
CLOCKTIME

FIGURE 2. EFFECT OF AN
IMPOSED 21 HR SLEEP-WAKE
CYCLE UPON TSH'S CIRCADIAN
RHYTHMICITY OF A NORMAL
YOUNG MAN. (Subject 305).
Details as per Figure 1.

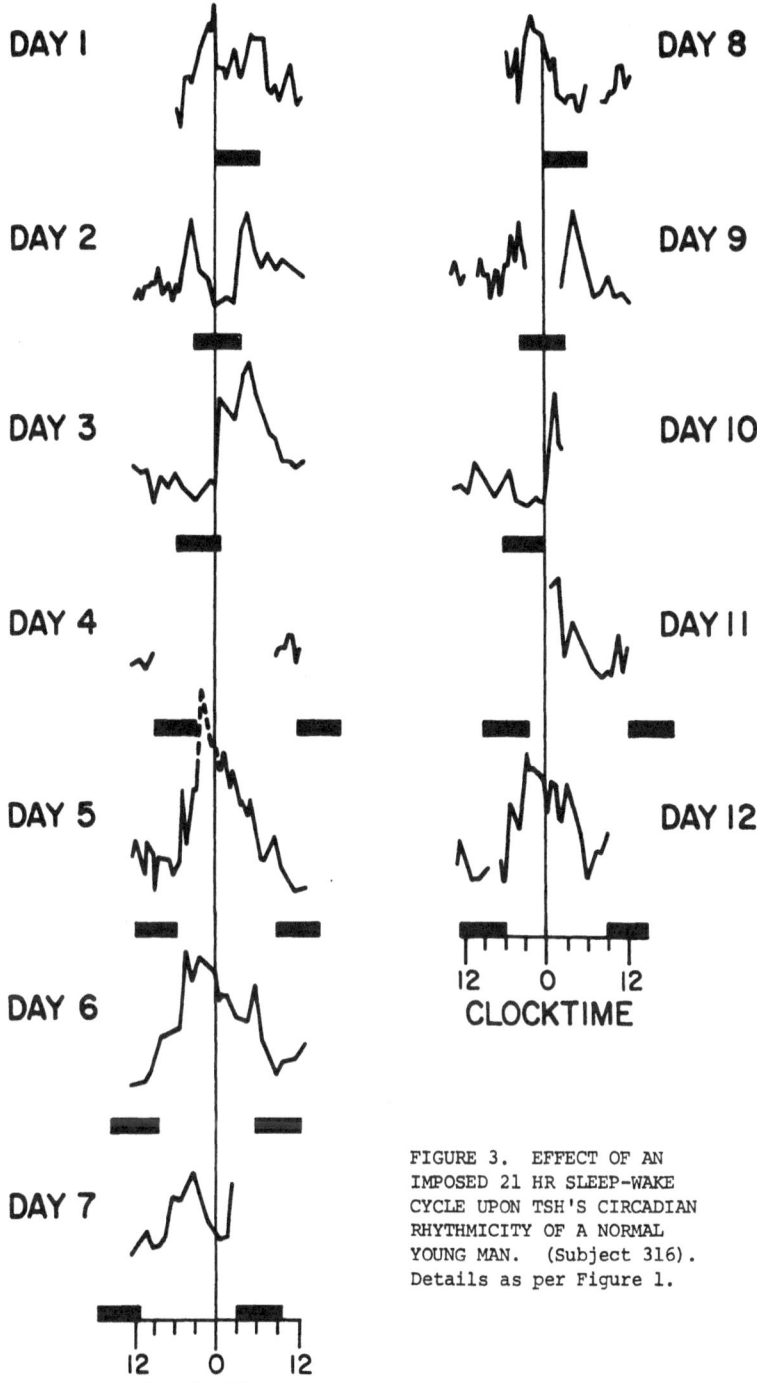

FIGURE 3. EFFECT OF AN
IMPOSED 21 HR SLEEP-WAKE
CYCLE UPON TSH'S CIRCADIAN
RHYTHMICITY OF A NORMAL
YOUNG MAN. (Subject 316).
Details as per Figure 1.

similarity suggests that their TSH rhythms were similarly synchronized across the study under our study's cueing conditions. Therefore, a free-running character was not assumed by any one subject's TSH pattern. The second point evidenced in all 3 TSH actigraphs was that a 21 hr period was not adopted by the usual basal pre-sleep maxima in TSH, as seen by glancing downward from Day 1's pre-sleep peak along the leading edge of the black sleep bars. Thus, the imposed (21 hr) sleep-wake period did not appear in any simple straightforward fashion to be the sole or major zeitgeber of the TSH rhythm. The third point uniformly evident in all 3 figures was that persistence of a strict 24 hr period to the TSH maxima was equally inapparent as one glances vertically down the actigraph along either the leading edge of the midnight line, (10, 11, 14, 15) or about the 0600 hr (9, 12, 13) loci. Thus, neither did the 24 hr period of L:D or social cues appear to be the simple, readily apparent zeitgeber to persistent circadian rhythmicity in TSH. However, of these 2 alternatives, in scanning figures 1-3 the eye was more prone to accept as explanation the persistence of a 24 hr period of TSH's nocturnal maxima than that of the assumption of a 21 hr period by these maxima. But, if one then looked at all closely, one saw that this also required acceptance of a range of 7-10 hr in the loci of the nocturnal maxima within even an individual. Such would be an unusually unstable character for a synchronized circadian oscillator.

In our estimate, the most conservative and realistic interpretation drawn from these 3 TSH actigraphs was that such simple explanations simply did not suffice and that a more complex situation was occurring. This led us to examine the serial change in each individual's maxima in search of a pattern to the changes. This was looked at by first rescanning the actigraphs and then by tabulating the loci of acrophases of 24 hr cosines fitted to serial 24 hr segments of each individual's TSH data (Table 1). From the actigraphs (figures 1-3) it was seen that any day's pattern was more similar amongst the 3 subjects than was the similarity of a subject's day to day pattern. It seemed to us that there was every reason to expect such a daily group change in pattern to result from a systematic effect. This systematic change may be descriptively generalized as an initial early evening pre-sleep peak on D_1 (e.g., the basal state TSH pattern) first becoming bifid and then delayed into the early

morning hours of Days 2 and 3, after which the peak then serially
advances back to its basal early evening locus during Days 4-7. This
pattern of change then began to reiterate upon Days 8-12. The serial
loci of acrophases of 24 hr fitted cosines are given in Table 1 and
confirmed this visual interpretation of plotted maxima: after rather
abrupt initial delays on D_{2-3}, the acrophases then returned to their
original locus by serial advances on D_{4-7} in each subject. Then on
D_8 it began to happen all over again so that the TSH patterns and
acrophases of Day 1 and 8, Day 2 and 9, etc., were surprisingly
faithful replicates in each subject. Note that Day 8 was a resonance
point of the sleep-wake schedule in 24 hr clocktime or in the natural
L:D schedule: sleep onset which had advanced by 3 hr every 24 hr
day, has gone full circle (in clocktime) to arrive back at its initial
starting point of midnight (e.g., eight 21 hr days = seven 24 hr days).
This indicated this latter (D_1 and D_8, etc.) replication of pattern
to be an effect of the imposed sleep-wake schedule, and that therefore
we should seriously consider the sleep-wake cycle as the source of
the rest of the witnessed similarity of patterns of serial change on
Days 1 through 7 and Days 8 through 12 in the 3 subjects.

Table 1. *Serial daily acrophases of 24 hr cosines fitted to 12:00-12:00 hr TSH segments*

	DAYS						
SUBJECT	1/8	2/9	3/10	4/11	5/12	6/	7/
301	332	32	64*	20	12	48	11
	54*	*	28	26	14		
305	331	43	131*	13	03	19	321
	358*	46	104*	04	03		
316	29	64*	69	*	357	344	311*
	290	01	93	301	357		

*Segment is < 8 hr long or a longer segment lacks a significant
cosinor fit. Acrophase is in degrees, 0° is midnight.

If this were to be the case, then a 21 hr effect upon TSH should exist in these patterns. Though we had not seen such a pattern to TSH maxima in the actigraphs of figures 1-3 and had not seen a consistent 45° (3 hr) advance in daily cosinor acrophases in Table 1, further evidence of such 21 hr effects was then sought in several other ways. The first was simply to stop looking at maxima in the actigraphs and look at minima. When we did this an immediate strong relationship of nadirs to sleep bars became readily apparent on virtually all the days plotted for the 3 subjects in figures 1-3. This persistence reaffirmed our previously reported "sleep-related inhibition of TSH release" (15). In order to extract this evidence of sleep-related inhibition for easier viewing, we selected 24 hr segments of data that were evenly balanced and weighted to represent all 3 subjects when their sleep was evenly distributed across the entire 24 hrs (e.g., the TSH data of the days on which sleep onset occurred at 0000, 1800, 1200 and 0600 were available in all 3 subjects). The hourly TSH data were pooled in 2 different ways. Firstly, from 4 hr before until 20 hr after sleep onset, each of the 3 subjects furnished an hourly TSH value from each of his four 24 hr segments to each of 24 hourly bins. The resultant mean TSH concentration plot was aligned by time from "sleep-onset" and more importantly was independent of clocktime of sleep. Secondly, the same data were arranged by clocktime from midnight so that averaging here yielded a TSH plot aligned by clocktime and independent of the effects of sleep since sleep was evenly dispersed in all 4 quadrants of the day. These 2 plots are shown in figure 4. The sleep-onset aligned plot shows that a sharp decline in TSH after sleep-onset followed by a rather prolonged nadir in TSH concentration during the 6 hr sleep period clearly characterized the pattern of TSH variation in sleep without regard to the time of day at which sleep occurred. This again represents in our view rather overwhelming evidence of the inhibitory effect upon TSH release into plasma that exists in sleep. We also believe this clearly and quite simply explains the presence of a 21 hr effect in the actigraph and explains why the effect is upon nadirs rather than maxima (figures 1-3) or even acrophases (Table 1). However, the clocktime-aligned TSH plot of figure 4 derived from the same data shows us an even more important and original result. Recollect that here in this plot the inhibitory sleep effects upon the release pattern of TSH have

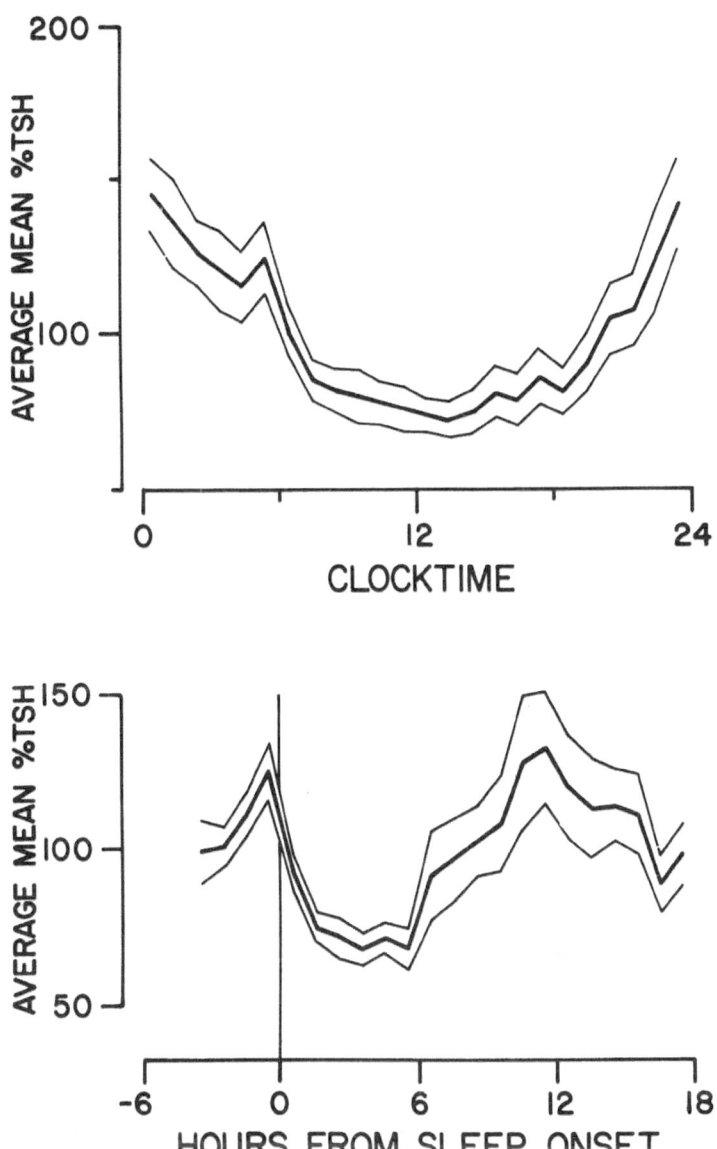

FIGURE 4. TOP: CIRCADIAN EFFECTS MADE DISTINCT FROM SLEEP-RELATED
EFFECTS. Clocktime aligned mean plot of group hourly TSH from 00:00 to
00:00 when sleep-related inhibitory effects upon TSH were minimized by
uniform dispersion of sleep onset across the day. BOTTOM: SLEEP-
RELATED TSH EFFECTS MADE DISTINCT FROM CIRCADIAN EFFECTS. Sleep-onset
aligned plot of the same TSH data used for binning in TOP plot, arranged
for averaging from 4 hr before until 20 hr after sleep onset on 4 days
when the 3 subjects' bedtimes were at 0000, 1800, 1200 and 0600 hr
respectively. This dispersed any persistently synchronized circadian
effects across the plot while focusing any sleep-related effects.

been largely negated by uniform dispersion of sleep across the 4
quadrants of the 24 hr day, so that a more clear view was permitted
of any synchronized circadian effect upon the daily TSH pattern that
might persist. Such a mean daily TSH plot (fig. 4 TOP) indeed showed
that a single daily maximum best represented the "clocktime-only
effect" upon the daily pattern in TSH and that this maximum's temporal
locus was around midnight. This indicates that TSH's average daily
maximum here indeed represented a persistent synchronized circadian
acrophase that we have allowed to stand out above the uniformly
dispersed inhibitory effects of sleep upon TSH release. This too
strongly supports our initial impression of the likelihood of
circadian character in TSH's rhythmicity (15).

Further evidence of the presence of both such a 21 hr sleep-wake
effect and a 24 hr synchronized circadian effect upon TSH rhythmicity
can be sought with the autocorrelation function and the variance
spectra (21). To yield a single time series of sufficient length, the
subjects' data were pooled and averaged across time to yield a single
continuous time series of hourly TSH concentrations over 12 days
(figure 5). The autocorrelation function that then resulted is shown
in fig. 5 also. Here one notes that the first major peak in positive
correlation significantly encompassed that of both the 21st [42] and
24th [48] lags. Thus, TSH samples both 21 and 24 hr apart were
significantly correlated. Such results were interpretable as
evidence of the occurrence of periodic components of both 21 and 24 hr
in the single 12 day long time series. The variance spectrum derived
from the Fourier transformation of the autocorrelation function is
shown in figure 5. Here line peaks at frequencies of both 1 (7/7)
and 1.14 (8/7) cycles/day were seen. Thus, once again evidence of
periodicities at both 24 and 21 hr confirmed our earlier suspicion
of the complexly engendered origin of our observed daily TSH patterns.

In figure 5, lesser peaks in the variance spectra were seen
which occurred at harmonic frequencies (16/7 or 2.3; 24/7 or 3.4 c/d,
etc.) of the fundamental (8/7 or 1.14 c/d). This fundamental
represented events witnessed to recur periodically every 21 hr like
sleep, TSH inhibition and TSH nadirs. There was also an interesting
significant variance peak at 1/7 c/d (at the beginning of the spectral
plot in figure 5) that might be considered a "subharmonic." If one
returns to the actigraphs (figures 1-3) one can see the amplitude of
the daily maxima wane before and after D_{4-5} and then wax again by

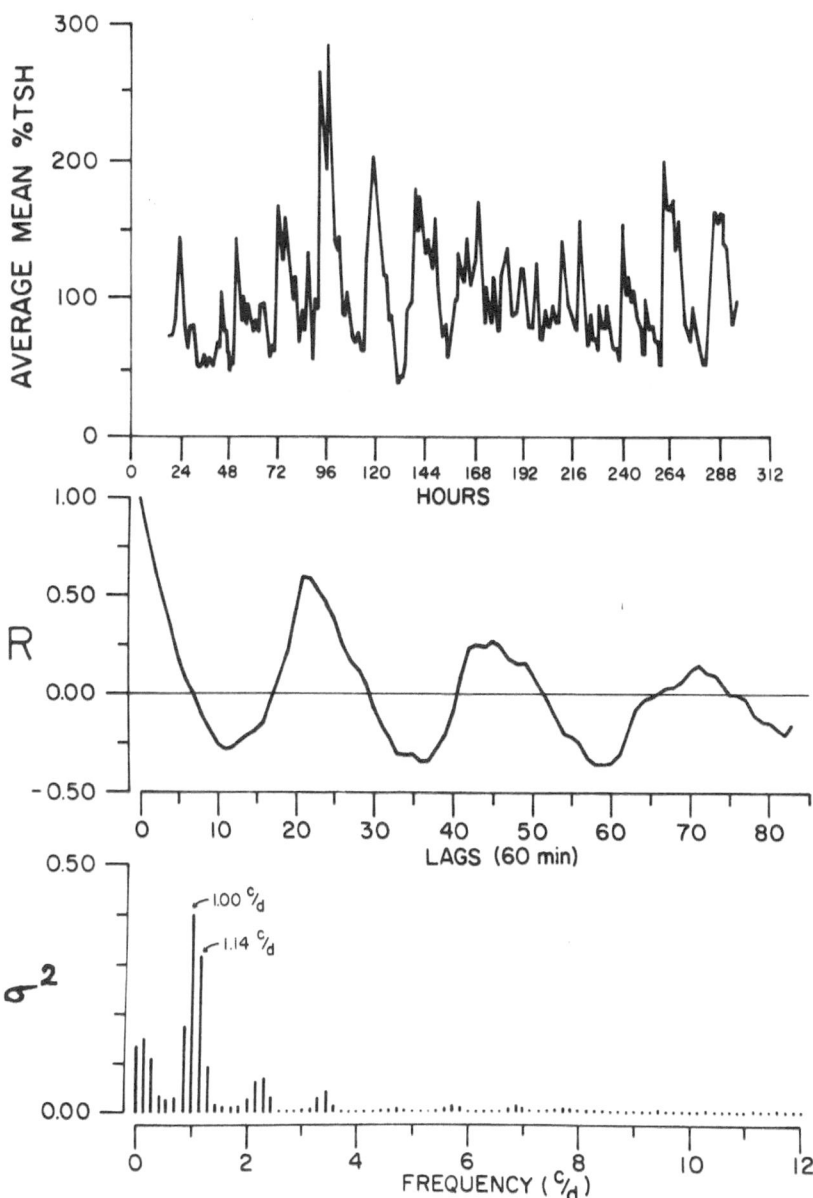

FIGURE 5. THE MEAN, (*top*) AUTOCORRELATION FUNCTION, (*middle*) AND
VARIANCE SPECTRUM (*bottom*) FOR THE ENTIRE 21 HR SLEEP-WAKE STUDY. The
group mean of hourly TSH from the TSH data shown in figures 1-3 was
calculated across the 12 days of the imposed 21 hr sleep-wake schedule.
This across subjects' mean was the time series used to calculate the
autocorrelation (R) function and variance spectrum (σ^2).

D_{11-12}. This 7 day-long pattern in variation of amplitude was the basis in reality of the rhythmic periodicity of 7 days identified by the spectral analysis and speaks strongly to the point of the great sensitivity of the variance spectra as an analytic technique. Only after these considerable analytic efforts were we finally confident that the observed complex patterns in TSH could be resolved into periodic components of both 21 and 24 hr.

It seems fairly certain that the identified 24 hr component can be safely attributed to an endogenous circadian character in TSH variation. The real issue seems to us to be in regard to exactly how the imputed circadian oscillator for TSH release was altered by the imposition of a 21 hr sleep-wake cycle. Certainly TSH did not adopt a 21 hr period that maintained the pre-sleep position of TSH maxima (figures 1-3) nor advance its daily acrophase by an equivalent 45° (Table 1), so that the sleep-wake zeitgeber was not accepted by the putative TSH oscillator. Neither was TSH rhythmicity so completely immune to 21 hr sleep-wake effects that it could maintain the strict 24 hr period of its other available zeitgebers (natural L:D, social) that would have been represented by persistent maxima and acrophases near midnight (figures 1-3) and 0° (Table 1) respectively across the 12 days. Instead there was an initial delay in both daily maxima and acrophases on D_{2-3} followed by an advance back toward original D_1 loci that occurred serially on D_{4-7}. Replication of this behavior began again across D_{8-12} (Table 1). In addition there was a 7-day periodicity seen in amplitudes of maxima (figures 1-3) and in the variance spectra (figure 5).

One potential explanation of this oscillation in phase is a phasing effect of some aspect of the imposed sleep-wake cycle upon the putative endogenous TSH oscillator. For example, the position of phase-response curve of this latter oscillator when stimulated by the initial advances in sleep on D_{2-3} would result in a delay in TSH phase. Further advances in sleep on D_{4-5} however would now fall in the phase-advance segment of the phase-response diagram for TSH so that the TSH acrophases would now return toward their starting loci by a series of advances. Further advances in sleep would result in lesser advances in TSH phase. Finally no movement would occur when the sleep cue to phase fell in the stable or insensitive portion of the TSH phase-response curve. On Day 8 the movement of the putative phasing effect of sleep across the TSH phase response curve would begin anew in a resonant fashion. Unfortunately this proposal is currently sui generis since no other real knowledge of any TSH phase-response curve exists at present. By inference however, other evidence may be the severe brief dampening of the daily TSH peak that occurs on D_2 of acute sleep-wake reversal (15). Here reversal would represent a 12 hr delay in imposed sleep cue on a phase-response curve. Similarly inferential was brief dampening out of the daily TSH peak seen on D_5 of imposition of a 30 hr sleep wake cycle if the latter were viewed as a series of 6 hr delays in imposition of sleep cues (19, 22). These suggest that an impressive "delay" in TSH phase was plausibly explained as a sleep-related phasing effect upon TSH release on these 2 occasions. The third supportive piece of inferential evidence is simply associative, in that cortisol clearly exhibits a major circadian peak whose phase is ultimately influenced by the locus of daily sleep (14, 23, 24). This thereby serves as a precedent for our expectations of effectors of the circadian phase of TSH.

One might consider as a more complex explanation that of competing phasers such as Light:Dark and Sleep:Wake. To account for the initial large delay in TSH phase both would be cooperatively effecting delay responses. Further advances in sleep in relation to L:D would then lead the phasing effect of sleep into an opposing segment of the phase-response curve, leading to serially smaller advances in TSH phase until finally balanced effects yielded a stably phased (basal) TSH again. Replication of the sleep advances then regenerates the cycle of cooperative and then competitive L:D and sleep-wake phasing effects resonantly.

However, in the current absence of further real evidence supportive of such a complexity of effects of a single phaser (sleep-wake) or competing (additional L:D or social) phasers, we prefer the following explanation as at least the most simple available. This views the inhibitory or suppressive effect upon TSH release during sleep as real, immediate, and noncircadian, since it appears wherever sleep is placed in the day (figures 1-3) without regard to clocktime (figure 4). This inhibitory effect disappears in the immediate absence of nocturnal sleep (figure 6) so that there is no day-long lag time for this inhibitory effect to occur nor does it persist 24 hr later (figure 6) unless sleep is also again immediately present

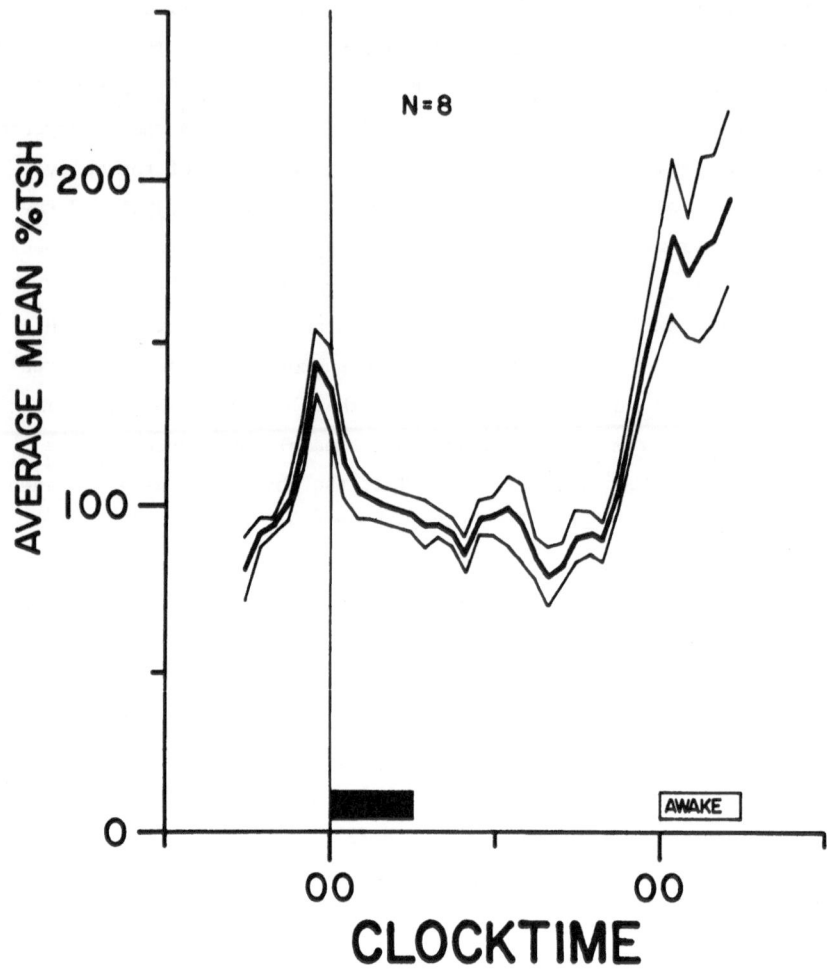

FIGURE 6. UNMASKING OF THE CIRCADIAN WAVEFORM OF BASAL STATE BY
SLEEP DELETION. Mean TSH of 8 other subjects across 24 hr in our
normally cued basal state environment where sleep was located from 00-
08 hr. This represents the usual daily basal-state TSH pattern that is
masked by sleep effects. This was followed on the second night by
deletion of usual sleep. As a result, this nocturnal segment of
circadian TSH demonstrates the waveform free of any inhibitory masking
effect of sleep and shows it to result in a remarkably greater and
delayed circadian peak in mean TSH.

at the same locus. Thus, much like the stimulatory "same-night" effects of sleep upon GH and PRL release, sleep's dampening effect upon TSH release is best viewed as a <u>state</u> effect of sleep, a point of view we have found both abstractly comfortable and practically helpful. With it one simply has to visualize imposing sleep as an "eraser" on the appropriate loci of circadian TSH pattern of figure 4 in order to model our actigraph plots. Thus, when sleep is advanced to 21-03 on D_2, only the 18-21 beginning and 03-09 termination of a circadian TSH peak remain. Then either a bifid peak of reduced amplitude must occur or a delayed peak must occur in which the entire onset of rise has been delayed and, pari passu, the peak. Similarly when sleep advances far enough to begin to approach the trailing edge of the circadian TSH peak (e.g., the sleep onsets of 0600 and 0300 hr on D_5 and D_6 of figures 1-3) one begins to see inhibition of the duration and then of peak loci and amplitudes as the inhibitory sleep block marches back through the underlying circadian peak. Again the circadian peak has been advanced and lessened by inhibitory attack, now from its trailing edge. Note that when the inhibitory effect of sleep is most antipodal to the nocturnal circadian TSH peak (e.g., on $D_{4,5}$ and $D_{11,12}$ where sleep onset are at 1500 and 1200) is when this TSH peak achieves its overall maximum in amplitude (e.g., the 7 day cycle of amplitudes noted in figures 1-3 and 5).

Here we have seen a unique and potentially very important biologic event - a state effect that can alter the shape, locus and amplitude (e.g., <u>the entire waveform</u>) of a circadian rhythm. This is indeed a very considerable masking effect (25, 26) that if unrecognized lends a dream-like quality to what we formerly thought we knew about daily TSH variation.

The important lesson to be learned from this is that one can't simply deal with the circadian rhythm of TSH like it were cortisol's; but instead one must pay equally careful attention to the masking effects of sleep upon its waveform and locus of acrophase. Only when this is done may we really begin to learn if there are indeed the additional phasing effects of the sleep-wake cycle that we suspect may also exist here. Thus, future studies of TSH rhythmicity will need to include studies of unmasking from the state effects of sleep. Our current hypothesis is that an endogenous circadian rhythm in TSH is modulated in its waveform by masking sleep-state effects and that there additionally will be shown to be phasing effects of the sleep-wake cycle upon the circadian oscillator underlying TSH rhythmicity.

REFERENCES

1. Utiger, RD, Radioimmunoassay of human plasma thyrotropin. J Clin Invest 44:1277-1286, 1965
2. Odell, WD, JF Wilber and RD Utiger, Studies of thyrotropin physiology by means of radioimmunoassay. Recent Prog Horm Res 23:47-85, 1967
3. Jaquet, P, P Franchimont, JP Rinaldi, JM Saintz, JL Codaccioni and J Vague, Le dosage radioimmunologique de h. TSH plasmatique. II. Resultats chez le Sujet Normal et en Pathologie. Ann Endocrinol (Paris) 32:495-507, 1971
4. Hershman, JM and JA Pittman, Utility of the radioimmunoassay of serum thyrotropin in man. Ann Intern Med 74:481-490, 1971
5. Webster, BR, AR Guansing and JC Paice, Absence of diurnal variation of serum TSH. J Clin Endocrinol Metab 34:899-901, 1972
6. Osterman, PO, G Wallin and L Wide, Nocturnal secretory patterns of FSH, GH, LH, and TSH. Upsala J Med Sci 79:55-62, 1974
7. Nicoloff, JT, DA Fisher and MA Appleman, The role of glucocorticoids in the regulation of thyroid function in man. J Clin Invest 49:1922-1929, 1970
8. Patel, YC, FP Alford and HG Burger, The 24 hr plasma thyrotropin profile. Clin Sci 43:71-77, 1972
9. Vanhaelst, L, E VanCauter, JP De Gaute and J Golstein, Circadian variations of serum thyrotropin levels in man. J Clin Endocrinol Metab 35:479-482, 1972
10. Alford, FP, HW Baker, HG Burger, DM deKretser, B Hudson, MW Johns, MP Masteron, YC Patel and GC Rennie, Temporal patterns of integrated plasma hormone levels during sleep and wakefulness. I. TSH, GH and cortisol. J Clin Endocrinol Metab 37:841-847, 1973.
11. Weeke, J, Circadian variation of the serum thyrotropin levels in normal subjects. Scand J Clin Lab Invest 31:337-342, 1973
12. VanCauter, E, R Leclercq, L Vanhaelst and J Golstein, Simultaneous study of cortisol and TSH daily variations in normal subjects and patients with hyperadrenalcorticism. J Clin Endocrinol Metab 39:645-652, 1974
13. VanCauter, E, J Golstein, L Vanhaelst and R Leclercq, Effects of oral contraceptive therapy on the circadian patterns of cortisol and thyrotropin (TSH). Eur J Clin Invest 5:115-121, 1975
14. Weitzman, ED, RM Boyar, S Kapen and L Hellman, The relationship of sleep and sleep stages to neuroendocrine secretion and biological rhythms in man. Rec Prog Horm Res 31:399-446, 1975
15. Parker, DC, AE Pekary and JM Hershman, Effect of normal and reversed sleep-wake cycles upon nyctohemeral rhythmicity of plasma thyrotropin: Evidence suggestive of an inhibitory influence in sleep. J Clin Endocrinol Metab 43:318-329, 1976

16. Rechtshaffen, A and A Kales, Manual of Standardized Terminology, Technique and scoring system for sleep stages of human subjects. National Institutes of Health Publication No. 204, U.S. Govt Printing Office, Washington, D.C., 1968

17. Pekary, AE, JM Hershman and AF Parlow, A sensitive and precise radioimmunoassay for human thyroid-stimulating hormone. J Clin Endocrinol Metab 41:676-684, 1975

18. Halberg, F, EA Johnson, W Nelson, W Runge and R Sothern, Autorhythmometry: Procedures for physiologic self-measurements and their analysis. Physiol Teach 1:1-11, 1972

19. Parker, DC, LG Rossman, DF Kripke, W Gibson and K Wilson, Rhythmicities in human growth hormone concentrations in plasma, In: Endocrine Rhythms, Krieger, DT (ed.), New York, Raven Press, 143-173, 1979

20. Halberg, F and HI Panofsky, Thermovariance spectra: Method and clinical illustrations. Exp Med Surg 19:284-309, 1961

21. Jenkins, GM and DG Watts, Spectral Analysis and its Applications. San Francisco, Holden-Day, 1968

22. Parker, DC, LG Rossman, E Pekary, J Hershman and DF Kripke, Effect of 30 hr. sleep-wake cycle on plasma thyrotropin (TSH) rhythmicity. Program, 60th Annual Meeting of the Endocrine Society, Abstract 674, page 414, 1978

23. Weitzman, ED, CA Czeisler and MC Moore-Ede, Relationship of cortisol, growth hormone, and body temperature to sleep in man living in an environment free of time cues. Program, 58th Meeting of the Endocrine Society, Abstract 390, page 252, 1975

24. Czeisler, CA, ED Weitzman, MC Moore-Ede and R Fusco, Phase angle and educed waveform relationships among the circadian rhythms of plasma cortisol, body temperature and sleep under free running conditions in man. Program, 59th Annual Meeting of the Endocrine Society, Abstract 389, page 251, 1976

25. Aschoff, J, Circadian rhythms: General features and endocrinological aspects, In: Endocrine Rhythms, Krieger, DT (ed.), New York, Raven Press, 1-61, 1979

26. Parker, DC, LG Rossman, DF Kripke, JM Hershman, W Gibson, C Davis, K Wilson and E Pekary, Endocrine rhythms across sleep-wake cycles in normal young men under basal conditions, In: Physiology in Sleep, Barnes, DC and J Orem (eds.), New York, Academic Press, 145-179, 1981

DISCUSSION

This discussion of Dr. Rossman's presentation was focused on the PRL data. The reports on the 24-h profile of TSH by Dr. Rossman, Dr. Golstein and Dr. Weeke were discussed simultaneously after Dr. Weeke's presentation.

VAN CAUTER: I would like to know whether your analysis of the relationship between REM - non-REM stages in sleep and PRL secretory episodes is based on tranverse means across subjects normalized for the time of occurrence of the REM period? I feel that if you consider individual rather than tranverse data, you might reach different conclusions. Using transverse means can sometimes bring up features which are characteristic of only a few individuals.

ROSSMAN: That the transverse mean is not demonstrative of each individual of the group is a well accepted fact. Some individuals in the group had two REM periods. We did not exclude them from our analysis. There are certainly differences at the individual level. All of the individual cross-correlation functions do not look like the average correlation function. Some of the individual functions have values at .95 for certain lags. But only one of the maximum in the cross-correlation was at the zero or -1 lag in all the studies.

VAN CAUTER: I would like to comment on the cross-correlation function. The cross-correlation function is a function which varies between +1 and -1. It is a standard theorem in time series analysis that spurious cross-correlations occur when one correlates two time series without filtering them to eliminate the time correlation within the series.

ROSSMAN: Our data were indeed regressed.

VAN CAUTER: Still, your average cross-correlation function varies between +.2 and -.2. Since estimations of cross-correlation are often severely skewed, I would feel

uncomfortable relying totally on cross-correlation estimations.

ROSSMAN: An individual cross-correlation of .2 would
not be significant but the concordance of individual cross-
correlations of .2 that we observed is significant. This .2
mean is significant at the group level when tested against
the hypothesis of a zero mean. Moreover, this is not the
only test we performed. We also calculated the phase angle
relationship in the Raleigh test.

DESIR: In your original paper in 1974, you used the
end of the REM period to investigate the relationship with
PRL secretory episodes. Your sampling interval was 20
minutes. When one looks at polygraphic records of sleep,
it can be seen that REM periods may last 15 minutes or 20
minutes or shorter or longer. How do you assign a given
sample to the end of a REM period when the REM period actually does not end at the time of blood sampling? We had
great difficulties to reproduce your methodology despite
the fact that our sampling interval was only of 15 minutes.

ROSSMAN: We had a computer program to perform this
operation. The end of REM was defined as the last 60
seconds of REM not followed by a REM episode in the next
20 minutes. It turned out that there was one 17 minute
REM episode and that all the other REM episodes lasted
less than 10 minutes. Non-REM samples were defined as
samples after the end of REM until the next REM. The
beginning of REM was defined as the first 60 seconds of
REM.

DESIR: You also mentioned in your original paper
that the individual profiles were different in what concerns the PRL- REM - non-REM cycle relationship from the
transverse mean. Now that you have a very large amount
of data, I would like to have a quantitative evaluation
of how many individual profiles are in accordance with
your hypothesis. Is it 25%? Is it 50%? Is it 75%?

ROSSMAN: I would like to know that too. We haven't looked at that yet.

WEITZMAN: The data from the two groups look so dissimilar that it is difficult to come to a conclusion. Why are they so different? One possibility would be that the sleep stage organization is not the same. If your sleep has a lot of multiple arousals, interruptions of REM episodes, different timing of stage IV distribution, these factors may distort the actual relationship between PRL secretion and REM - non-REM cycles. We know that the sleep-wake cycle is a powerful control of PRL secretion. Before we conclude that the data from the two groups are really different, we should compare the internal organizations of sleep in terms of percent of REM, number of awakenings, percent of stage IV, stage IV distribution, etc.

BARDIN: In my laboratory, I had a young fellow running a PRL assay using a standard N.I.H. kit. He did an experiment which I told him not to do since it had been done many times before. He did it anyway and measured PRL across the normal menstrual cycle in a woman. He found a mid-cycle PRL peak which no one else had observed before. We thought it was an artefact but he repeated the experiment and obtained the same results. So we started a systematic analysis of the available PRL assays. I can tell you that two different N.I.H. kits and two different commercial kits are all measuring something different in the female. We cannot tell yet what they are measuring. We have now progressed to a point in radioimmunoassay technology that we use the reagents without checking them. From time to time, we should look at the standard, the first antibody and the second antibody. Such assay problems could be involved in the discrepancies you observed.

ROSSMAN: Can I ask you which kit is the disturbing one?

BARDIN: I can't remember the exact details right now but I will gladly send them to you.

ROSSMAN: I would appreciate it. I am using the first antibody and the first standard made by Dr. Lewis and provided by the N.I.H.

BARDIN: I was referring to a later N.I.H. kit.

Further discussion of Dr. Rossman's presentation took place after the paper by Dr. Weeke.

PHYSIOLOGICAL FACTORS INFLUENCING THE NYCTOHEMERAL PATTERN OF TSH

J. Golstein[*], L. Vanhaelst[**] and E. Van Cauter[*]

[*]Institut de Recherche Interdisciplinaire en Biologie Humaine et Nucléaire (L.M.N.) and [**]Division of Endocrinology, Akademische Ziekenhuis, School of Medicine, Universities of Brussels.

INTRODUCTION

Many studies describe the nyctohemeral pattern of TSH, but important variations in the times of occurrence of circadian maxima have been reported (1-5). These studies generally involve young male subjects and the circadian rhythms are examined regardless of season. Here are reported data obtained when sex and seasons are taken into account.

SUBJECTS AND METHODS

Six normal males were investigated in summer and in winter. Two of them were investigated during 2 consecutive winter periods. Blood samples have been collected at 15- or 30-min intervals during a 24-hour span. Serum TSH levels were measured in duplicate by radioimmunoassay (6).

The low (e.g. circadian) and high (e.g. episodic) frequency components of the 24-hour variation of TSH were evaluated separately. The methodology of analysis of the low frequency variation has been described in detail elsewhere (7). Briefly, a best-fit pattern is built using repeated periodogram calculations. The periodogram method consists of fitting a sum of sinusoid functions on the series of data and selecting the terms which contribute significantly ($p < .10$) to the observed variation. Only significant com-

ponents of periods longer than 6 h are retained for inclusion in the best-fit pattern which may be unimodal, bimodal
or trimodal. The acrophases are the times of occurrence of
maxima in the best-fit pattern. The value of the best-fit
pattern at the acrophase was expressed in per cent of the
24-h mean. Acrophases were classified in four sub-sections
of the 24-hour span, the sleep period itself (from sleep
onset to final morning awakening), a pre-sleep period (3
hours preceding sleep onset), a post-sleep period (3 hours
following final morning awakening) and the remainder of the
24-hour span, referred to as "mid-day" period. The acrophases were plotted on a polar graph and the hypothesis of
their uniform distribution over the 24-hour cycle was tested
using the Rao   test (8).

The same analysis was also applied to the TSH profiles published by Parker et al. (4) for purposes of comparison.
To compare profiles obtained in males and in females, data
previously collected in 9 normal females, investigated regardless of season, were similarly reprocessed (1, 9, 10).

In all profiles obtained at 15-min intervals, the number of
peaks occurring during the 24-hour span, during the sleep-
wake cycle and during the night-day cycle (night : from sunset to sunrise; day : from sunrise to sunset) was estimated
using an analytical procedure detailed in this volume (11).
The duration and the magnitude of each peak were calculated.
The average intra-assay coefficient of variation (5 %) was
taken into account to establish the significance of the
peaks.

RESULTS

Fig. 1 illustrates the transverse mean profiles obtained in
males in both seasons. Despite the artefactual smoothness
introduced by the averaging across individuals, differences
between the 24-hour TSH secretory pattern in summer and
in winter seem to emerge. In summer, the TSH levels declined
during the morning hours and were higher during the night.
Two phases seemed to be present during the night. In winter,
lower levels were also found in the morning hours but they

started to increase earlier than in summer and remained
higher throughout the night.

Fig. 2 illustrates some individual profiles. The times of
observed maxima and the acrophases did not always coincide
since an acrophase corresponds to consistently elevated
values rather than to isolated maxima. In the case of subject 1, no best-fit pattern was found significant in winter
because of the asymmetry of the profile while in summer, the
best-fit pattern was monomodal, with an acrophase during
sleep.

Table 1 lists for each season and across all subjects, the
numbers of acrophases found in each sub-section of the 24-
hour span together with their average value expressed in
per cent of the 24-hour mean. No seasonal variation was
found for the mean values and both sets of data were pooled.
A total of 31 acrophases were counted. Though, on the average, the pre-sleep acrophase had the largest value, it occurred rather infrequently (only one subject in winter, only
half of the subjects in summer). Sleep acrophases were
most commonly found.

Fig. 3 illustrates the distribution of the acrophases plotted on a polar graph. In summer, the acrophases appeared
concentrated into 3 separate well-defined periods of the
24-hour span : a pre-sleep period (21.30 to 22.30), a late
sleep period (03.00 to 07.00) and a mid-day period, confined to the afternoon hours (15.00 to 16.30). The Rao test
allowed to reject the hypothesis of uniform distribution of
the acrophases over the 24-hour span with a probability
level of .07. In contrast, in winter the acrophases were randomly
distributed throughout the 24-hour span. When a sleep
phase was present in winter, it occurred generally earlier
than in summer.

Fig. 4 illustrates the best-fit patterns calculated for the
18.00 to 18.00 portion of the profiles reported by Parker
et al. (4) for subjects 1 and 3. Subject 1 (lower part)
exhibited a trimodal pattern, with acrophases at 24.00,
08.30 and 15.00 while subject 3 (top) presented a bimodal
best-fit pattern with acrophases at 22.00 and 06.00.

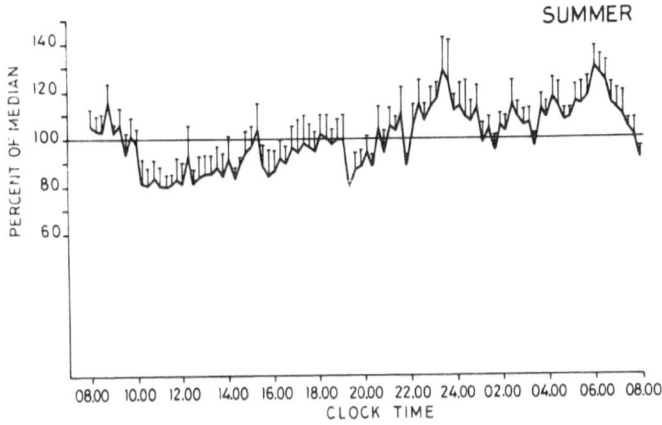

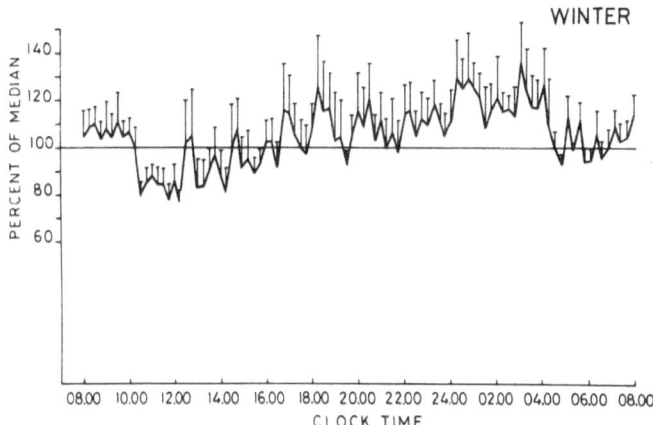

Figure 1 : Transverse mean profiles obtained in summer (top) and in winter (lower panel) for the 6 male subjects. The data have been expressed in per cent of the median. The standard errors of the mean are also shown.

Table 2 gives the number and the average values, in percent of the 24-hour mean, of the TSH acrophases obtained in profiles recorded in females. In 8 of the 9 profiles, a sleep acrophase was dominant, with highest value. Significant acrophases with generally lower values, were found outside the sleep period and classified under "post-sleep", "mid-day" or "pre-sleep" according to their time of occurrence.

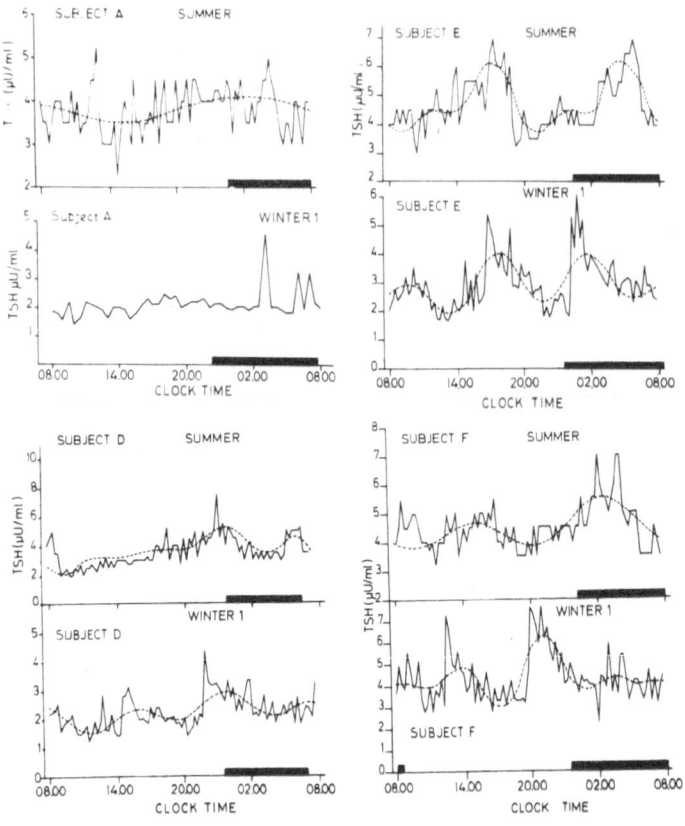

Figure 2 : Individual TSH profiles of subjects A, D, E and F in summer and in winter. Best-fit patterns are illustrated in dotted line. The sleep period is indicated by a black bar.

Fig. 5 illustrates the distribution of the acrophases on a polar plot for female subjects, investigated regardless of season (left) and for male subjects for which acrophases detected in summer and winter profiles have been pooled. In females, the major circadian increase occurred during the early morning hours and a clear concentration of the acrophases into 3 separate zones was observed. The Rao test rejected the hypothesis of uniform distribution with a pro-

Table 1. Distribution and average value of TSH acrophases in four periods of the 24-hour span; n denotes the number of individual best-fit patterns under consideration

TSH acrophases	Post-sleep	Mid-day	Pre-sleep	Sleep
SUMMER (n = 6)				
Average value ± SEM	113 %	98 % ± 9 %	130 % ± 9 %	121 % ± 7 %
Number	1	4	3	5
WINTER (n = 7)				
Average value ± SEM	113 % ± 6 %	111 % ± 5 %	136 %	121 % ± 5 %
Number	4	6	1	7
BOTH SEASONS (n = 13)				
Average value ± SEM	113 % ± 5 %	106 % ± 5 %	131 % ± 7 %	121 % ± 4 %
Number	5	10	4	12

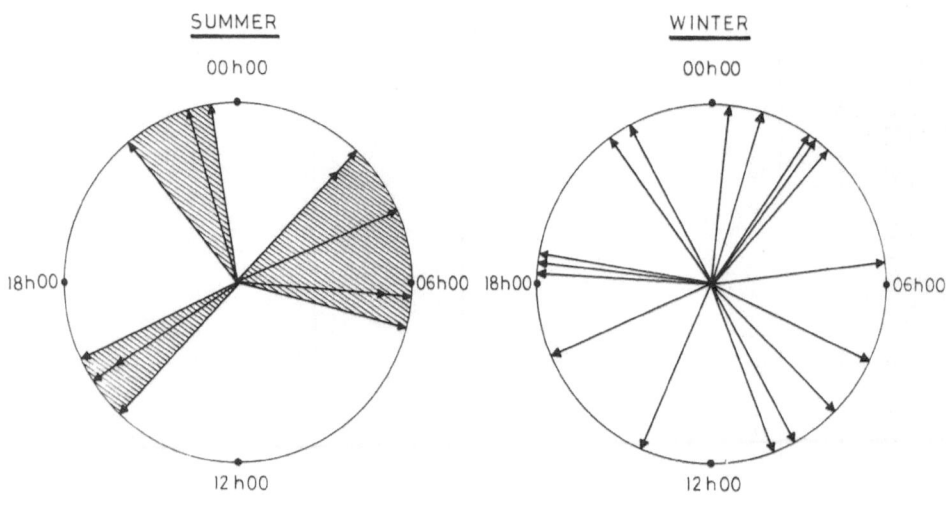

Figure 3 : Polar plots of acrophases for the profiles obtained in males in summer (left) and in winter (right). Each arrow represents an acrophase of the best-fit pattern. When more than one acrophase occurred at the same clock time, it was illustrated by a double or triple arrow. The hatched areas show the zone of concentration of acrophases.

bability level of .01. In contrast, in males, the acrophases seemed to be randomly distributed over the 24-hour span and the hypothesis of uniform distribution was accepted.

Table 3 gives the average characteristics of the episodic fluctuations of TSH levels.

Table 2. Number of acrophases and average ± SEM values at the acrophases expressed in percent of the 24-hour TSH mean for 9 female subjects investigated regardless of season

		Post-sleep	Mid-day	Pre-sleep	Sleep
FEMALES	Average value ± SEM	180%	105% ± 6%	115% ± 13%	140% ± 15%
	Number of acrophases	1	5	4	8

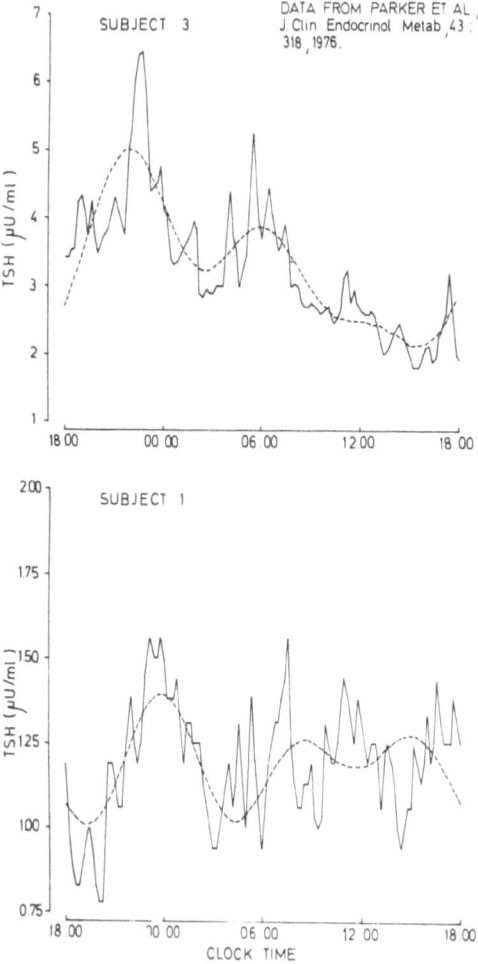

Figure 4 : TSH profiles reported by Parker et al. (4) for subjects 3 and 1 of their study. The best-fit patterns calculated according to the method described here and elsewhere ( ) are illustrated in dotted line.

The total number of significant TSH peaks over the 24-hour span varied little within and among subjects (range : 17-26). The range of variation of mean durations and magnitudes was wider (durations : 45 min-69 min; magnitudes : 28 %-48 %). For magnitudes, no difference between night and day or sleep and wake could be demonstrated. When the number of peaks occurring during the night and during the day as well as during sleep and during wakefulness were weighed, respectively, according to the length of night and day or sleep and wake, no night-day or sleep-wake differences in the frequency of occurrence of TSH episodic peaks were found. However, peaks occurring during the day lasted longer than

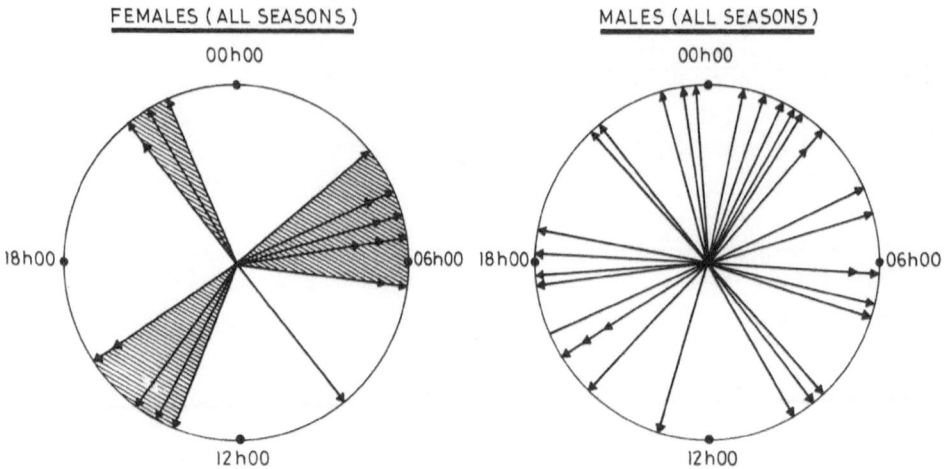

Figure 5 : Polar plot for the profiles obtained in females (left) investigated regardless of season and in males (right) when summer and
winter investigations were pooled. Symbols are as in Fig. 3.

peaks occurring during the night; this was true in summer as
well as in winter (p < .02). No similar sleep-wake difference was found. No seasonal effect could be demonstrated
for any of the parameters reported in Table 3. When all
the data on episodic TSH fluctuations were pooled, a total
of 233 peaks were detected and 77 % of them lasted one hour
or less.

DISCUSSION

In a given 24-hour profile, one to three significant acrophases were observed in males (except subject 1, winter).
Parker et al. (4) characterized their profiles by an increase occurring generally before sleep onset. However,
when best-fit patterns were calculated for their profiles,
more than one acrophase was also found. Differences in methodology of statistical analysis may partially account for

Table 3. Averages, across all profiles obtained at 15-min intervals, of the individual means for the number of episodic TSH peaks, their magnitude and their duration. Results are given for the night-day cycle, the sleep-wake cycle and the entire 24-hour span for both summer and winter seasons

	SUMMER					WINTER				
	24-h span	night	day	sleep	wake	24-h span	night	day	sleep	wake
Number of peaks	20	7	13	5	15	23	15	8	9	14
duration (minutes)	59	51	65	60	60	50	48	55	50	51
magnitude (% increment over prececing trough)	36	36	35	32	36	44	43	46	43	45

the discrepancies in the reported times of occurrence of
TSH circadian maxima. The finding of acrophases outside the
sleep period also suggests that factors other than sleep
could play a role in the regulation of the TSH nyctohemeral
pattern. The present data suggest a difference in the temporal organization of the TSH secretion related to seasons.
It could be speculated that this apparent season modulation
is related to the dark-light cycle since the hypothesis of
darkness as initiator of inhibitory events in TSH secretion
has already been proposed (4). In studies involving male
subjects, the geographical latitude of the laboratory where
the samples are collected, as well as the fact that generally subjects are not matched for season, could account for
the differences observed in the times of occurrence of circadian maxima.

Few data are available on normal females (3, 5). The comparison presented here shows that the characteristics of the
24-hour profile of TSH levels depend on the sex of the subjects. In males, the times of occurrence of circadian maxima appeared to be under seasonal modulation. In females,
the major increase occurred in the early morning hours, regardless of the season of the investigation. The existence
of such sex differences was already suggested by Azukizawa
et al. (5) who observed "pre-sleep" peaks in male subjects
but an "early morning" peak in their only female subject.
Thus, it is important to match subjects for sex when circadian rhythms are compared in different situations, either
physiological or pathological. As far as the episodic variations were concerned, no seasonal difference was found
suggesting the existence of different mechanisms controlling
circadian variations on the one hand and short-term fluctuations on the other. Different authors have described episodic TSH peaks. The mean durations reported varied from 30
min to 100-200 min (14, 3). They are unlikely to result
from feedback by thyroid hormones. The fact that 77 % of the
peaks lasted less than 1 hour does not support the concept
of entrainment of TSH episodic release by 100 min REM-non REM
cycles during sleep or by a basic "rest-activity" cycle of
similar period during wakefulness. It has been proposed

that central serotonin could be involved in the regulation of the TSH diurnal rhythm in rats (13). Administration of cyproheptadine, a drug with antiserotonin properties, significantly increased the number of episodic variations in male subjects (14), suggesting a possible serotoninergic control of the episodic fluctuations of TSH secretion.

130

REFERENCES

1. Vanhaelst, L, E Van Cauter, JP Degaute and J Golstein, Circadian variations of serum thyrotropin. J Clin Endocrinol Metab 35:472, 1972

2. Weeke, J, Circadian variation of serum thyrotropin levels in normal subjects. Scand J Clin Lab Invest 31:337, 1973

3. Alford, FP, HWG Baker, HG Burger, DM de Kretser, B Hudson, HW Johns, JP Masterton, YC Patel and GC Rennie, Temporal patterns of integrated plasma hormone levels during sleep and wakefulness. Thyroid-stimulating hormone, growth hormone and cortisol. J Clin Endocrinol Metab 37:841, 1973

4. Parker, DC, AE Pekary and JH Hershman, Effect of normal and reversed sleep-wake cycles upon nyctohemeral rhythmicity of plasma thyrotropin. Evidence suggestive of an inhibitory influence of sleep. J Clin Endocrinol Metab 43:318, 1976

5. Azukizawa, M, AE Pekary, JM Hershman and DC Parker, Plasma thyrotropin, thyroxine and triiodothyronine relationships in man. J Clin Endocrinol Metab 43: 533, 1976

6. Golstein, J and L Vanhaelst, Influence of thyrotropin-free serum on the radioimmunoassay of human thyrotropin. Clin Chim Acta 49:141, 1973

7. Van Cauter, E, Method for the characterization of the 24-hour temporal variation of blood components. Amer J Physiol 237:E255-E264, 1979

8. Batschelet, E, Recent statistical methods for orientation data, In:Animal Orientation and Navigation, Galler, SR et al (eds.), NASA Symposium 1970, US Government Printing Office, 1972

9. Van Cauter, E, J Golstein, L Vanhaelst and R Leclercq, Effects of oral contraceptive therapy on the circadian patterns of cortisol and thyrotropin (TSH). Europ J Clin Invest 5:115, 1975

10. Van Cauter, E, R Leclercq, L Vanhaelst and J Golstein, Simultaneous study of cortisol and TSH daily variations in normal subjects and patients with hyper-

adrenalcorticism. J Clin Endocrinol Metab 39:645, 1974

11. Van Cauter, E, Quantitative methods for the analysis of circadian and episodic hormone fluctuations. In this volume

12. Weeke, J and HJG Gundersen, Circadian and 30 min-variations in serum TSH and thyroid hormones in normal subjects. Acta Endocrinol 89:659, 1978

13. Jordan, D, P Pigeon, A McRae-Degueurce, JF Pujol and R Mornex, Participation of serotonin in thyrotropin release. II. Evidence for the action of serotonin on the basic release of thyrotropin. Endocrinology 105:975, 1979

14. Golstein J, L Vanhaelst, OD Bruno and M L'Hermite, Effect of cyproheptadine on thyrotropin and prolactin secretion in normal man. Acta Endocrinol 92: 205, 1979

CIRCADIAN AND ULTRADIAN VARIATIONS IN SERUM TSH AND THYROID HORMONES IN NORMAL MAN AND IN PATIENTS WITH TREATED AND UNTREATED PRIMARY HYPOTHYROIDISM

Jørgen Weeke

Second University Clinic of Internal Medicine, Kommune-hospitalet, 8000 Aarhus C, Denmark.

This study was supported by the Danish Research Council.

The thyroid activity is effectively regulated via the plasma concentration of thyrotropin (TSH) in normal man. The pituitary secretion of TSH is under the influence of both stimulatory and inhibitory factors. The primary control of TSH secretion is believed to be mediated through the interaction between the negative feedback effects of thyroxine (T_4) and triiodothyronine (T_3) and the stimulatory effect of thyrotropin releasing hormone (TRH) secreted by the hypothalamus (1). The peptidergic neurons releasing TRH are then in turn regulated by bioaminergic neurons connected with higher brain centers involved in the relay of stress and temperature influences and possibly also with a brain center with circadian oscillator activity. The regulatory system is, however, more complex. It has recently been shown that both somatostatin (2) and dopamine (3) have an inhibitory effect on TSH secretion, probably of physiological significance for the regulation. Estrogen, growth hormone, and glucocorticoids can also influence the TSH secretion at least when pharmacological doses or pathological states are considered.

DIURNAL TSH VARIATIONS IN NORMAL MAN

Diurnal variation in serum TSH in euthyroid subjects is now well documented (4-11). There is general agreement that the levels are highest at night and lowest during the day. Serum

TSH increases from the low and rather stable day level after 2000 hours and it reaches the day level again after 1100 hours. The patterns of the reported TSH variation during the night have, however, varied a great deal. Parker et al. (9) have shown that the displacement of sleep is associated with alterations in the shape and amplitude of the pattern of nyctohemeral TSH release and as pointed out by these authors this may explain, at least in part, the different patterns reported.

The diurnal TSH variation is reflected in the TSH response to TRH given intravenously. The absolute peak TSH levels as well as the increase in serum TSH after TRH stimulations are higher at 2300 hours than at 1100 hours, but there is, however, no difference in the increase expressed in percentages (12). This is in accordance with the direct relationship which we have shown exists between basal serum TSH and the degree of TSH release after TRH given intravenously to normal subjects (13, 14). The TSH response to TRH probably reflects the size of the readily releasable TSH pool which may be proportional to basal TSH levels (3).

THE RELATION BETWEEN SERUM TSH AND THYROID HORMONES IN NORMAL MAN

Since a considerable amount of the daily T_3 production derives from peripheral monodeiodination of T_4 to T_3 (15-19) the possibility exists that some of the variations observed in serum TSH levels could be generated through a negative feedback on the hypophyseal TSH secretion from this T_3 produced in peripheral tissues. The following observation throws some light on this problem. In an investigation on the dose response relationship between TRH given intravenously and serum TSH and T_3 (20), a direct relationship between basal TSH and T_3 was found in the four subjects studied (Fig. 1). TRH tests were done with 3 days interval 8 to 10 times in each of four young subjects. The tests were started in the morning between 0700 and 0730 hours and the subjects were supine from 30 minutes before the first blood sample was drawn. At this particular time of day,

134

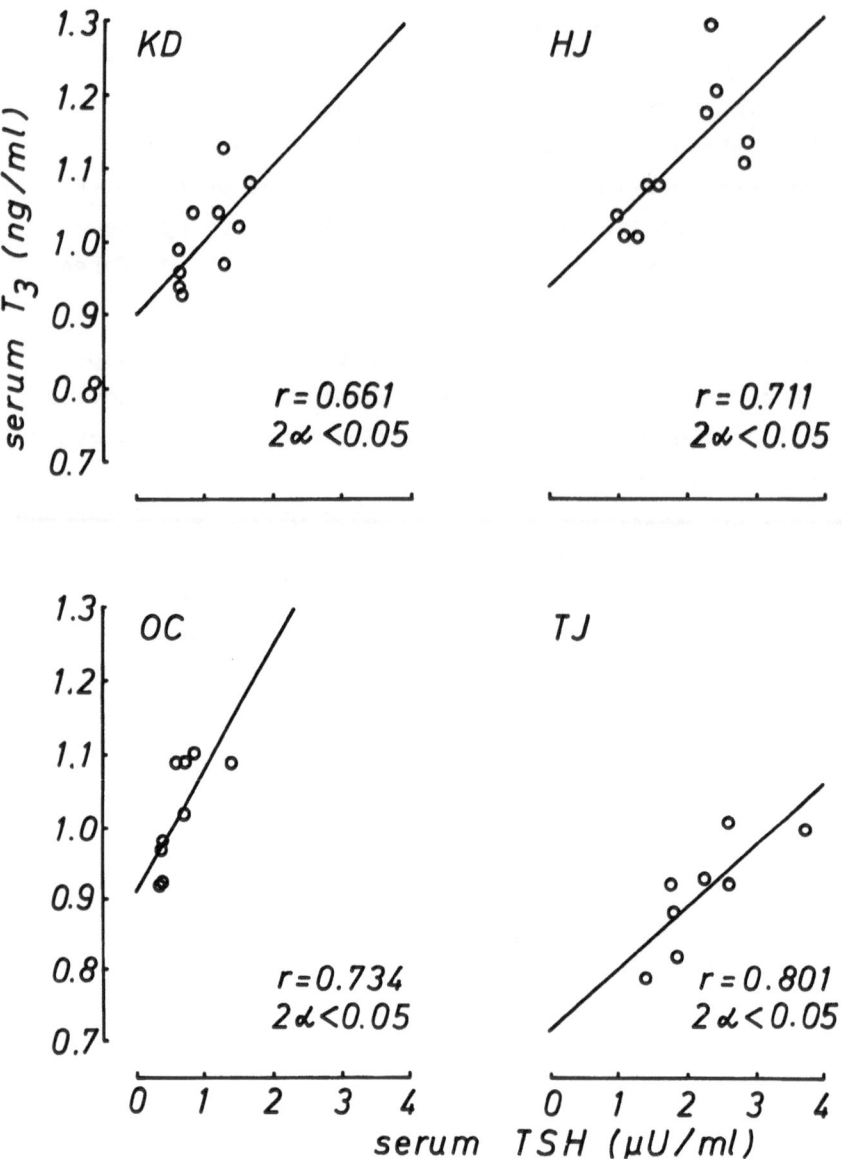

Figure 1 : Correlation of basal serum TSH and basal serum T₃ in four normal subjects.

where serum TSH is declining in most subjects, a negative feedback is thus not determining the TSH variation. This finding encouraged us to investigate the diurnal variation of circulating thyroid hormones in more detail. Diurnal variations in total T_4 and total T_3 have been investigated by several authors (8, 10, 11, 21-24). Generally, hormone levels have been found to be rather stable during the day with a tendency towards higher levels in the morning and low levels in the afternoon and at night. The trend towards lower total thyroid hormone levels observed during the sleeping period, when the subjects were supine, has been explained by changes in the binding capacities of serum known to occur concomitant with postural changes (25, 26). In order to evaluate the importance of such an alteration in protein binding of circulating thyroid hormones we have studied the diurnal variation of serum free T_4 and free T_3 in five normal young male subjects (24). We found that serum free T_3 and to a lesser degree free T_4 were indeed higher at night than during the day period, varying in parallel with serum TSH (Fig. 2). The mean increase from day to night was 140 per cent for TSH and 15 and 7 per cent for free T_3 and free T_4, respectively. Since equilibrium between extracellular and the large cellular compartments for T_3 and T_4 occurs within 3 to 4 h (27) the maximal diurnal variation in T_3 and T_4 is mainly determined by their biological $T1/2$ of 0.97 and 6.6 days, respectively (28, 29). The limit to the diurnal variation, calculated under the assumption that secretion only occurs during night, would then be 30 and 5.1 per cent for the two thyroid hormones. If, however, we assume that 50 per cent of the T_3 is produced in peripheral tissues by a constant monodeiodination from T_4 and the other 50 per cent is secreted from the thyroid gland during night, then the above limit to the diurnal variation of T_3 is reduced to 14 per cent. The observed values compare well to these theoretical limits and the observed pattern is consistent with a predominant thyroid secretion at night. However, other possible mechanisms may also be operative, e.g. diurnal variations in the amount of T_3 generated in peripheral tissues from T_4. In order to evaluate whether such a diurnal variation in peripheral monodeiodination of iodothyronines takes place, we have also measured rT_3 and 3,3'-diiodothyronine

per cent of mean

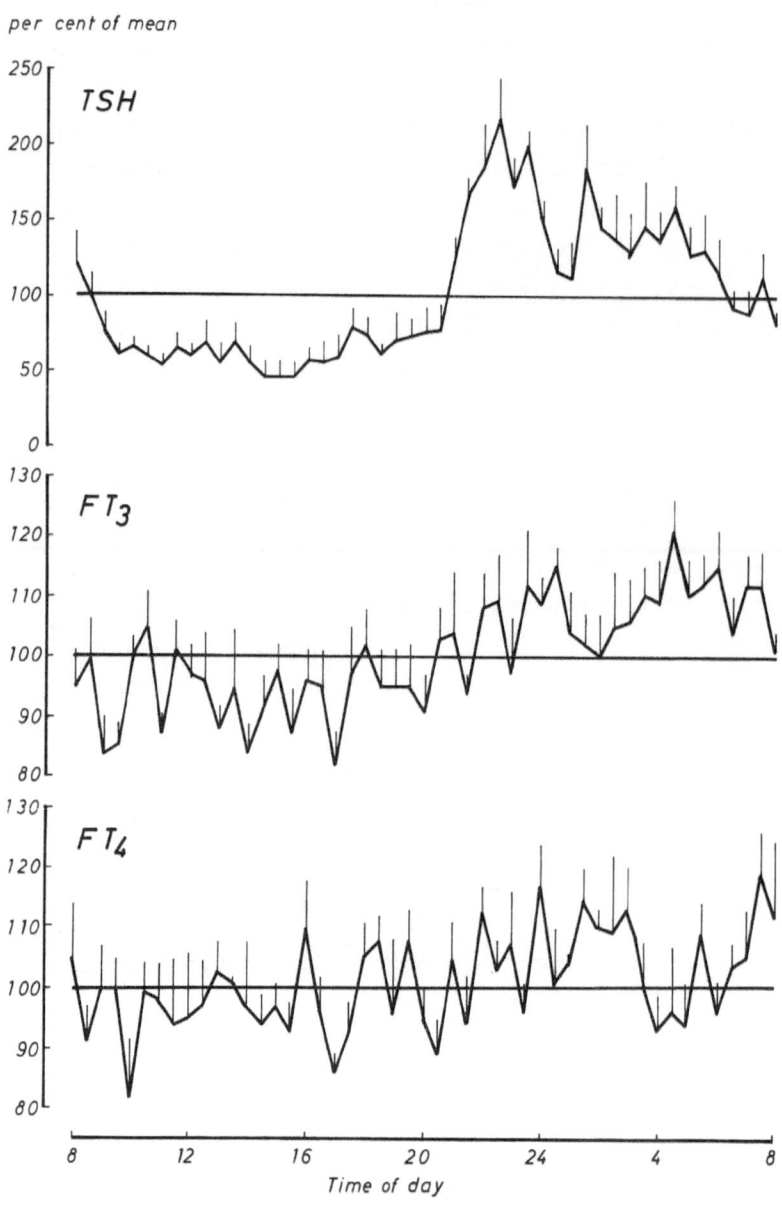

Figure 2 : Diurnal variations of serum TSH, free T₃ and free T₄ in five normal male subjects. Average curves of values relative to the 24 hour mean (+ SE).

$(3,3'-T_2)$ in the serum samples from the five normal sub-jects (30). Both rT_3 and $3,3'-T_2$ are primarily generated in peripheral tissues by deiodination (19, 31). We found constant levels of these two iodothyronine metabolites in serum during a 24-hour period which suggests that no major diurnal change in peripheral iodothyronine deiodination occurs. Thus, these processes are probably not involved in the night increase in serum free T_3. The concept that thyroid secretion in normal man is higher at night than during the daytime was originally set forth by Nicoloff (4) who observed an increase in the excretion of thyroidal iodide in urine at night.

DIURNAL TSH VARIATIONS IN HYPOTHYROIDISM

We have studied the diurnal rhythm of TSH in hypothyroidism, especially taking into account the various degrees of hypothyroidism (32). The diurnal variation in serum TSH was preserved in patients with hypothyroidism of a moderate degree, i.e. serum TSH below 2 µU/ml and serum T_3 and T_4 levels at the lower limit of the normal range. The patients with severe hypothyroidism showed no significant diurnal variation in TSH whereas the diurnal rhythm of serum TSH was restored after partial thyroid hormone replacement with thyroxine. This is illustrated in Fig. 3, where the 24-hour serum TSH variation studied three times in one patient is depicted. First, in a state of mild untreated hypothyroidism due to an infiltrative neoplasm in the thyroid gland, then 1 month after total thyroidectomy and finally 25 months after the initiation of T_4 substitution.

The existence of a diurnal rhythm of TSH in patients treated for myxoedema with thyroxine gives further evidence for a central mechanism underlying the diurnal rhythm. The central mechanism is further supported by the finding of Fukuda and Greer (33), that basal hypothalamic deafferentation abolished the nyctohemeral rhythm of plasma TSH in rats. The reason why the rhythm disappears in patients with severe hypothyroidism might simply be that the hypothalamic stimulation of the pituitary TSH secretion under this condition is near maximal and therefore not sensitive to the input from a circadian oscillator. There is in fact some

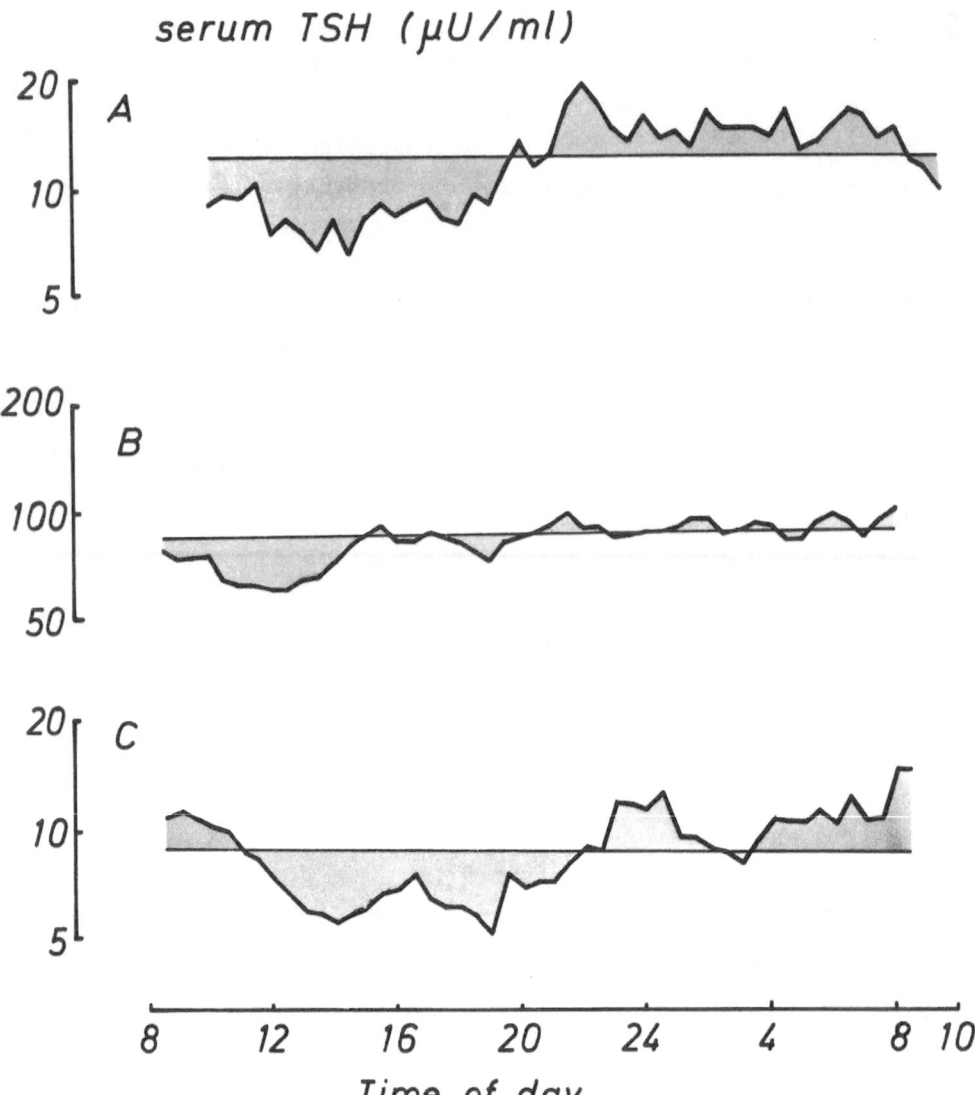

serum TSH (μU/ml)

Figure 3 : Serum TRH measured in three complete 24-hour periods in the same patient in a state of A : mild hypothyroidism, B : severe hypothyroidism, and C : after substitution with thyroxine.

evidence that serum TSH is increased in patients with thyrogenic myxoedema (34).

SOMATOSTATIN, A THYROTROPIN INHIBITING HORMONE

It is possible that there is a dual hypothalamic control of
TSH regulation. The physiological importance of somatostatin as an inhibitor of TSH secretion has been investigated in animal experiments both in vitro and in vivo providing strong evidence of a physiological inhibitory role for
somatostatin in the control of TSH secretion (35-38). Direct evidence for a physiological role of somatostatin in
the regulation of the hypophyseal-thyroid system in man is
not available.

The influence of presumably pharmacological doses of somatostatin on serum TSH in human subjects has been investigated
in a number of studies. The TRH induced increase in serum
TSH is suppressed by somatostatin infusions both in normal
man (39-41) and in patients with untreated primary myxoedema (42). The high basal serum TSH in patients with primary
myxoedema is also partially suppressed by somatostatin (43).
In normal subjects the high basal serum TSH level at night
is also suppressed. We have studied the effect of 1 mg
somatostatin given over a 2 h period from 0100 to 0300 to
six normal young men (2). The subjects were supine and
awake during the experimental procedure. Somatostatin induced a clearcut inhibitory effect on the nocturnal elevated basal TSH level (Fig. 4). The serum concentrations of
T_3 and T_4 were unchanged as could be expected due to the
long half lives of these hormones in serum. Similar results
have been presented by Azukizawa et al. (8). Controversy
exists, however, concerning the influence of somatostatin
on the low basal TSH level in the daytime. Copinschi et
al. (44) studied the effect of somatostatin infusion for
1 hour on serum TSH after insulin injection and Siler et al.
(45) studied the effect of somatostatin infusion for 45 min
on serum TSH during infusion of arginine or after administration of L-Dopa. Neither of these studies revealed any
effect of somatostatin on the low daytime serum TSH. In
a subsequent study Copinschi et al. (46) infused somatostatin in normal subjects for one hour and found a significant fall in serum TSH. However, this study was performed

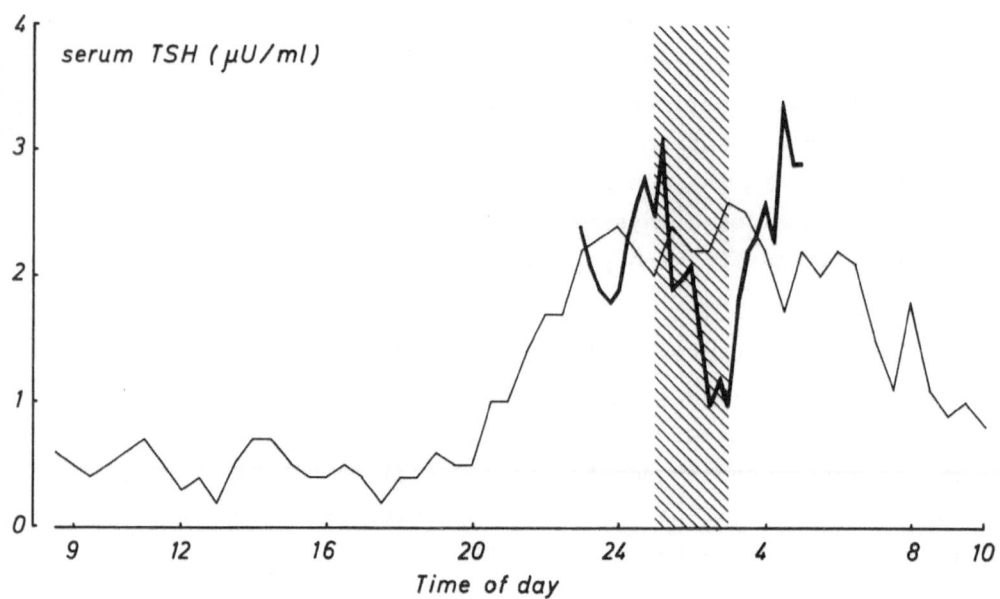

Figure 4 : Serum TSH level before, during and after a 2-h infusion of 1 mg somatostatin (shaded area) and serum TSH level during a 26-hour control period in 1 of the 6 normal subjects.

in the morning and the observed variation in serum TSH was probably the normal diurnal variation. We have investigated the effect of 24-hour somatostatin infusion in five normal subjects, seven juvenile type diabetic patients receiving a fixed daily insulin dose and in five patients treated with thyroxine for primary myxoedema (47). Blood samples were obtained every hour for 51 hours. During the first 24 hours saline was infused and during the following 24 hours cyclic somatostatin 2 to 6 mg was infused. As expected, somatostatin obliterated the night increase in serum TSH in all three groups. The daytime serum TSH was, on the other hand, nearly unaltered (Fig. 5). Since somatostatin inhibits the TSH secretion induced by TRH, our findings may suggest that the high TSH levels at night are induced by a hypothalamic TRH stimulation -rendering the night levels of TSH suppressible by somatostatin- while the lower daytime level of TSH is somehow independent on hypothalamic TRH, and therefore

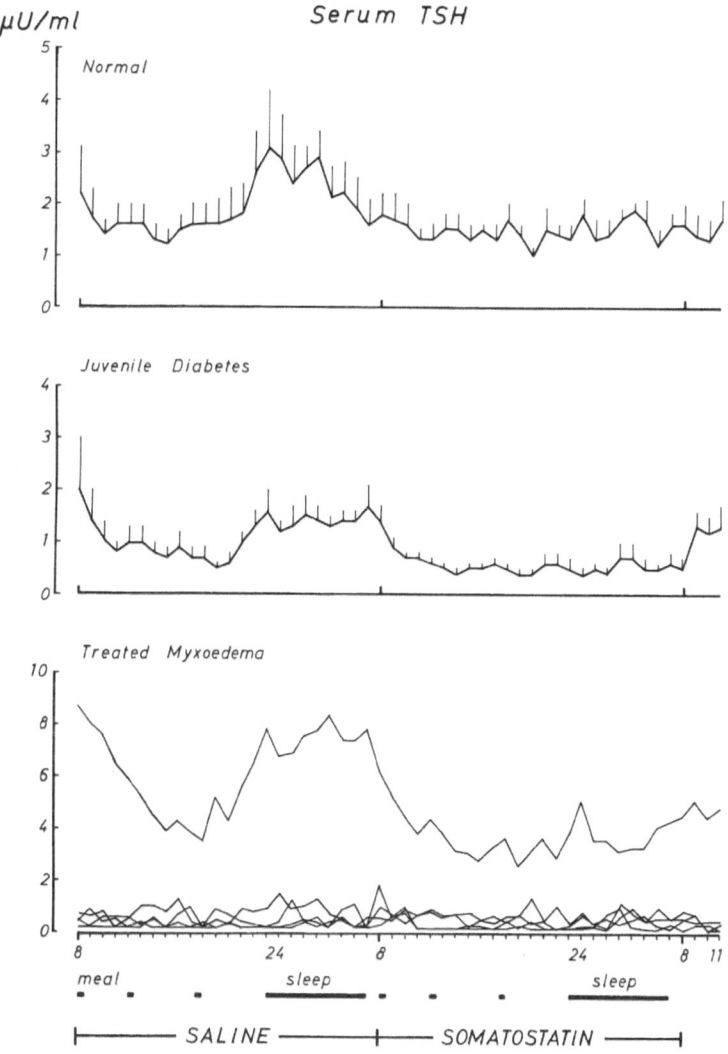

Figure 5 : Serum TSH in five normal subjects, seven juvenile type diabetics and in five patients treated for primary myxoedema. The total experiment lasted for 51 hours : a 24-h period with saline infusion, followed immediately by 24-h of somatostatin. During the final three hour period no somatostatin was given. Average curves of values relative to the mean of the 24-h saline period (+ SE).

not suppressed by somatostatin. However, other hypothetical models could explain the lack of suppressibility of the low daytime TSH, e.g. it has been suggested by Snow et al. (48) that a maximal somatostatinergic tone could be present in the daytime. The 24-hour somatostatin infusion induced a clearcut decrease in serum T_3 and free T_3 in normal subjects and diabetic patients. Serum free T_3 fell 23 ± 6 % and 25 ± 6 % in the two groups, respectively. In contrast, serum free T_3 was unaltered after somatostatin infusion in patients with treated myxoedema. This difference in effect of somatostatin suggests that the main mechanism behind the fall in serum T_3 in normal subjects and diabetics is a decrease in thyroidal secretion of T_3 and not inhibition of peripheral monodeiodination of T_4 to T_3.

ULTRADIAN VARIATIONS IN SERUM TSH, FREE T_3 AND FREE T_4

Besides the diurnal variation in serum TSH and thyroid hormones, small short-term fluctuations have also been observed (7, 8, 49). We have studied these short-term variations in five normal subjects (24). During the experiments, the subjects rested in armchairs. Blood was sampled every 5 min in a 6 to 7 h period. The experiments were started in the interval from 1915 to 2200 h. A considerable short-term variation in the serum TSH, free T_3 and free T_4 was found (Fig. 6). No regularity in there variations is apparent by simple inspection of the curves. To disclose hidden periodicities, data analyses were performed. This has been described in detail elsewhere (24). In short, first the variation due to the 24-hour rhythm was isolated using a smoothing procedure. Then a new time series was formed by the differences at each point of time between the original time series and the smoothed one. The variation of this new time series is mainly due to sources of short duration. The presence of regular variation was then looked for by calculation of the autocorrelation of the time series. The autocorrelation was then evaluated by its transformation to the power-spectrum which expresses the amount of variation in the time series that is attributable to a regular (cyclic) variation. The cycle- length corresponding to the peak value of the power-spectrum is taken as the estimate of the cycle length. Significant short-term variations were found for all three hormones, the estimated cycle-lengths varied

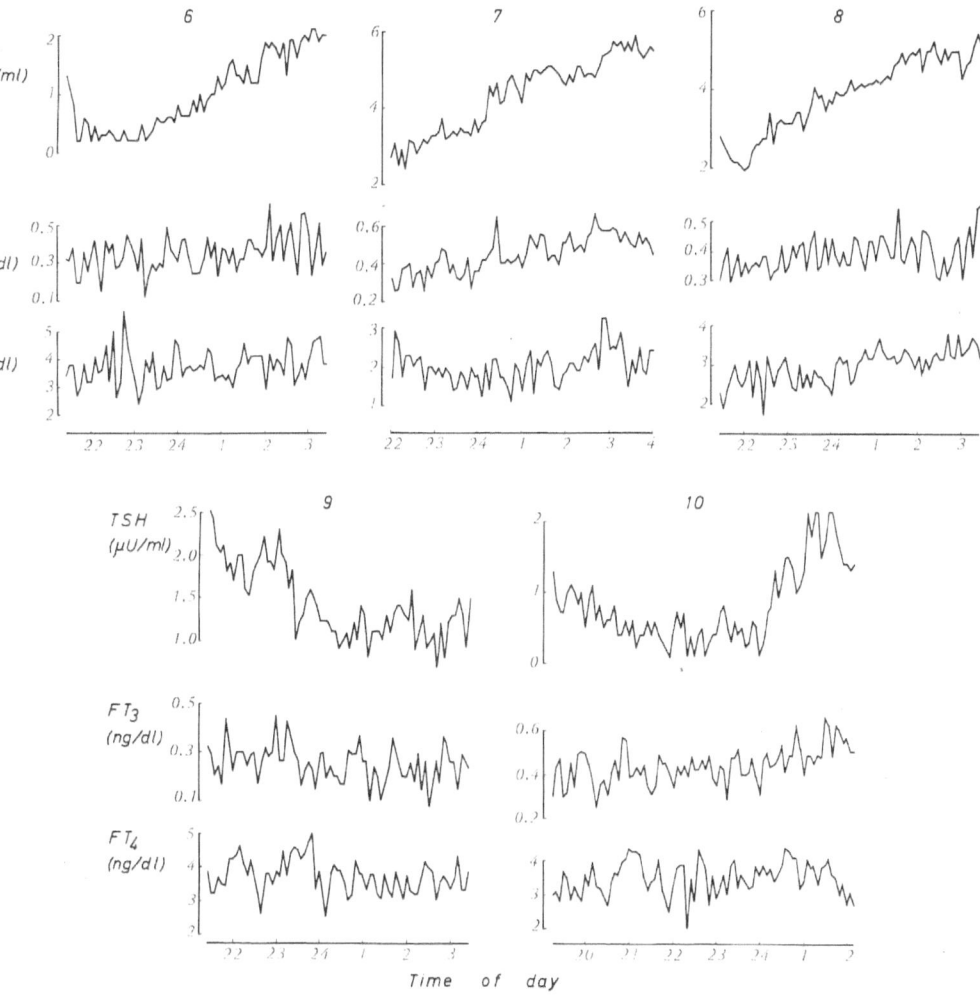

Figure 6 : Short-term variation of serum TSH, free T_3 and free T_4 in five male subjects for 6 to 7 h periods with a sampling interval of 5 min.

between 27-35 min. When the frequency of the short-term periodicity is estimated, the absolute amplitude of this variation in the time-series can be calculated (Fig. 7). The mean amplitude of the short-term variation was 13, 15, and 11 per cent of the mean level of TSH, free T_3 and free T_4, respectively.

A regular variation with a cycle-length of 30 minutes can

144

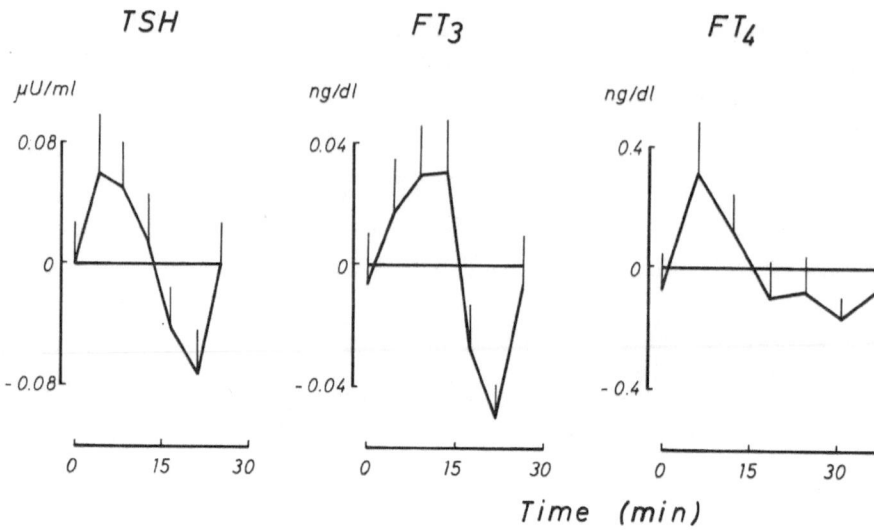

Figure 7 : Estimates of the absolute variation in one mean short-term cycle of TSH, free T_3 and free T_4 (mean + SE).

thus account for a significant part of the total variation in the serum levels of the three hormones.

The mechanisms underlying these short-term variations are unknown. Since both serum TSH and thyroid hormones exhibit the same short-term variation one might envisage that the mechanism was a hypothalamic mediated pulsatile TSH secretion which in turn leads to pulsatile secretion of T_3 and T_4 from the thyroid gland. This mechanism is, however, inconceivable. If a total daily production of T_4 of about 100 µg was secreted as 48 separate pulses, then the maximal amplitude of the variations in serum would have been one per cent at most and not 11 per cent as we found. Another speculative mechanism for the short-term variation in serum T_3 and T_4 could be rapid changes of the distribution space of intracellular thyroid hormones. The concomitant TSH rhythm then has to be explained. A feedback from T_3 and T_4 on the pituitary TSH secretion is less likely, since this process in comparison is rather slow (50-52), and there is no evidence for the other possibility that TSH has a direct influence on the intracellular distribution space of thyroid hormones. Finally, one might speculate that the thyroid gland both absorb thyroid hormones from the serum pool and secrete them to the serum pool. In this case TSH could regulate secretion of both T_3 and T_4, giving rise to the relatively large variation in serum concentrations without a corresponding de novo synthesis of T_3 and T_4 in the thyroid gland.

None of the three mechanisms mentioned above are immediately evident. Investigation of this puzzling question is presently under progress in our laboratory.

REFERENCES

1. Martin, JB, S Reichlin, and GM Brown, Clinical neuroendocrinology contemporary neurology series, F.A. Davis Company, Philadelphia, 1977

2. Weeke, J, AaP Hansen, and K Lundbaek, Inhibition by somatostatin of basal levels of serum thyrotropin in normal men. J Clin Endocrinol Metab 41:168-171, 1975

3. Scanlon, MF, DR Weightman, DJ Shale, B Mora, M Heath, MH Snow, M Lewis, and R Hall, Dopamine is a physiological regulator of thyrotropin (TSH) secretion in man. Clin Endocrinol (Oxf) 10:7-15, 1979

4. Nicoloff, JT, DA Fisher, and MD Appleman, The role of glucocorticoids in the regulation of thyroid function in man. J Clin Invest 49:1922-1929, 1970

5. Vanhaelst, L, E Van Cauter, JP Degaute, J Golstein, Circadian variations of serum thyrotropin levels in man. J Clin Endocrinol Metab 35:479-482,1972

6. Patel, YC, FP Alford, and HG Burger, The 24-hour plasma thyrotrophin profile. Clin Sci Mol Med 43:71-77, 1972

7. Weeke, J, Circadian variation of the serum thyrotrophin level in normal subjects. Scand J Clin Lab Invest 31:337-342, 1973

8. Azukizawa, M, AE Pekary, JM Hershman, and DC Parker, Plasma thyrotropin, thyroxine and triiodothyronine relationships in man. J Clin Endocrinol Metab 43: 533-542, 1976

9. Parker, DC, AE Pekary, and JM Hershman, Effect of normal and reversed sleep-wake cycles upon nyctohemeral rhythmicity of plasma thyrotropin : evidence suggestive of an inhibitory influence in sleep. J Clin Endocrinol Metab 43:318-329, 1976

10. Lucke, C, R Hehrmann, K Mayersbach, and A Mühlen, Studies on circadian variations of plasma TSH, thyroxine and triiodothyronine in man. Acta Endocrinol (Kbh) 86:81-88, 1977

11. Chan, V, A Jones, P Liendo-Ch, A McNeilly, J Landon, and GM Besser, The relationship between circadian variations in circulating thyrotrophin, thyroid hormones and prolactin. Clin Endocrinol (Oxf) 9:337-349, 1978

12. Weeke, J, The influence of the circadian thyrotropin rhythm on the thyrotropin response to thyrotropin-releasing hormone in normal subjects. Scand J Clin Lab Invest 33:17-20, 1974

13. Weeke, J, Thyrotropin response to thyrotropin releasing hormone in normal subjects. Eur J Clin Invest 4:29-32, 1974

14. Sawin, CT, and JM Hershman, The TSH response to thyrotropin-releasing hormone (TRH) in young adult men : intraindividual variation and relation to basal serum TSH and thyroid hormones. J Clin Endocrinol Metab 42:809-816, 1976

15. Pittman, CS, JB Chambers, and VH Read, The extrathyroidal conversion rate of thyroxine to triiodothyronine in normal man. J Clin Invest 50:1187-1196, 1971

16. Surks, MI, AR Schadlow, JM Stock, and JH Oppenheimer, Determination of iodothyronine absorption and conversion of L-thyroxine (T_4) and L-triiodothyronine (T_3) using turnover rate techniques. J Clin Invest 52:805-811, 1973

17. Braverman, LE, A Vagenakis, P Downs, AE Foster, K Sterling, and SH Ingbar, Effects of replacement doses of sodium-L-thyroxine on the peripheral metabolism of thyroxine and triiodothyronine in man. J Clin Invest 52:1010-1017, 1973

18. Inada, M, K Kasagi, S Kurata, Y Kazama, H Takayama, K Torizuka, M Fukase, and T Soma, Estimation of thyroxine and triiodothyronine distribution and of the conversion rate of thyroxine to triiodothyronine in man. J Clin Invest 55:1337-1348, 1975

19. Chopra, IJ, An assessment of daily production and significance of thyroidal secretion of 3,3',5'-triiodothyronine (reverse T_3) in man. J Clin Invest 58:32-40, 1976

20. Weeke, J, The response of thyrotropin and triiodothyronine to various doses of thyrotropin releasing hormone in normal man. Eur J Clin Invest 5:447-453, 1975

21. De Costre, P, U Buhler, LJ DeGroot, and S Refetoff, Diurnal rhythm in total serum thyroxine levels. Metabolism 20:782-791, 1971

22. O'Connor, JF, GY Wu, TF Gallagher, and L Hellman, The 24-hour plasma thyroxine profile in normal man. J Clin Endocrinol Metab 39:765-771, 1974

23. Balsam, A, CR Dobbs, and LE Leppo, Circadian variations in concentrations of plasma thyroxine and triiodothyronine in man. J Appl Physiol 39:297-299, 1975

24. Weeke, J, and HJG Gundersen, Circadian and 30 minutes variations in serum TSH and thyroid hormones in normal subjects. Acta Endocrinol (Kbh) 89:659-672, 1978

25. Judd, SJ, JN Carter, and JM Corcoran, Circulating thyroid hormone concentrations and posture and venous compression. Br Med J 4:735-736, 1975

26. Vernikos-Danellis, J, CS Leach, CM Winget, PC Rambaut, and PB Mack, Thyroid and adrenal cortical rhythmicity during bed rest. J Appl Physiol 33:644-648, 1972

27. Oppenheimer, JH, MI Surks, and HL Schwartz, The metabolic significance of exchangeable cellular thyroxine. Recent Prog Horm Res 25:381-414, 1969

28. Oddie, TH, DA Fisher, JH Dussault, and CS Thompson, Triiodothyronine turnover in euthyroid subjects. J Clin Endocrinol Metab 33:653-660, 1971

29. Gregerman, RI, GW Gaffney, and NW Shock, Thyroxine turnover in euthyroid man with special reference to changes with age. J Clin Invest 41:2065-2074, 1962

30. Weeke, J, and P Laurberg, 24-hour profile of serum rT_3 and $3,3'-T_2$ in normal man. To be published

31. Gavin, LA, ME Hammond, JN Castle, and RR Cavalieri, $3,3'$-diiodothyronine production, a major pathway of peripheral iodothyronine metabolism in man. J Clin Invest 61:1276-1285, 1978

32. Weeke, J, and P Laurberg, Diurnal TSH variations in hypothyroidism. J Clin Endocrinol Metab 43:32-37, 1976

33. Fukuda, H, and MA Greer, The effect of basal hypothalamic deafferentation on the nyctohemeral rhythm of plasma TSH. Endocrinology 97:749-752, 1975

34. Mitsuma, T, Y Hirooka, and N Nihei, Radioimmunoassay of thyrotrophin releasing hormone in human serum and its application. Acta Endocrinol (Kbh) 83:225-235, 1976

35. Ferland, L, F Labrie, M Jobin, A Arimura, and AV Schally, Physiological role of somatostatin in the control of growth hormone and thyrotropin secretion. Biochem Biophys Res Commun 68:149-155, 1976

36. Arimura, A, A Gordin, and AV Schally, Increase in basal and thyrotropin-releasing hormone-stimulated secretion of thyrotropin and the effects of triiodothyronine in rats passively immunised with antiserum to somatostatin. Fed Prod 35:782, 1976

37. Tanjasiri, P, X Kozbur, and WH Florsheim, Somatostatin in the physiologic feedback control of thyrotropin secretion. Life Sci 19:657-660, 1976

38. Terry, LC, JO Willoughby, P Brazeau, JB Martin, and YC Patel, Antiserum to somatostatin prevents stress-induced inhibition of growth hormone secretion in the rat. Science 192:565-567, 1976

39. Hall, R, GM Besser, AV Schally, DH Coy, D Evered, DJ Goldie, AJ Kastin, AS McNeilly, GH Mortimer, C Phenekos, WMG Tunbridge, and D Weightman, Action of growth-hormone-release inhibitory hormone in healthy men and in acromegaly. Lancet II:581-584, 1973

40. Siler, TM, SSC Yen, W Vale, and R Guillemin, Inhibition by somatostatin on the release of TSH induced in man by thyrotropin-releasing factor. J Clin Endocrinol Metab 38:742-745, 1974

41. Weeke, J, AaP Hansen, and K Lundbaek, The inhibition by somatostatin of the thyrotropin response to thyrotropin-releasing hormone in normal subjects. Scand J Clin Lab Invest 33:101-103, 1974

150

42. Carr, D, A Gomez-Pan, DR Weightman, VCM Roy, R Hall, GM Besser, MO Thorner, AS McNeilly, AV Schally, AJ Kastin, and DH Coy, Growth hormone release inhibiting hormone. Actions on thyrotropin and prolactin secretion after thyrotropin-releasing hormone. Br Med J 3:67-69, 1975

43. Lucke, C, B Höffken, and A von zur Mühlen, The effect of somatostatin on TSH levels in patients with primary hypothyroidism. J Clin Endocrinol Metab 41:1082-1084, 1975

44. Copinschi, G, E Virasoro, L Vanhaelst, R Leclercq, J Golstein, and M L'Hermite, Specific inhibition by somatostatin of growth hormone release after hypoglycemia in normal man. Clin Endocrinol (Oxf) 3:441-445, 1974

45. Siler, TM, G Vandenberg, SSC Yen, P Brazeau, W Yale, and R Guillemin, Inhibition of growth hormone release in humans by somatostatin. J Clin Endocrinol Metab 37, 632-634, 1973

46. Copinschi, G, V Leclercq-Meyer, E Virasoro, M. L'Hermite, L Vanhaelst, J Golstein, R Leclercq, F Fery and C Robyn, Pituitary and extrapituitary effects of somatostatin in normal man. Horm Metab Res 8:226-231, 1976

47. Weeke, J, SE Christensen, AaP Hansen, P Laurberg, and K Lundbaek, Somatostatin and the 24 hour levels of serum TSH, T_3, T_4, and reverse T_3 in normals and patients treated for myxoedema. Acta Endocrinol (Kbh) in press

48. Snow, MH, MF Scanlon, B Mora, M Heath, R Hall, and A Gomez-Pan, Pituitary actions of somatostatin. Ann Clin Res 10:145-150, 1978

49. Alford, FP, HWG Baker, HG Burger, DM de Kretser, B Hudson, MW Johns, JP Masterton, YC Patel, and GC Rennie, Temporal patterns of integrated plasma hormone levels during sleep and wakefulness. I. Thyroid stimulating hormone, growth hormone and cortisol. J Clin Endocrinol Metab 37:841-847, 1973

50. Saberi, M, and RD Utiger, Serum thyroid hormone and thyrotropin concentrations during thyroxine and triiodothyronine therapy. J Clin Endocrinol Metab 39:923-927, 1974

51. Azizi, F, AG Vagenakis, GI Portnay, SH Ingbar, and LE Braverman, Effect of a single oral dose of tri-iodothyronine on the subsequent response to TRH in normal individuals. J Clin Endocrinol Metab 40:157-159, 1975

52. Wartofsky, L, RC Dimond, GL Noel, AG Frantz, and JM Earll, Effect of acute increases in serum triiodo-thyronine on TSH and prolactin responses to TRH and estimates of pituitary stores of TSH and prolactin in normal subjects and in patients with primary hypo-thyroidism. J Clin Endocrinol Metab 42:443-458, 1976

DISCUSSION

The TSH data of Drs. Parker and Rossman and the reports by Drs. Golstein and Weeke were discussed simultaneously after Dr. Weeke's presentation.

VAN CAUTER: From the presentations of Drs. Rossman, Golstein and Weeke, one can conclude that the reproducibility of the 24-h pattern of TSH is rather poor. When one looks at individual profiles, the three groups observe essentially the same characteristics. In Dr. Weeke's individual data, sometimes an early morning peak is dominant, sometimes elevated values are observed throughout sleep. However, the first slide showed a mean TSH profile where continually elevated values were present during sleep. On another slide, comparing T3, T4 and TSH, another transverse mean TSH profile was shown and instead the TSH levels were decreasing during sleep. In a third slide, where 3 individual profiles were shown and blood samples were drawn every 5 minutes during the night only, these subjects had an increase of TSH during sleep. Since Dr. Golstein observed seasonal differences in the temporal organization of TSH secretion over the 24-h span, I wonder whether your subjects were studied at a specific time of the year and whether, when individual profiles were incorporated in a transverse mean, they were matched for season?

WEEKE: The first 13 subjects of our initial study were studied in 1971. As far as I remember, the 6 males were studied in the early winter and the 7 females in the early spring. Of course, we did not think of possible seasonal differences at that time. The next study was designed to investigate the variations in the thyroid hormones and to relate them to TSH variations and the experiments were conducted in the month of May.

WEITZMAN: We also have some data on TSH circadian rhythm and, in general, they agree with Drs. Parker's and Rossman's data. When the subject goes to sleep, there is a peak that precedes the onset of sleep and that turns off

dramatically after sleep. I think their data are very
strong in this regard and cannot be ignored.

ROSSMAN: We have more than 75 sleep periods in our
data and in only one instance, a female subject, was there
a peak in the early morning that was almost as important
as the pre-sleep peak.

WEITZMAN: The question is: way is there an apparent
discrepancy? When we think of season of the year, we should
think of it in terms of what happens to people in different
seasons. People live on schedules and these schedules vary
from one season to another, not only the subjects, but also
the technicians and the experimenters. Therefore, the timing
of when a person goes to sleep, of when you record the persons' going to sleep and how long they sleep in the laboratory under these artificial conditions, must take into account the schedule that the subjects had for weeks prior
to the investigation. If indeed, TSH has an endogenous circadian rhythm which is in some way phase-locked to the
sleep-wake cycle that has been going on for weeks, if you
superimpose sleep on that rhythm, you may get a rise at
the end of sleep if you superimpose it too early, at the
beginning if you superimpose it too late, or you may get
no rise or very little rise is you superimpose it at the
same time. So the key is knowing what the individual's
sleep-wake cycle is and where you superimpose the sleep-
wake schedule of the investigation in relationship to this
actual sleep-wake cycle.

KRIEGER: Considering the factors that are responsible
for TSH circadian rhythm rather than the exact time of the
peak, the GH and the TSH rhythms seem to have some common
regulatory mechanism involving respectively somatostatin
and serotonin. My question to Dr. Weeke is: in the experiments where the TSH circadian peak was suppressed by somatostatin, were you able to investigate the effect of somatostatin on the GH pattern?

WEEKE: Dr. Hansen will talk about that tomorrow. There was an effect of somatostatin of the GH peak.

KRIEGER: You compare TSH levels at 11.00 and 23.00 and obtain a maximal TSH peak at 23.00 which is the time of minimal ACTH-cortisol release. It seems that the circadian rhythm of TSH is 12 hours out of phase with the ACTH-cortisol periodicity. Would you comment on that?

WEEKE: To make a valid comparison of different hormonal rhythms, one must consider individual profiles rather than mean curves. It is quite clear that these mean curves give a wrong picture of the individual results. Unfortunately, we were not allowed by the referees at the time to show individual curves.

KRIEGER: I would like to ask Dr. Golstein what was the schedule of administration of cyproheptadine? Was it administered throughout the 24-h period or at a specific time prior to sleep onset?

GOLSTEIN: It was administered during 3 days, 4 mg four times a day, at 08.00, 14.00, 20.00 and midnight.

DUMONT: It is striking, in the data of Dr. Weeke trying to relate TSH variations and thyroid hormone variations, that thyroid hormone variations are observed at all. When you take into account the huge buffering capacity of the binding proteins and the half-life, which for T3 is one day, and for T4 7 days, I am really wondering what the physiologic significance of these variations is? Are they significant at all?

WEEKE: Yes, I think these variations are significant. Their physiologic significance is a puzzling question. These variations cannot result from the secretion from the thyroid gland because of these long half-lives. They could result from shifts between the intra- and extracellular spaces. However, then, one has to explain why the TSH rhythm is so similar to the thyroid hormone rhythms since they are all components of such a close feedback system. Maybe the thyroid gland could take up some thyroid hormone and excrete it again without de novo synthesis. There is little evidence for such a process at the present time. The fact that we still observe these T3 and T4 short term variations concomitantly with the TSH variations is most interesting.

DUMONT: Such parallel variations could also be produced by artefacts. For instance, if I leave some of my tubes on the table, there may be some evaporation and that will create a parallel increase in the concentration of the 3 hormones. If a drop of water falls in the tube, a parallel decrease will be observed. I don't see any physiological explanation for these variations. Another question I wanted to ask concerns your data in the hypothyroid patients who, when their TSH is high enough, have no nycthemeral variation. Did I understand correctly that you implied that this observation could result from lack of negative control of the thyroid hormones on the hypothalamus? Do you have any data to support such a concept?

WEEKE: There could be very high TRH levels in hypothyroid patients and then small superimposed TRH variations resulting from the circadian rhythm could not be transmitted.

DUMONT: If that were true, that would imply that you have a negative feedback of the thyroid hormone on the hypothalamus. There are no data at the present time to support such a concept. In fact, a positive feedback was postulated a few years ago but this hypothesis has been dropped since.

VIGNERI: There are data available in the literature showing that sleep deprivation would increase significantly T3 and T4 levels and that would agree with maintenance of

high TSH levels during sleep deprivation. Regarding the
cross-correlation of TSH, T3 and T4 short-term variations,
in addition to the problems of binding proteins and half-
lives mentioned by Dr. Dumont, it has recently been demonstrated that the feedback mechanism is dependent on the
intracellular concentrations of these hormones and on the
intracellular deiodination of these hormones and these
processes do take time. I would also like to ask Dr. Golstein what was the phase of the menstrual cycle when her
female subjects were studied? The oestrogen variations may
interfere in the assay and differences in sleep organization between the follicular and luteal phases of the menstrual cycle have been reported.

GOLSTEIN: All subjects were young women. We did not
form sub-groups of subjects according to the phase of the
menstrual cycle.

VIGNERI: Can Dr. Weeke give us some information on
the treatment of your myxedematous patients? Did they
recover the TSH rhythm when they were treated? Which drug
did they receive and how many times a day?

WEEKE: They received thyroxine one time a day.

VAN CAUTER: Regarding the amplitude of the episodic
TSH fluctuations, you showed that the average fluctuation
around the mean ranged from -.08 to .08 µU/ml. What was
the sensitivity of your assay ?

WEEKE: It was .2 µU/ml.

VAN CAUTER: I did not understand how fluctuations
which occurred in a range of concentration where your
assay was not sensitive can finally turn out to be statistically significant when averaged among subjects.

WEEKE: The statistical method used was the Monte-
Carlo procedure.

VAN CAUTER: Let us assume that the fluctuations are significant. Your estimation of the average period of recurrence of the fluctuation is 25 minutes. Is that right?

WEEKE: 30 minutes.

VAN CAUTER: When Dr. Golstein evaluated the episodic TSH variations in her studies using 15-minute blood sampling, there was a linear relationship between the average magnitude of the peak and its duration. Thus, higher peaks lasted longer. This was an expected result. However, if the actual rate of change of TSH level is faster, as you seem to imply, then with 15 minute sampling we should have missed many peaks and this linear correlation between duration and magnitude should not be observed. Is it your impression that sampling at 15 minute intervals is not frequent enough to evaluate the episodic fluctuations of TSH?

WEEKE: Yes. It depends on what you are looking for. If you are looking at the long-term variations, then 15 minute blood sampling is frequent enough. If you are looking at the short-term variations, then you need more frequent blood sampling.

ROSSMAN: When Dr. Van Cauter showed us this morning her slide on the transverse mean, the variance around the point corresponding to the sleep elevation was not shown and that would have made the experimenter suspicious of the results. I prefer to see raw data and raw means and make my decisions after looking at the data rather than making sophisticated mathematical operations.

ASCHOFF: If seasonal variations influence night-time TSH levels, I would think that such influences are very different in Aarhus, Denmark and Southern California. I would also like to ask a question to Dr. Rossman regarding his experiments on dissociation of sleep and dark

periods. You said that the TSH values were higher when
sleep did not occur. However, my impression was that, over
the 7 days, the amplitude between the nadir and the maximum
seemed to be constant.

ROSSMAN: I don't think that the phenomenon is that
marked. It is a single event occurring in a single individual on which I don't like to comment.

VAN HAELST: To try to reconciliate the views of the
different groups, I would like to make a comment. Everybody agrees that there is a drop of TSH in the morning
so the level must have been higher sometimes before that.
Sleep appears to be superimposed to the rhythm and exert
an inhibitory effect. Depending on the length of sleep,
there might be 2 peaks, a pre-sleep peak and a post-sleep
peak, or only an early morning peak or only a pre-sleep
peak. The results of the 3 groups can probably be explained by the hypothesis of inhibitory influence in sleep.
Therefore, we have to monitor sleep before, during and
after the experiment very carefully.

ASCHOFF: If one accepts the idea that sleep exerts
a masking effect, despite the fact that we don't know the
mechanisms of masking, the masking effect depends on the
circadian phase. I would like to know whether the sleep
times of Aarhus and San Diego subjects were different with
regard to the rest of the circadian system. If so, we
should expect different masking effects in the two groups.
Unfortunately, neither group has recordings of body temperature which would have given a reference for the rest of
the circadian system. Secondly, whereas the concept of
negative masking is well accepted, there are also positive
masking effects. For instance, the triggering of the
secretion of some hormones has been referred to as a positive masking effect. However, in most cases, the more
masking, the more difficult to speak of any circadian phase
since the true phase is masked.

ROSSMAN: We can explain all our data in terms of masking effects if we do not look too closely at it. What I do not understand is why the peak values appear to be advanced or delayed.

WEITZMAN: We begin to have differences in meaning of the words. "Masking" implies that the effect is not too important, since the rhythm goes on, whereas the word "inhibition" is very strong. The habitual sleeping time will set the phase of the endogenous oscillation of TSH if it exists, and this phase is inter-related with the time of "masking" or "inhibition". So that if the subject is living according to his own clock (the environmental clock is not important), a difference in TSH rhythm should be expected, depending on the life style. I know that, in Scandinavia, the life style is very different in winter and in summer. All these factors have to be taken into account when we try to understand the differences in wave-shape.

ASCHOFF: I think you were referring to the 21 or 20-hour day experiment of Dr. Rossman. It is my impression that the subjects were free-running with a period longer than 24 hours. Superimposed on the free-running rhythm, you see the masking effects and, thus, some decreases and increases in amplitude. I would not be surprised that if the data were submitted to a periodogram or a spectral analysis, a 24.5 hour rhythm would emerge.

VAN CAUTER: The data presented today also suggest that the dark-light cycle and the natural daylight may be other components of the control of the TSH circadian rhythm. First, Dr. Rossman presented a study where a slight shift of the pre-sleep peak occurred when the dark-light cycle was manipulated. Second, Dr. Golstein's data suggest that seasonal variations may be partly responsible for the poor reproducibility of the TSH circadian rhythm in males. Also, Dr. Weeke, when asked about the components of his transverse mean, said that they were obtained

at different seasons. Now, Denmark is not much further
north than Brussels, but between San Diego, on the one
hand, and Aarhus and Brussels on the other hand, there
is an important latitude difference which results in a
seasonal difference of daylight duration of 100% (the day
in summer lasts twice as long as the day in winter) in
Brussels and Aarhus but only of 30% in San Diego. We have
thus a variable factor in the environment which may play
a role.

CONTROL OF PITUITARY-ADRENAL PERIODICITY

D.T. Krieger

Department of Medicine, Division of Endocrinology,
Mount Sinai School of Medicine, New York, New York 10029,
USA

The present report will review studies of the pituitary-adrenal periodicity in the animal and the human and consider some of the possible factors involved in its regulation.

Initial studies of the circadian periodicity of human plasma corticosteroid concentrations using a 4-6 hour blood sampling paradigm described a pattern in which peak concentrations occurred in the early morning hours followed by a gradual decline during the rest of the 24-hour span (1,2). When a half-hourly blood sampling schedule is used to measure simultaneously the variations of plasma ACTH and cortisol, it is apparent that superimposed upon the smooth circadian pattern observed with the 4-hour blood sampling protocol are a series of periods of episodic secretion (3, 4) (Fig. 1). An amazingly good concordance between the peaks of immunoreactive ACTH and cortisol can be seen despite the considerable differences in half-life times of these two substances. With 5-min sampling periods, the same overall 24-hour periodicity is evident; episodic secretion is especially prevalent during the active portion of the day and minimal during the quiescent period, from 2000 to 2300. In these studies (5) there were periods where ACTH appeared to be secreted with very little resultant response in plasma corticosteroid concentrations. However, bioassay of ACTH yielded values and patterns which were similar to those obtained by immunoassay, excluding the possibility that the immunoassay was measuring biologi-

162

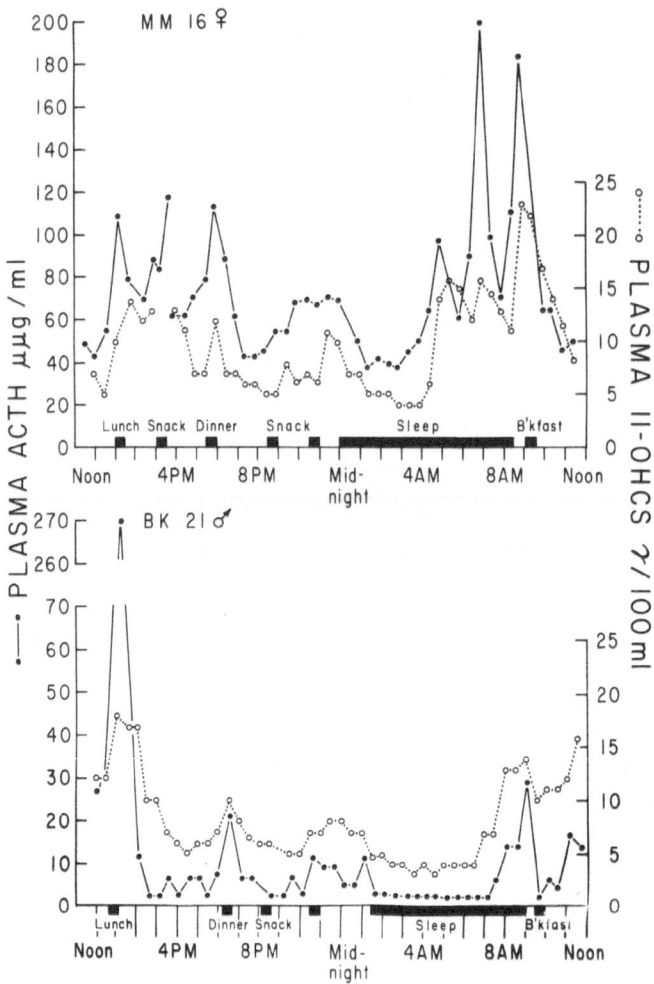

Figure 1 : Circadian periodicity of plasma corticosteroid and ACTH concentrations determined by half-hourly sampling over a 24-h period. Meal times and sleep as indicated.

cally inactive fragments of the ACTH molecule. The reason for such dissociation of ACTH and corticosteroid concentrations remains so far unclear. Lack of priming of the adrenal glands by a previous dose of ACTH does not seem to be involved since peaks of ACTH associated with no or very little corticosteroid response may be preceded by large ACTH secretory spikes. The circadian variation of ACTH and cortisol can be suppressed by an 0.5 mg dose of dexamethasone administered in the early morning hours (i.e. 0800); the

episodic secretion will be markedly damped but not completely suppressed. A normal circadian rise reappears the next
day (between 0400-0800). If the same dose of dexamethasone
is given around midnight prior to the onset of the circadian rise, suppression is observed throughout the ensuing
c. 28-hour period till the next circadian rise, but minor
secretory episodes will still appear (3). This would seem
to suggest that dexamethasone acts mostly on the mechanism
controlling the major circadian rise but that is does not
completely suppress episodic secretion. The reproducibility within a subject of the level and amplitude of the circadian variation of plasma cortisol is excellent as has been
shown in 24-hour studies carried out in the same subjects
at 4-month intervals. Aging does not seem to affect the
level or the amplitude since normal corticosteroid rhythmicity was found in older subjects with intact CNS function
up to 90 years of age (6).

In the rat, which is active in the evening period rather
than during daytime, the time of corticosteroid peaking is
immediately prior to or at the time of lights off with a
greater amplitude in females than in males (7). Circadian
variation in responsiveness of the adrenals to ACTH has
been reported and it has been implied that the adrenal
periodicity reflected the variation in responsiveness of
the adrenals to ACTH and did not require circadian periodicity of ACTH levels (8). There have been very few studies
where the circadian periodicity of ACTH was measured in the
rat. However, in all studies presently available, a circadian variation of plasma ACTH with higher levels in the
afternoon, preceding the peak of corticosteroid concentration,was found (8-11).   The circadian periodicity
of corticosteroid concentrations is also paralleled by variation in pituitary ACTH content (11). Available data on the
variation in hypothalamic content of the still elusive corticotropin releasing factor (CRF) (as estimated by bioassay
on the ability of hypothalamic material to release pituitary ACTH) also indicate that a rise in CRF precedes that
of plasma corticosteroids. Hiroshige (12, 13) reported a

male-female difference at the time of the peak, the CRF peak
preceding by several hours the corticosteroid peak in females. Vasopressin has been suggested to be a CRF or to have
CRF-like activity. However, in Brattleboro rats, in an investigation where plasma ACTH concentration was measured on
tail vein samples obtained serially in a given animal
(samples obtained within 45 seconds after initial venipunc-
ture to avoid stress effects) a circadian periodicity was
still found, in both homozygote and heterozygote animals
(14). This suggests that, if CRF is involved in the regulation of the circadian periodicity of ACTH and corticosteroids, such a CRF is not vasopressin, since the homozygote
animals studied were deficient in vasopressin.

A hierarchy of controls at various levels seems to regulate
the circadian periodicity of corticosteroids. As noted
above, some reports indicate that adrenal glands cultured
in vitro have a circadian variation in corticosterone output (15). One study reported a circadian variation of
corticosteroid concentration in hypophysectomized animals
with even a phase-reversal of the rhythm (16). Thus far
these results have not been confirmed. At the adrenal level, a circadian variation in responsiveness of the glands
to ACTH has been demonstrated. Ungar and Halberg (17)
showed that, when adrenals are taken out from rats at different points of the 24-hour cycle and incubated with concentrations of ACTH of 0.4 units and 4 units, a circadian
periodicity in the output of the glands is observed. Previously, Perkoff, using infusion of ACTH over a 6-hour
period between either 0800-1400, or 1600-2200, or midnight-
0600, showed evidence of decreased adrenal responsiveness
in the period midnight-0600 in the human. However, when the
study was repeated with infusion from midnight-0800 after
administering a very small priming dose of ACTH from 1700-
2300, the sensitivity of the adrenals was restored and a
normal response obtained (1). Thus, it seems that decreased adrenal responsiveness in the early morning hours in
the human results from lack of priming of the glands by an
adequate amount of ACTH. Another possible control exerted

on the circadian periodicity of corticosteroid at the adrenal level consists of the circadian variation in metabolic clearance rate. However, the reported data are diametrically opposed to what would have been expected if the diurnal variation in metabolic clearance rate were to be responsible for the circadian periodicity of corticosteroid concentration. Indeed, the metabolic clearance rate of cortisol is greater in the early morning hours, around 0800, when the plasma concentration is highest, than it is during the quiescent period (18).

Evidence for control of the circadian periodicity of corticosteroid concentrations at the pituitary level is provided by studies on the adrenalectomized animal in humans with adrenal insufficiency. The periodicity of plasma ACTH concentrations is present and even enhanced because of the absence of feedback in patients with Addison's disease, taken off their maintenance medication (19). Plasma corticosteroid concentrations in such patients are very low and there is no evident periodicity. Studies on the response to pyrogen administration at different points of the 24-hour cycle in human subjects show that a greater increment in corticosteroid response is obtained when the administration takes place just before the major circadian increase, at about 2300 (20). This result is even more impressive when one remembers that the sensitivity of the adrenals to ACTH is decreased at this particular time. Studies where the actual amounts of ACTH released at different points of the 24-hour cycle are measured and related to the amount of corticosteroids secreted are presently in progress.

Several factors support the hypothesis of CNS regulation of pituitary-adrenal periodicity. In addition to the demonstration of a circadian rhythm in CRF mentioned above, each of the neurotransmitters norepinephrine, dopamine and serotonin undergoes a circadian variation of concentration in some area of the brain (21, 22). The areas of the brain where a periodicity is present, as well as the time of maximal concentration, differ from one neurotransmitter to another. Therefore, to relate a circadian periodicity of a

neurotransmitter to a specific endocrine event, experiments
where the measurements are carried out in the whole brain
should be avoided since the relevant periodicity may be
blunted or even obscured.

Evidence with regard to CNS regulation of the pituitary-
adrenal periodicity is also provided by the fact that, in
all species studied so far, the development of the circadian periodicity is age-related. In the human, a definite
circadian periodicity of plasma cortisol apppears somewhere
between two and 13 years of age (23). In the rat, the circadian periodicity of plasma corticosteroid concentrations
appears around 30 days of age (24) and can be advanced, by
early handling of the animal, to 20-22 days of age (25).
In rats studied from birth to days 55-66, a 24-hour variation in brain serotonin and norepinephrine develops roughly
at about 33 days of age, coincidentally with the time of
appearance of the periodicity of corticosteroid concentration in plasma (26). Hiroshige (27), studying the postnatal development of the circadian periodicity in CRF,
showed evidence of appearance of the periodicity around 21
days of age, roughly one week prior to the appearance of
the circadian periodicity of corticosteroids.

Assuming that the CNS regulation of the corticosteroid periodicity constitutes the highest level of the hierarchy
of its control, we will now consider questions pertaining
to the nature of this periodicity such as whether it is endogenous or exogenous, what are its zeitgebers, which anatomical pathways and which neurotransmitters are involved
in its regulation.

Abnormal circadian periodicity of plasma ACTH and corticosteroids is found in 60-70 percent of patients with hypothalamic disease. Patients with hypothalamic tumor without
evidence of hypercortisolism can have a totally random pattern of episodic ACTH and cortisol secretion (28). In many
cases of hypothalamic disease, absence of circadian periodicity of ACTH and cortisol concentration may be one of
the first endocrine abnormalities which can be observed.
In animals, neuro-anatomical studies showed that lesions in

the anterior hypothalamus (anterior hypothalamic deafferentation or complete deafferentation) will obliterate the circadian rhythm (29-32). Section of the fornix also causes
alteration of the periodicity but this seems to be only a
transitory effect, since the normal rhythm is restored
several weeks post lesion (33). In the human, two studies
have indicated that one can modify the corticosteroid
periodicity by administering drugs presumably affecting
neurotransmitter concentrations. When infused during the
onset of sleep, cyproheptadine, primarily an anti-serotoninergic agent, has absolutely no effect on the circadian
rhythm of cortisol, but if the infusion takes place between
0400-0700, thus just prior to the time of the circadian rise,
the circadian rise is suppressed (34). The circadian periodicity could also be obliterated by a banthine derivative,
an anti-vagal compound if administered between 1600 and midnight, but not at all other times (35). Thus, the time of
administration of the drug affecting the neurotransmitter is
important as to whether or not it alters the circadian periodicity. In the animal, a number of drugs affecting serotonin concentration, atropine, an anti-vagal drug, and pheno-
barbital have been shown to markedly depress the circadian
amplitude, whereas thus far none of the drugs affecting the
adrenergic system seemed to have any effect on the circadian
rhythmicity of plasma corticosteroids (36, 37).

In a study of Orth et al., human subjects were allowed to
sleep (in the dark) during two 4-hour periods of the 24-
hour cycle. Each of the sleep periods was associated with
a rise in plasma corticosteroid concentrations at the end of
sleep or at the time of lights-on, thus resulting in two
corticosteroid peaks over the 24-hour cycle. In these experiments, possible effects of the light-dark cycle, on the
one hand, and of the sleep-wake cycle, on the other hand,
could not be dissociated (38). Weitzman et al. reported
that, in subjects maintained on a 3-hour sleep-wake cycle
schedule with one hour of sleep and two hours of wake, circadian periodicity of plasma cortisol was unaltered (39).
Thus, it seems that there is a time framework within which

corticosteroid periodicity can be manipulated by varying
the sleep-wake and light-dark cycles but that extreme changes of these schedules will not affect the periodicity.
Subsequently, Orth et al. kept the sleep period constant but
prolonged darkness by 4 hours after awakening and observed
a delay in the time of occurrence of the circadian rise of
plasma corticosteroids. When a period of darkness with no
sleep was inserted in the middle of the day, there was a
short spurt of corticosteroid activity at the time of
lights-on. When the subjects were kept in constant dark
except for one hour of light, normal periodicity persisted,
with a superimposed burst of secretory activity at the
time of lights-on. In all these studies, subjects were
adapted to the experimental condition for 10-14 days prior
to the investigative day (40). Thus, despite the fact
that observations in sleep-deprived patients and phase-shift
experiments support the concept of an endogenous component
in the circadian periodicity of plasma corticosteroids,
manipulations of sleep-wake parameters and spurts of dark-
light can, within a certain time framework, influence the
periodicity. In blind subjects, whether blindness is congenital or acquired, there is an essentially normal but
free-running periodicity of plasma cortisol concentration
(41, 42). The periodicity was also unaltered in subjects
maintained in constant light for a 2-week period (43).
When these subjects were then submitted to sleep reversal,
the circadian rhythm of cortisol phase-reversed completely.

Recently, we have studied feeding as a zeitgeber for corticosteroid circadian periodicity. Rats maintained under
normal ad lib feeding conditions will consume most of their
food during the dark period. If the time of lights-off is
maintained, but access to food and water is restricted to
a 2-hour period in the morning (food shift), when normally
the rat does not eat, the circadian periodicity of plasma
corticosteroids is inverted by 12 hours. Under ad lib feeding conditions, serotonin concentrations in various areas
of the CNS (except for the median eminence and the suprachiasmatic nucleus) are highest in the early morning and

then drop over the rest of the 24-hour period. In the
areas of the brain which showed a circadian variation, food-
shifted animals had a shift of the neurotransmitter rhythm
suggesting that one of the mechanisms whereby the food
shift alters the corticosteroid periodicity may be by modi-
fying the neurotransmitter periodicity within the CNS (44).

Sham suprachiasmatic nuclear lesions do not alter the observed circadian corticosteroid periodicity in ad lib or
food-shifted animals. Lesions of the suprachiasmatic nucleus in rats on ad lib feeding obliterate the circadian
rhythm of body temperature and plasma corticosteroid concentrations. However, if an animal that has been food-
shifted undergoes a suprachiasmatic nuclear lesion, the
food-shifted rhythm is not obliterated. Moreover, if an
animal with suprachiasmatic lesion on ad lib feeding is put
on the restricted A.M. food regimen, a food-shift rhythm
appears (45) (Fig. 2). The food-shift rhythm even takes
precedence over some of the effects of dark and light.
When the dark period is shifted to 0800 to 2000 instead of
2000 to 0800 and ad lib feeding is allowed, the animals eat
from 0800-2000 and phase reversal of the rhythm of plasma
corticosteroids occurs. However, in such animals if a
restricted food presentation is then enforced, with access
to food during the night time (2000-2200), their normal
time of eating, the phase reversal resulting from the dark-
light shift cannot be maintained and the corticosteroid
rhythm is in phase with the time of food presentation.
Animals maintained in constant dim lighting conditions under ad lib feeding conditions become arrhythmic with regard
to corticosteroid variation and feeding. However, if access
to food in such animals is then restricted to a 2-hour
period, a food-shift rhythm appears, synchronous with the
time of food presentation (46). These studies would indicate that the presence of food may serve to some degree as
a zeitgeber which may even, in some cases, override the
effects of the light-dark zeitgeber in the rat.

Additional studies were performed in obese animals (who
also exhibited aperiodic feeding) in order to locate the

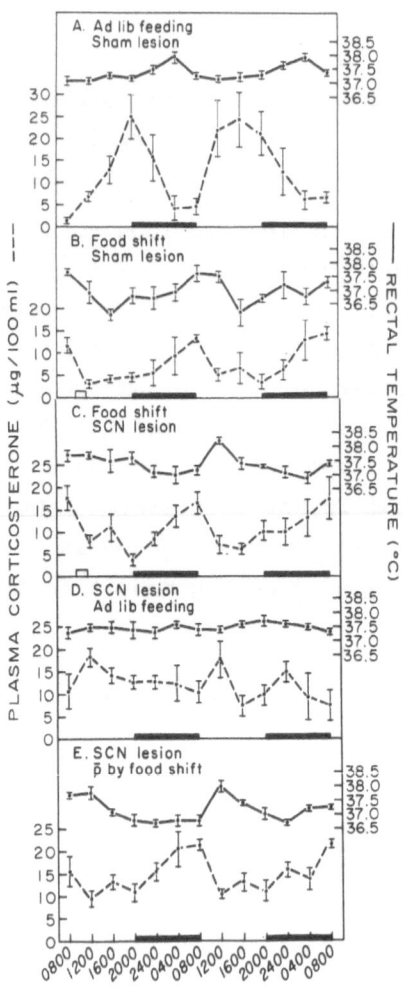

Figure 2 : Circadian periodicity over a 48-hr period of body temperature and plasma corticosteroid concentrations in adult female Sprague-
Dawley rats. A/ rats given unrestricted access to food and water;
periodicity studied 2 weeks after sham lesions were made. B/ rats on
restricted-feeding schedule studied 2 weeks after sham lesions were
made. C/ rats on restricted-feeding schedule studied 2 weeks after
suprachiasmatic nuclear (SCN) lesions were made. D/ rats on unrestric-
ted-feeding schedule studied 2 weeks after SCN lesions were made. E/
the same rats as in D studied 2 weeks later when they had been changed
to the restricted feeding schedule. Vertical bars indicate ± standard
error of the mean. Solid horizontal black bars indicate darkness.
Open horizontal bars indicate time of daily access to food and water
of animals on restricted-feeding schedule. B and C show that SCN
lesions do not change shifts in circadian patterns of body temperature
and plasma corticosteroid concentrations induced by the restricted-
feeding schedule. The arrhythmic pattern in animals with SCN lesions
on the unrestricted schedule D is shifted by restricted feeding to a

pattern E almost identical to that in the animals shown in B and C.
Patterns of body temperature and plasma corticosterone concentrations
obtained from individual animals in A, B, C and E were similar to those
depicted for the group.

site of action of this zeitgeber. The circadian periodicity of corticosteroids is obliterated in obese rats on an ad
lib feeding regimen, once the obesity is well established.
However, if a food-shift restriction regimen is imposed,
the arrhythmic obese rat acquires a circadian periodicity
in plasma corticosteroid concentrations, the peak occurring
at the time of food presentation (47). The ventral median
nucleus is thought to be involved to some extent in the control of the eating rhythm. Lesions of the ventral nucleus
will obliterate corticosteroid rhythmicity in rats fed ad
lib, and also (in contrast to what was observed for animals
with lesions of the suprachiasmatic nucleus) in animals
with previously imposed food-shift rhythms. Moreover, the
food-shift rhythm of plasma corticosteroid concentrations
cannot be restored in aperiodic animals with lesions of
the ventral medial nucleus, in contrast to the above noted
findings in animals with lesions of the suprachiasmatic
nucleus (48). These results imply that the anatomical locus
whereby food can serve as a zeitgeber for the corticosteroid
circadian periodicity is in the area of the ventral medial
nucleus and thus in an area different from the presumed
locus of maintenance of the dark-light zeitgeber, the
suprachiasmatic nucleus.

In summary, in the human, the circadian periodicity of corticosteroids can be altered by phase-shifts, by sleep-wake
and dark-light cycles (within a certain time framework), by
changes in the day length, by metabolic abnormalities, such
as liver diseases in which the clearance of corticosteroids
is decreased, and in Cushing's disease and CNS disease affecting the hypothalamic limbic system, in diffuse CNS disease characterized by coma, but not by CNS disease outside
the hypothalamic limbic system. The only drugs found so
far to alter the circadian periodicity of plasma corticosteroids in man have been anticholinergic and presumably
anti-serotoninergic medications. Constant light, constant

darkness, blindness, prolonged wakefulness, as well as a number of other drugs acting on the CNS, will not alter this circadian periodicity. Data in the animal are mostly confirmatory of data in the human except for a few differences. For instance, blinding in the experimental animal at a neonatal age does seem to alter the circadian periodicity of corticosteroids. Also, constant light conditions will alter the rhythm. Finally, it has been shown that neonatal animals given corticosteroids will have a delay in the appearance of the circadian periodicity. Experiments in the rat regarding the role of food shifts have not, at the moment, been performed in human subjects in comparable conditions.

In conclusion, there is evidence for circadian periodicity in various parts of the CNS-pituitary adrenal axis. The predominant control is probably on a CNS substrate and multiple pacemakers responding to external stimuli can synchronize the periodicity of corticosteroids.

REFERENCES

1. Perkoff, GT, K Eik-Nes, CA Nugent, HL Fred, RA Nimer, L Rush, LT Samuels and FH Tyler, Studies of the diurnal variation of plasma 17-hydroxycorticosteroids. J Clin Endocrinol Metab 16:432-443, 1959

2. Migeon, CJ, FH Tyler, JP Mahoney, AA Florentin, H Castle, EL Bliss and LT Samuels, The diurnal variation of plasma levels and urinary excretion of 17-hydroxycorticosteroids in normal subjects, night workers and blind subjects. J Clin Endocrinol 16: 622-633, 1956

3. Krieger, DT, W Allen, F Rizzo and HP Krieger, Characterization of the normal pattern of plasma corticosteroid levels. J Clin Endocrinol Metab 32:266-284, 1971

4. Gallagher, RF, K Yoshida, HD Roffwarg, DK Fukushima, ED Weitzman and L Hellman, ACTH and cortisol secretory patterns in man. J Clin Endocrinol Metab 36:1058-1073, 1973

5. Krieger, DT and W Allen, Relationship of bioassayable and immunoassayable ACTH and cortisol concentration in normal subjects and in patients with Cushing's disease. J Clin Endocrinol Metab 40:675-687, 1975

6. Silverberg, AI, F Rizzo and DT Krieger, Nyctohemeral periodicity of plasma 17-OHCS levels in elderly subjects. J Clin Endocrinol Metab 28:1661-1663, 1968

7. Critchlow, V, RA Liebelt, M Bar-Sela, W Mountcastle and HS Lipscomb, Sex difference in resting pituitary-adrenal function in the rat. Am J Physiol 205: 807-815, 1963

8. Dallman, MF, WC Engeland and J Shinsako, Circadian changes in adrenocortical responses to ACTH. Prog 58th Meeting Endo Soc 58:4, 1976 (abstract)

9. Cheifetz, P, N Gaffud and JF Dingman, Effects of bilateral adrenalectomy and continuous light on the circadian rhythm of corticotropin in female rats. Endocrinology 82:1117-1124, 1968

10. Rees, LH, DM Cook, JW Kendall, CF Allen, RM Kramer, JG Ratcliffe and RA Knight, A radioimmunoassay for rat plasma ACTH. Endocrinology 89:254-261, 1971

11. Retiene, K, E Zimmerman, WJ Schindler, J Neuenschwander and HS Lipscomb, A correlative study of endocrine rhythms in rats. Acta Endocrinol (Kbh) 57:615-622, 1968

12. Hiroshige, T, and M Sakakura, Circadian rhythm of corticotropin releasing activity in the hypothalamus of normal and adrenalectomized rats. Neuroendocrinology 7:25-36, 1971

13. Hiroshige, T, M Sakakura and S Itoh, Diurnal variation of corticotropin releasing activity in the rat hypothalamus. Endocrinol Jpn 16:465-467, 1969

14. Krieger, DT, A Liotta and MJ Brownstein, Corticotropin releasing factor distribution in normal and Brattleboro rat brain, and effect of deafferentation, hypophysectomy and steroid treatment in normal animals. Endocrinology 100:227-237, 1977

15. Shiotsuka, R, J Jovonovich and JA Jovonovich, Circadian and ultradian corticosterone rhythms in adrenal organ cultures, In:Chronological aspects of endocrinology, Schattauer, FK (ed.), New York, Springer-Verlag, 255-267, 1974

16. Meier, AH, Daily variation in concentration of plasma corticosteroid in hypophysectomized rats. Endocrinology 98:1475-1479, 1976

17. Ungar, F and F Halberg, Circadian rhythm in the *in vitro* response of mouse adrenal to adrenocorticotropic hormone. Science 137:1058-1059, 1962

18. Delacerda, L, A Kowarski and CJ Migeon, Diurnal variation of the metabolic clearance rate of cortisol. Effect of measurement of cortisol production rate. J Clin Endocrinol Metab 36:1043-1049, 1973

19. Krieger, DH and GP Gewirtz, The nature of the circadian periodicity and suppressibility of immunoreactive ACTH levels in Addison's disease. J Clin Endocrinol Metab 39:46-52, 1974

20. Takebe, K, C Setaishi and M Hirama, Effects of a
    bacterial pyrogen on the pituitary-adrenal axis and
    various times in the 24 hours. J Clin Endocrinol
    Metab 26:437-442, 1966

21. Reis, DJ, A Corvelli and J Conners, Circadian and
    ultradian rhythms of serotonin regionally in cat
    brain. J Pharmacol Exp Ther 167:328-333, 1969

22. Reis, DJ, M Weinbren and A Corvelli, A circadian
    rhythm of norepinephrine regionally in cat brain.
    Its relationship to environmental lighting and to
    regional diurnal variations in brain serotonin.
    J Pharmacol Exp Ther 164:135-145, 1968

23. Franks, R, Diurnal variation of plasma 17-OHCS in
    children. J Clin Endocrinol Metab 27:75-78, 1967

24. Allen, C, and JW Kendall, Maturation of the circadian
    rhythm of plasma corticosterone in the rat.
    Endocrinology 80:926-930, 1967

25. Ader, R, Early experiences accelerate maturation of
    the 24-hour adrenocortical rhythm. Science 163:
    1225-1226, 1969

26. Asano, Y, The maturation of the circadian rhythm of
    brain norepinephrine and serotonin in the rat.
    Life Sci 10:883-894, 1971

27. Hirosnige, T and T Sato, Postnatal development of
    circadian rhythm of corticotropin releasing activi-
    ty in the rat hypothalamus. Endocrinol Jpn 17:1-6,
    1970

28. Krieger, DT and HP Krieger, Circadian variation of the
    plasma 17-OHCS in the central nervous system disease.
    J Clin Endocrinol Metab 26:929-940, 1966

29. Halasz, MA Slusher and RA Gorski, Adrenocorticotrophic
    hormone secretion in rats after partial or total
    deafferentation of the medial basal hypothalamus.
    Neuroendocrinology 2:43-55, 1967

30. Moore, RY and VB Eichler, Loss of a circadian adrenal
    corticosterone rhythm following suprachiasmatic
    lesions in the rat. Brain Res 42:201-206, 1972

31. Palka, A, D Coyer and V Critchlow, Effects of isolation
    of medial basal hypothalamus on pituitary-adrenal

and pituitary-ovarian functions. Neuroendocrinology
5:333-349, 1969

32. Slusher, MA, Effect of chronic hypothalamic lesions on
    diurnal and stress corticosteroid levels. Am J
    Physiol 206:1161-1164, 1964

33. Lengvari, I and B Halasz, Evidence for a diurnal fluc-
    tuation in plasma corticosterone levels after
    fornix transection in the rat. Neuroendocrinology
    11:191-196, 1973

34. Chihara, K, Y Kato, K Maeda, S Matsukura and H Imura,
    Suppression by cyproheptadine of human growth hor-
    mone (GH) and cortisol secretion during sleep. J
    Clin Inv 57:1393-1402, 1976

35. Ferrari, E, PA Bossolo, A Vailati, I Martinelli, A
    Rea and I Nosari, Variations circadiennes des
    effets d'une substance vagolytique sur le système
    ACTH-sécrétant chez l'homme. Annales d'Endocrinologie
    (Paris) 38:203-213, 1977

36. Krieger, HP and DT Krieger, Chemical stimulation of
    the brain : effect of adrenal corticoid release.
    Am J Physiol 218:1632-1638, 1970

37. Scapagnini, U, Moberg GP, GR Vanloon, J DeGroot and
    WF Ganong, Relation of brain 5-hydroxytryptamine
    content to the diurnal variation in plasma cortico-
    sterone in the rat. Neuroendocrinology 7:90-96,
    1971

38. Orth, DN, DP Island and GW Liddle, Experimental al-
    teration of the circadian rhythm in plasma cortisol
    concentration in man. J Clin Endocrinol Metab 27:
    549-555, 1967

39. Weitzman, ED, C Nogeire, M Perlow, D Fukushima, J
    Sassin, P McGregor, TF Gallagher and L Hellman,
    Effects of a prolonged 3-hour sleep-wake cycle on
    sleep stages, plasma cortisol, growth hormone and
    body temperature in man. J Clin Endocrinol Metab
    38:1018-1030, 1974

40. Orth, DN, DP Island and GW Liddle, Light synchroniza-
    tion of the circadian rhythm in plasma cortisol
    concentration in man. J Clin Endocrinol Metab 29:

479-486, 1969

41. Orth, DN, GM Besser, PH King and WE Nicholson, Free-running circadian plasma cortisol rhythm in a blind human subject. Clin Endocrinol 10:603-618, 1979

42. Miles, LEM, DM Raynal and MA Wilson, Blind man living in normal society has circadian rhythms of 24.9 hours. Science 198:421-423, 1977

43. Krieger, DT, J Kreuzer and F Rizzo, Constant light : effect on circadian pattern and phase reversal of steroid and electrolyte levels in man. J Clin Endocrinol Metab 29:1634-1638, 1969

44. Krieger, DT, Food and water restriction shifts corti-costerone, temperature, activity and brain amine periodicity. Endocrinology 95:1195-1201, 1974

45. Krieger, DT, H Hauser and LC Krey, Suprachiasmatic nuclear lesions do not abolish food shifted circa-dian adrenal and temperature rhythmicity. Science 197:398-399, 1977

46. Krieger, DT and H Hauser, Comparison of synchroniza-tion of circadian corticosteroid rhythms by photo-period and food. Proc Natl Acad Sci 75:1577-1580, 1978

47. Krieger, DT, Restoration of corticosteroid periodicity in obese rats by limited AM food access. Brain Res 171:67-75, 1979

48. Krieger, DT, Ventromedial hypothalamic lesions abolish food-shifted circadian adrenal and temperature rhythmicity. Endocrinology 106:649-654, 1980

178

DISCUSSION

WEITZMAN: Your data on the food induced shift of the cortisol rhythm are of great interest and importance. However, I am concerned about the concept of a zeitgeber for a rhythm and the concept of establishing the phase of a rhythm in your analysis. If you impose a food schedule on these animals, you induce a timing of cortisol release. If you then stop the restricted food regimen, does the food shift rhythm continue ?

KRIEGER: No. The rhythm will continue for only about 2 days and then the animal will resume a normal rhythm.

WEITZMAN: Then, your concept of a rhythm being established or synchronized is really dependent on the time of the behavioral event you have imposed.

KRIEGER: It is similar in terms of behavioral timing to what happens in light-dark shifts experiments, except that the food shift is established a little quicker.

WEITZMAN: The key experiment is the study of the suprachiasmatic nucleus. If you make a lesion of the suprachiasmatic nucleus, the animal become arrhythmic. If you then give the animal access to food only at a critical time of day you re-establish the rhythm. Have you re-establish a rhythm or have you produced a stimulus-response to the timing of meals ?

KRIEGER: You have induced a very specific stimulus-response to the timing of meals. If you would take another stimulus-response such as stressing the animal at a given time of day, you could not have induced a rhythm.

WEITZMAN: You use the term "zeitgeber" for the food shift. A zeitgeber establishes the phase of an already existing rhythm, it does not produce the rhythm. The concept of establishing a food shift rhythm, particularly in arrhythmic animals, is not the same as the concept of

establishing the phase of a rhythm in the sense of endogenous periodicity.

KRIEGER: You establish a timing of stimulus-response
which is dependent on a certain neural locus probably involving here the ventral median nucleus. You obtain a
timing of a stimulus-response in a situation where previously no rhythmicity was even seen. The terminology may
not be correct. You might call it "zeitgeber" or "stimulus-response". As far as I am aware, there has been no
precedent for taking a totally arrhythmic animal and conditioning it, if you want to use that term, to a stimulus
that produces a reproducible rhythm.

WEITZMAN: But the concept of conditioning implies,
that if you stop the stimulus, the system continues.

KRIEGER: Any kind of conditioning wears out whether
you consider passive avoidance, active avoidance, etc.
This type of conditioning extinguishes itself fairly
rapidly.

WEITZMAN: I thing that this is a conceptual problem
rather than a question of terminology. What does it mean
to establish a timed relationship to a stimulus and to
assume that you have an endogenous biological rhythm? The
other way to look at your data is to presume that food
timing is a powerful determinant of the time of sleep onset
and awakening within the light-dark cycle and indirectly
causes a shift of the rhythm.

KRIEGER: That is perfectly true. The food shift
changes the activity cycle and the temperature cycle and a
number of other parameters.

WEITZMAN: In order for the animal to survive a shift
of sleep time must occur since it has to eat at a time
when it normally would be sleeping.

REINBERG: We deal with a very complex situation involving two types of synchronizers, the light-dark cycle and the feeding schedule. There is a competition between two zeitgebers. The way to solve this problem is to do experiments in continuous light or continuous darkness and thus manipulate only one zeitgeber.

KRIEGER: This is what we did in the constant light studies and we were able to show that under those conditions the food schedule was able to serve as an entrainer of the rhythm. There are indeed a number of factors that are in competition for entrainment. What our experiments seem to show is that the food is a more powerful stimulus to entrainment than the dark-light cycle.

REINBERG: At least in rats.

KRIEGER: I have no comment about what happens in man. Such experiments would be extremely difficult since man is such a social animal.

JAQUET: Regarding the periodicities you observed in hypothalamic pathology, what type of disease did you study besides Cushing's disease? Is it possible to modify the circadian periodicity under these conditions, for example by administering corticosteroids? Last, do you have any data on the endorphin variations in these types of pathologies? Are they parallel or superimposed to the ACTH fluctuations?

KRIEGER: The hypothalamic diseases that we studied were in patients who had no evidence of endocrine dysfunction as evaluated by a battery of baseline and stimulated tests. The hypothalamic disease was usually diagnosed by radiographic procedures, pneumoencephalography or arteriography. Occasionally, it was confirmed by surgery. We

studied about 30 patients with localized hypothalamic
tumors and, in about 70% of those patients, we found
abnormal circadian periodicity. If we study patients
with CNS disease outside the hypothalamic limbic area, we
may find about a 10% incidence of abnormal periodicity,
which is comparable to what may be observed in normal subjects where some abnormalities in periodicity may also occur. We have not studied the effect of corticosteroids or
of any medication on the periodicity under these conditions.
I cannot comment on the endorphin rhythm in these subjects
because the endogenous endorphin levels are so low in normal
man that we have not been able to perform a good systematic
study in normal subjects. In patients with Nelson's syndrome who have high ACTH levels with abnormal periodicity,
we have found that the endorphin concentration has the
same abnormal periodicity. We think however that the
pituitary is shifting the processing of the molecule so
that more endorphin is produced.

JAQUET: In the patients with hypothalamic tumors,
was the mean ACTH level normal or elevated?

KRIEGER: We have seen such patients with normal ACTH
level and patients with elevated level. We wondered why
in the patients with high ACTH we did not see any associated
endocrine abnormalities. A tentative suggestion is that the
disease had not been present for a long enough period of
time to be able to see the hypercorticoid manifestations.

JAQUET: Another explanation might be possible. There
might be secretion of a form of ACTH precursor, rather than
ACTH itself. We have, in such a case, shown that there
was an excess of precursor and also of LPH and endorphin.
The ratio of ACTH to big ACTH, which is difficult to evaluate because the position of these molecules on the dilu-
tion diagram is the same, and also the ratio of ACTH to
LPH and endorphin were decreased as compared to normal.
Thus, maybe your patients with high ACTH levels have some

disease of the pre-hormones of the ACTH or LPH systems.

KRIEGER: Was this a patient with hypothalamic
disease?

JAQUET: Yes.

KRIEGER: We have seen a dissociation in a patient with
Cushing's disease who had a large suprasellar extension.
In this patient, there was a marked discrepancy between
ACTH measured by RIA and ACTH measured by bioassay. We
have not looked for such discrepancies in hypothalamic
diseases.

VAN CAUTER: If the food shift experiments could be
reproduced in humans, it would have interesting clinical
and social implications. For instance, such food shifts
could fasten the adaptation to jet lag. I remember a
study by Dr. Reinberg where healthy volunteers having a
single daily meal in the morning were loosing weight
whereas they were gaining weight when the meal was taken
in the evening. Did Dr. Reinberg obtain data on cortisol
periodicity in these patients?

REINBERG: In a later study with Dr. Apfelbaum, we
were not able to confirm the temporal dependence of weight
loss when the caloric intake was normal rather than a highly
caloric diet. On the other hand, there is a small phase
shift of one to two hours of the plasma cortisol rhythm
in these conditions. I do not consider this shift as
significant whereas Dr. Halberg does.

VAN CAUTER: Regarding the circadian rhythm of sensitivity of the adrenals to ACTH in vitro, would you interpret this result as a direct consequence of receptor occupancy or do you think that there is an endogenous rhythm
of sensitivity of the glands?

KRIEGER: It probably is more related to the rate of receptor occupancy. The infusion studies in humans as well as the studies on hypophysectomized individuals suggest strongly that priming of the gland is an essential factor. There may be some intrinsic rhythmicity but I think that the major part of the variation results from the priming.

INFLUENCE OF DRUG ADMINISTRATION ON ACTH CIRCADIAN RHYTHM

F. Ceresa

Clinica Medica Generale e Terapia Medica B, Università di
Torino, Via Genova 3, 10126 Torino, Italy.

Among many other oscillatory phenomena the circadian rhythm
of the ACTH-cortisol secreting system is by far the most
studied, both under physiological and pathological conditions.

At present the most current view is that in conscious subjects conforming to a regular sleep/wake and rest/activity
schedule both ACTH and cortisol levels in the plasma increase rapidly during the early morning hours and reach
their maximum at about the time of waking. During the ensuing hours circulating ACTH and cortisol decrease reaching
a minimal plateau in the late evening and in the nocturnal
hours preceding midnight (1-3).

If plasma concentrations of ACTH and cortisol are estimated
every 15-20 minutes, rapidly occurring oscillations of the
respective levels can be noted so that an "episodical" activity of the ACTH-cortisol secreting system in form of episodic bursts of secretion has been postulated (4-6).
However, if the integrated area of the curve traced by the
secretory bursts during the day is considered, the existence of a circadian rhythm of the overall 24-hour secretion
is easily detected by "macroscopic" examinations as well
confirmed by "microscopic" analyses according to the
Cosinor procedures (3). The circadian rhythmicity of circulating ACTH and cortisol can be accounted for neither by
variations of the adrenal responsiveness to ACTH (2, 7) nor
by variations in the metabolic clearance rate (8) or in the
plasma corticosteroid binding (9), although rhythmic patterns along the 24-hour cycle have been described for all
three variables (8, 10, 11).

It is generally taken for granted that the circadian rhythm
of ACTH secretion is driven by a circadian rhythm of hypothalamic corticotrophin releasing hormone (CRH) secretion
(12, 13) according to a programmed sequence under central
nervous sytem (CNS) control, so that the circadian variation of the pituitary-adrenal function can be regarded as a
reflection of the rhythmic variations in the CNS mechanisms
involved in the regulation of hypothalamic CRH secretion
(14).

Among the effects induced by drugs on ACTH-cortisol secreting system, we must first take into consideration the
effects of corticoids.

Much evidence has been collected of variations in the sensitivity of the ACTH-secreting system to corticoid inhibition
throughout the 24-hour day. Synthetic corticoids given
during, or just prior to the nocturnal circadian rise of
ACTH and cortisol secretion display a greater inhibitory
effect than compounds given at other times of the day (15-
17). Ceresa et al. (18-20) studied these differences by
intravenously infusing different doses of corticoids and
estimating the 17-hydroxycorticosteroid (17-OHCS) urinary
output as an index of the ACTH and cortisol secretions.

Ceresa et al. (18) taking into   account both the
fact that at the end of any intravenous infusion a certain
amount of corticoid was still present at the CNS level acting conceivably longer and the time of the cortisol transformation into 17-OHCS metabolites, could prove that the
ACTH-cortisol secreting system can not be affected at all
by moderate doses of corticoids for a rather long period
of time lasting from about 08.00 to about midnight. Moderate doses of 6-methylprednisolone and dexamethasone corresponded to about 0.7 mg/hour and, respectively, to 50 µg/
hour. A total inhibition of the system was reached at any
time of the day only when i.v.   infusing doses of corticoids were 2 or 3   times greater than those above mentioned (Fig. 1).

By contrast, the ACTH-cortisol secreting system showed a
very high sensitivity during a rather short and temporarily

186

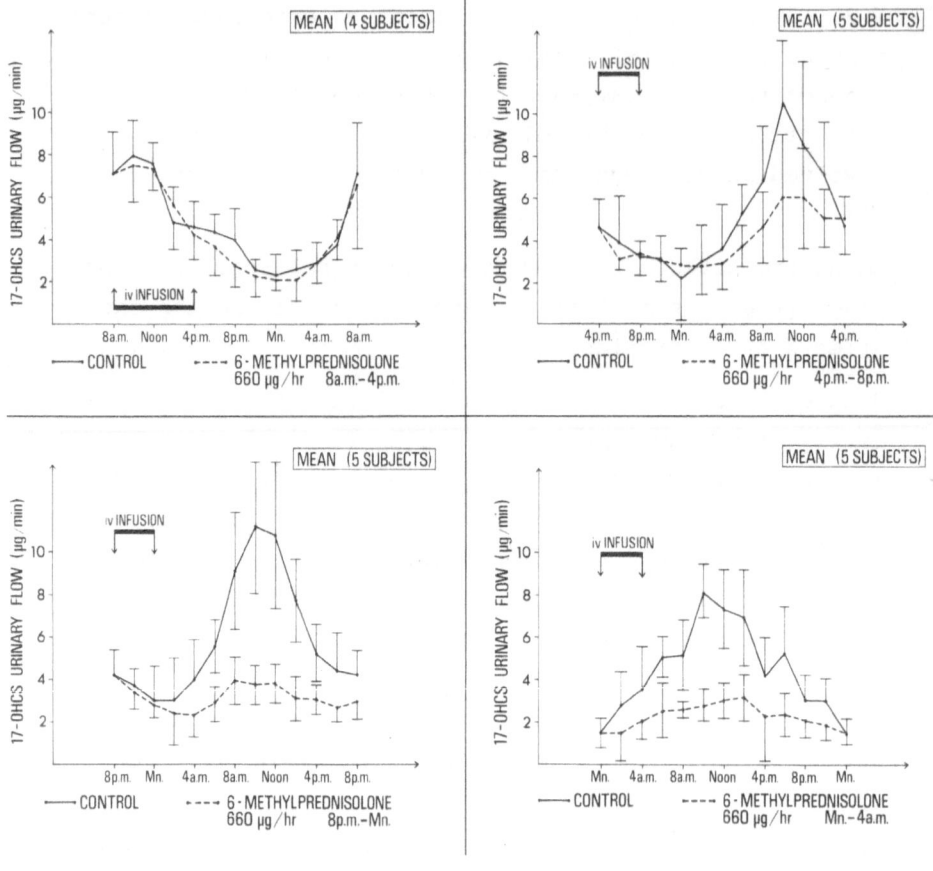

Figure 1: Effect of 6-methylprednisolone 660 µg/h iv infused in normal subjects during different time-spans of the 24-h cycle on the 17-hydroxycorticosteroid (17-OHCS) urinary flow. The curves show mean + 1 SD values. Continuous line : flow curve recorded during the control day. Dashed line : flow curve recorded during the 24-h day following the start of the corticoid infusion. (Adapted from Ceresa et al. (18)).

well defined time-span of the 24-hour cycle, being located from midnight till approximately 07.30. During these nocturnal-early morning hours the doses of 0.7 mg/hour of 6-methylprednisolone and, respectively, of 50 µg/hour of dexamethasone intravenously infused showed a partial but definite inhibitory effect resulting in the disappearance of the wave of increasing activity that characterizes ACTH-cortisol secretion in the hours ensuing midnight till a maximum just at time of waking (approximately at 07.30 in subjects conforming to a normal rest/activity schedule)(Fig.1).

According to Ceresa et al. (18) two different phases of activity of the system exist. The "basal" secretory phase lasts the 24-hour day long and shows a rather weak sensitivity to the inhibiting effect of corticoids; the "impulsive" phase overimposed to the basal phase lasts a limited time-span of the 24-hour day (approximately from midnight to 7-8 a.m.) and shows a very high sensitivity to the corticoid inhibition. The thesis of two secretory phases even if differently called is at present shared by many authors : "circadian" and "basal" phases (21), "phasic" and "tonic" phases (22).

Ceresa et al. (19) showed that when a dose of 50 µg/hour of dexamethasone was infused from 22.00 to 04.00 on the night following that during which total suppression of the steroid output had been obtained by infusing a dose of 100 µg/hour of dexamethasone, the secretory morning peak of the second day was suppressed : in spite of this suppression the "basal" 17-OHCS output reappeared during the course of the day. Such a behaviour is consistent with the concept that the drive eliciting during the nocturnal-early morning hours the "impulsive" secretory activity is not necessary to reestablish the basal secretion (Fig. 2).

On the basis of their findings, Ceresa et al. (18-20) put forth the hypothesis that in humans the neuroendocrine mechanisms responsible for the circadian rhythmicity of the ACTH-cortisol secreting system during the last part of the night's sleep are qualitatively different from those responsible for the secretion during the remainder of the 24-

188

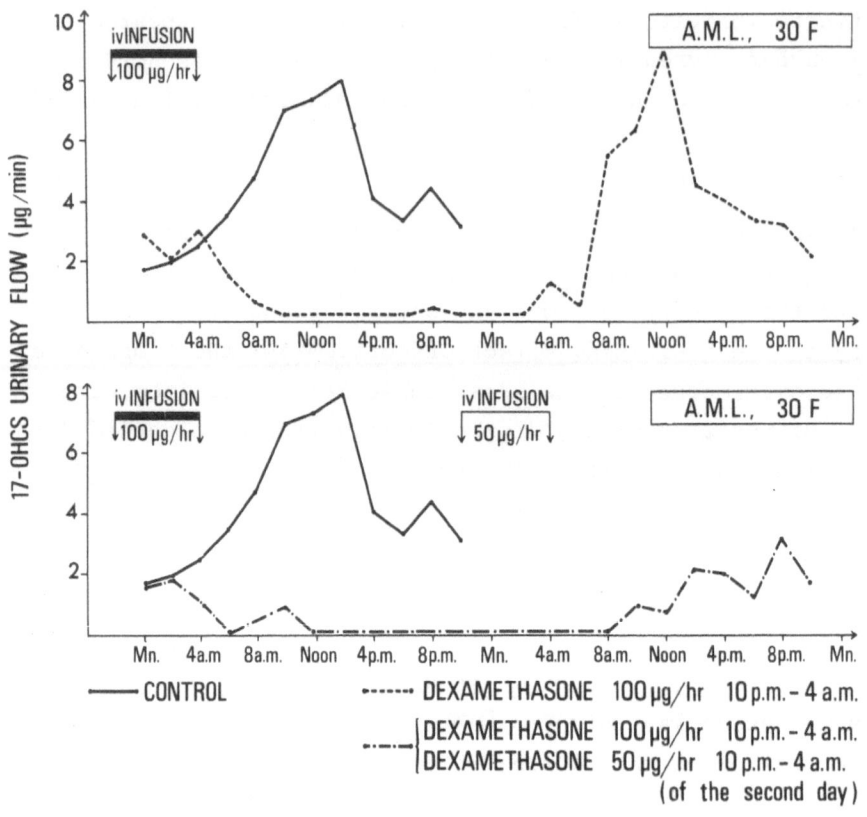

Figure 2: *Resumption of the 17-OHCS urinary flow after total suppression of ACTH-glucocorticoid secretion achieved by iv infusing dexamethasone 100 μg/h from 10 p.m. to 4 a.m. in a normal subject. Continuous line : flow curve recorded during the control day. Dashed line : the normal pattern reappears with the following-morning "impulsive" phase.*
Pecked line : the "basal" phase reappears spontaneously in spite of a second infusion (dexamethasone 50 μg/h) suppressing the following-morning wave (from Ceresa et al. (19)).

hour day. A similar suggestion has been made after experiments in animals (13).

The inhibiting effect displayed by exogenous corticoids on ACTH-cortisol secretion requires a certain degree of anatomical and functional integrity of the CNS. Our group (23) has recently studied the circadian profile of plasma cortisol in patients suffering from severe cerebral injury (traumatic accident) and presenting conditions of deep coma (III-IV degree). Six patients entered the study : serial measurements of plasma cortisol were carried out throughout three consecutive 24-hour cycles in the week immediately following trauma with the patients receiving 12 mg/daily of dexamethasone-21-phosphate. This high dose of the corticoid derivative did not succeed in totally inhibiting ACTH-cortisol secretion as it always does in normal subjects. The rather poor response of the system appeared more striking since it was found that also the more sensitive "impulsive" phase of secretion was but partially affected. The circadian rhythm of plasma cortisol was maintained and appeared to be normally synchronized; the mean cosinor evaluation according to Halberg et al. (24) could confirm the presence of a significant circadian oscillation even if the mean mesor appeared to be reduced in comparison with that of the normal subjects (Fig. 3-4).

The persistence of a rhythmic pattern of the glucocorticoid secretion in the face of the lack of consciousness and of the pharmacological administration of dexamethasone is an intriguing finding. Failure to suppress circadian cortisol profile by dexamethasone administration has already been reported in depressed patients; interestingly enough, the normal responsiveness to corticoid administration was restored after recovery (25). Acute head injury with post-traumatic coma and depression are clearly not comparable conditions, and at present no simplistic explanation can be sought for the observed escape of cortisol rhythm from the glucocorticoid suppression. It is worth noting, however, that this abnormal escape is shared by two different disorders of the CNS function.

190

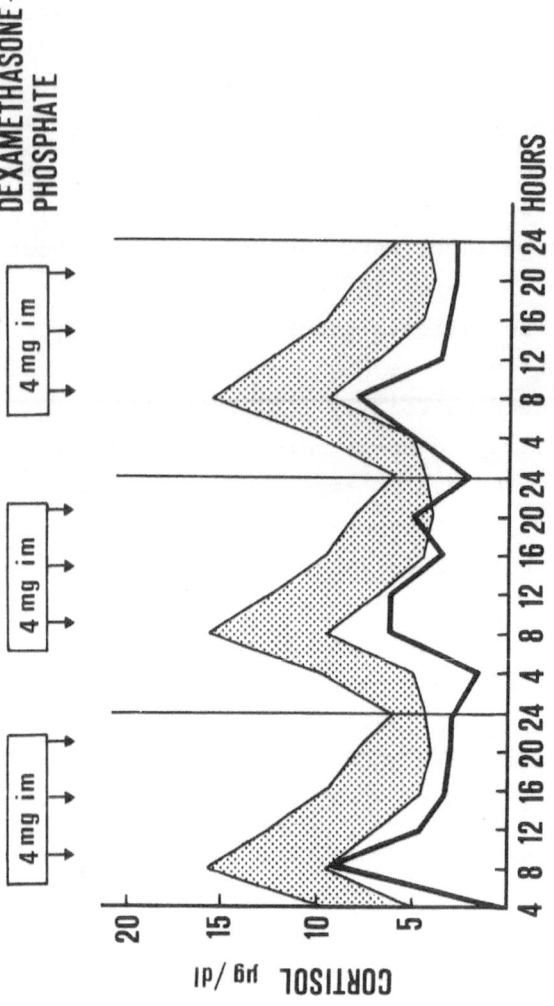

Figure 3: Plasma cortisol levels recorded at 4-h intervals during days 3-4-5 following acute head injury (road accident) in a male comatose patient receiving dexamethasone-21-phosphate 12 mg im daily. Arrows indicate the timing of corticoid injection (4 mg). The shaded area represents the normal circadian pattern (mean ± 1 SD).

A: comatose patients
B: normal subjects

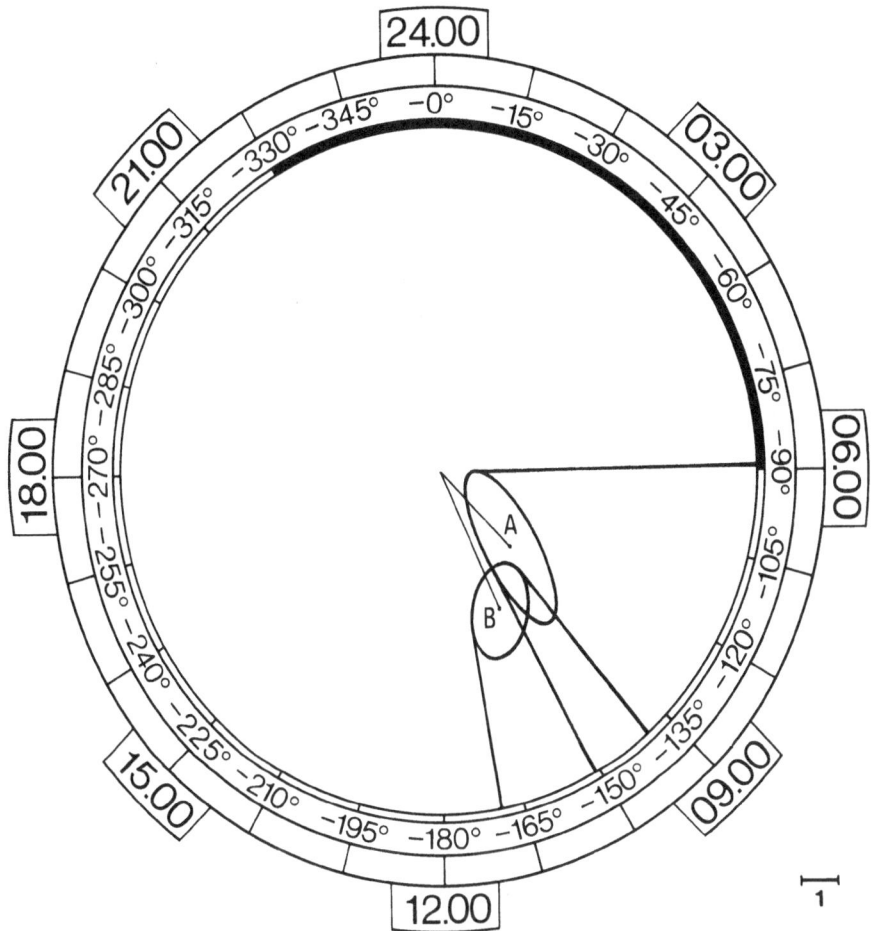

Figure 4:Mean Cosinor display of the circadian rhythm in plasma cortisol levels for data obtained at 4-h intervals throughout one 24-h cycle
in twenty normal adult subjects of both sexes and for data obtained at
4-h intervals throughout three consecutive 24-h cycles in six comatose
patients from acute head injury receiving dexamethasone-21-phosphate
12 mg im daily. Amplitude is expressed as µg/dl.

Since ACTH secretion appears to be controlled by two separate mechanisms showing a different sensitivity to corticoid inhibition it is worth to consider the problem of the glucocorticoid effect by the opposite approach, i.e. by studying the behaviour of the ACTH-secreting system after metyrapone administration.

The drug is assumed to block the 11-β-hydroxylase activity in the adrenal steroidogenesis, thereby preventing the synthesis of cortisol causing the fall of plasma cortisol levels, removing the endogenous glucocorticoid inhibition and thus enhancing release and secretion of ACTH by the pituitary gland. This increased corticotrophic activity results in a further stimulation of the adrenal steroidogenesis and in a rise of 17-OHCS in blood and urine mainly represented by 11-deoxycortisol and its metabolites. Therefore metyrapone can be regarded as a drug producing an opposite condition as compared with corticoids : it removes glucocorticoid inhibition of the ACTH-cortisol secreting system, hence it enhances, instead of suppressing, ACTH secretion.

Metyrapone seems to exert a different effect according to the timing of its administration. A greater pituitary-adrenal response with higher elevation of plasma 11-deoxy-cortisol and of 17-OHCS output was observed when the administration occurred just prior to or during the circadian rise of ACTH-cortisol secretion as compared with other administration times far from this particular time-period of the 24-hour day (26-28). Angeli et al. (29, 30) have studied the rhythmic pattern of ACTH-adrenal secretion along a 48-hour time-span during and after a sustained oral administration of metyrapone started at two opposite times of the 24-hour day (at 08.00 and at 20.00). They found a greater output of 17-OHCS during the first 24-hour cycle in the 20.00-test, whereas the output was greater during the second 24-hour cycle in the 08.00-test; moreover, they demonstrated the occurrence of a normally-synchronized circadian rhythm in 17-OHCS output during the two 24-hour cycles examined, both in the 20.00-test and in the 08.00-test, i.e. during metyrapone-induced ACTH release. An interesting finding of this investigation was the demonstration of a highly significant circadian rhythm in 17-OHCS output after metyrapone administration also in cases of anorexia nervosa who were lacking the "impulsive" rise of ACTH-cortisol secretion during the control day. The mechanisms whereby a rapid restoration of the circadian ACTH pattern occurs in these patients after administration of metyrapone are not clear; anyway, the finding seems to fit well with our assumption (31) that abolition of the circadian rise of glucocorticoid secretion in anorexia nervosa represents a mechanism of adaptation to the nutritional status rather than an expression of primitive derangements of ACTH secretion. The overall data of Angeli et al. (29, 30) are in agreement with previously published findings (26) and support the view that the effect of metyrapone is primarily confined to the "impulsive" phase of ACTH secretion. It is tempting to think that the endogenous circulating levels of cortisol play their regulatory role of negative feedback just on the easily-suppressible "impulsive" secretion and therefore are centrally active only during a limited time-span of the 24-hour cycle when the CNS mechanisms responsible for the "impulsive" ACTH secretion are operating (approximately from midnight to 7-8 a.m.). According to this view (29, 32), the negative feed-back mechanism mainly acts when the CNS drive promoting the periodic oversecretion of ACTH shows the highest sensitivity to corticoid inhibition while the other factors responsible for the basal adrenocorticotropic activity lasting the whole 24-hour day and showing a poor sensitivity to inhibition may substantially ignore the signal of endogenous physiological levels of cortisol. If this is true, an exceeding amount of 11-deoxycortisol (compound S) will be secreted by the adrenal glands as a consequence of a metyrapone-induced enhancement of the "impulsive" ACTH secretion, hence the circadian rhythmicity of the 17-OHCS output will be preserved, as it was found (29).

Angeli et al. (33) provided additional support to this

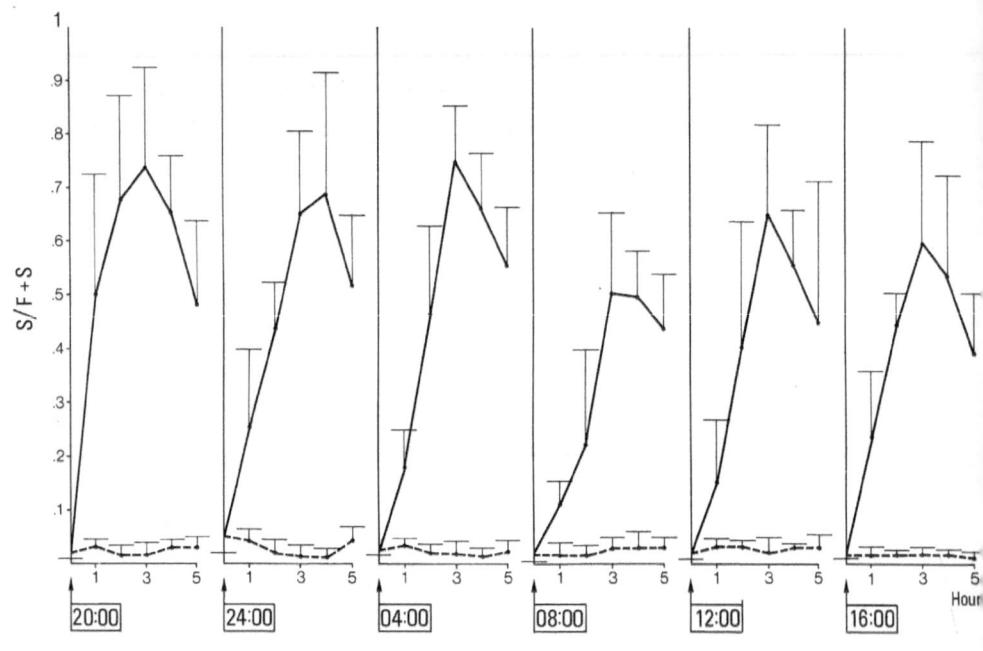

Figure 5: Effects of metyrapone (750 mg) and placebo orally administered at different times of the 24-h cycle on the relationship between circulating cortisol (compound F) and 11-deoxycortisol (compound S) in normal adult volunteers. The curves show mean ± 1 SD values of the ratio plasma S/plasma F + plasma S, calculated on blood samples drawn at 1-h intervals for 5 consecutive hours following administration. Continuous line : metyrapone administration. Dashed line : placebo administration. (from Angeli et al. (33)).

viewpoint. Metyrapone was orally administered at the dose
of 750 mg to five normal subjects in separate experiments
with one-week intervals at the following hours : 20.00,
00.00 (midnight), 04.00, 08.00, 12.00 and 16.00. Total
glucocorticoid, cortisol and 11-deoxycortisol concentrations
were measured on blood samples drawn every one hour for
five hours from the administration time. The degree of
11-β-hydroxylase inhibition was estimated by calculating
the ratio deoxycortisol/deoxycortisol + cortisol plasma
concentrations. Total glucocorticoid levels in the plasma,
which represented an indirect measure of the ACTH release
hence of the pituitary response did clearly rise when the
metyrapone administration was at 00.00 and at 04.00. Mean
percent increments over control values at 3, 4 and 5 hours
after administration at these nocturnal hours were significantly higher than those observed after placebo administration. On the contrary the curve of the total glucocorticoid plasma levels after metyrapone was overimposable to
the curve after placebo when both were administered at any
other time examined (Fig. 5-6).

The finding that the removal of cortisol feed-back inhibition ensuing metyrapone administration results in a significantly enhanced ACTH release only during a limited time-
span independently from temporal variations in 11-β-hydro-
xylase suppression seems to fit rather well with the assumption that the action of the endogenous feed-back mechanism
is mainly confined to the "impulsive" phase secretion and
that it acts only during the limited time-span when this
secretion is present. The system is hardly affected by the
physiological concentrations of cortisol during the other
portion of the 24-hour cycle when the only basal secretion
is active.

Recent studies in different laboratories have suggested that
5-hydroxytryptamine (5-HT) systems are involved in the feedback control of the pituitary-adrenal axis in unstressed
animals (22, 34, 35). In the human, the point remains
controversial, although it has been reported that methergo-
line, an anti-serotoninergic drug, may affect metyrapone-

196

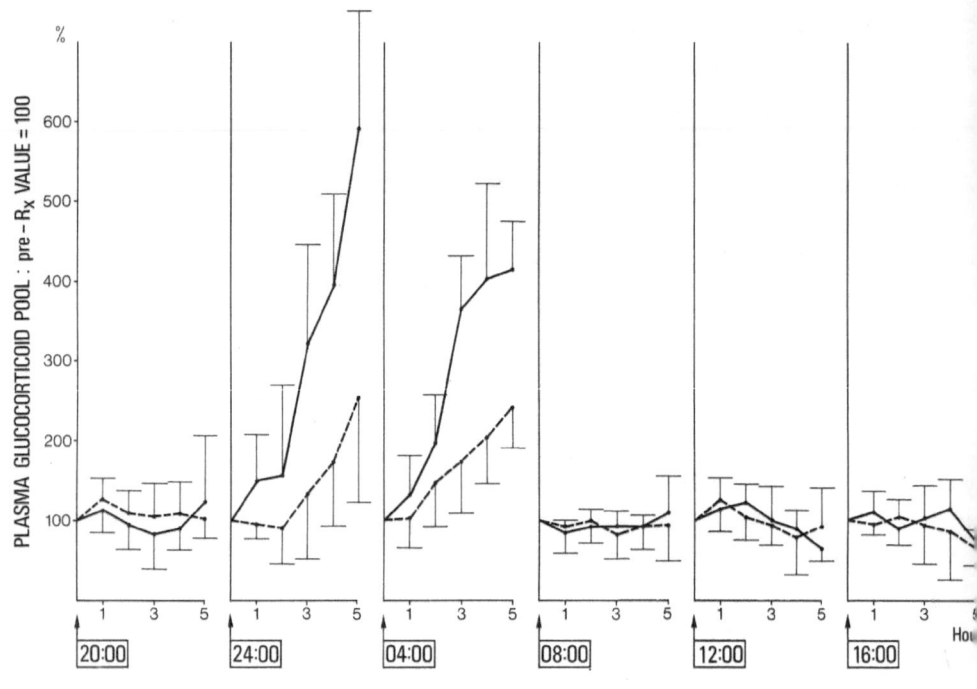

Figure 6:Effects of metyrapone (750 mg) and placebo orally administered at different times of the 24-h cycle on "total" plasma glucocorticoid levels in normal adult volunteers. The curves show mean ± 1 SD values of the steroid concentrations measured on blood samples drawn at 1-h intervals for 5 consecutive hours and plotted as percent of the respective pre-administration values, which were taken as 100 %. Continuous line : metyrapone administration. Dashed line : placebo administration (from Angeli et al. (33)).

induced ACTH release (36). It is admittedly difficult to study the effects of changed brain serotoninergic tone on the pituitary hormone secretion. Previous results on a decline of plasma cortisol due to L-tryptophan treatment (37) have not been confirmed (38). Hyyppä et al. (39) have most recently pointed to the ineffectiveness of L-tryptophan on cortisol levels when the serotonin precursor is given during the diurnal hours following 08.30. This would not be surprising if one hypothezes that serotoniner-gic mechanisms are specifically involved in the regulation of the nocturnal ACTH rise ("impulsive" phase) as it has been suggested to occur in rats (40, 41).

Information is yet lacking to get out of conjectures; research is needed to evaluate how the activity of 5-HT systems in the brain may be affected by glucocorticoids and how its role in the control of ACTH secretion is cir-cadian-stage dependent.

REFERENCES

1. Migeon, CV, FH Tyler, JP Mahoney, AA Florentin, H
   Castle, FL Buss and LT Samuels, The diurnal variation of plasma level and urinary excretion of 17-
   hydroxycorticosteroids in normal subjects, night
   workers and blind subjects. J Clin Endocrinol
   Metab 16:622-633, 1956

2. Perkoff, WH, K Eik-Nes, CA Nugent, HL Fred, RA Nimer,
   L Rush, LT Samuels and FH Tyler, Studies of the
   diurnal variation of plasma 17-hydroxycorticoste-
   roids in man. J Clin Endocrinol Metab 19:432-443,
   1959

3. Halberg, F, Chronobiology. Ann Rev Physiol 31:675-
   725, 1969

4. Hellman, L, F Nakada, J Curti, ED Weitzman, J Kream,
   H Roffwarg, S Ellman, DK Fukushima and TF
   Gallagher, Cortisol is secreted episodically by
   normal man. J Clin Endocrinol Metab 30:411-422,
   1970

5. Krieger, DT, W Allen, F Rizzo and HP Krieger, Characterization of the normal temporal pattern of plasma
   corticosteroid levels. J Clin Endocrinol Metab
   32:266-284, 1971

6. Weitzman, ED, D Fukushima, C Nogeire, H Roffwarg, TF
   Gallagher and L Hellman, Twenty-four hour pattern
   of the episodic secretion of cortisol in normal
   subjects. J Clin Endocrinol Metab 33:14-41, 1971

7. Martin, MM and DH Mintz, Effect of altered thyroid
   function upon adrenocortical ACTH and methopyrapone
   (SU-4885) responsiveness in man. J Clin Endocrinol
   Metab 25:20-27, 1966

8. De Lacerda, L, A Kowarski and CJ Migeon, Diurnal
   variation of the metabolic clearance rate of cortisol. Effect on measurement of cortisol production
   rate. J Clin Endocrinol Metab 36:1043-1049, 1973

9. De Moor, P; K Heiwegh, JF Heremans and M Declercq-
   Raskin, Protein binding of corticoids studied by
   gel filtration. J Clin Invest 41:816-827, 1962

10. Ferrari, E, PA Bossolo, A Rea, A Vailati, I Martinelli
    M Tamborini, S Dematte and C Bertulessi, La rispos-
    ta corticosurrenalica agli stimoli farmacologici
    specifici in ore diverse della giornata, In:
    Giornate Endocrinologiche Pisane, Tronchetti, F,
    and GF Menchini-Fabris (eds.), Pisa, Pacini
    Editore, 431-443 (vol. I), 1978

11. Angeli, A, R Frairia, F Agrimonti, L Richiardi, G
    Boccuzi and F Ceresa, Circadian variations of cor-
    tisol binding capacity by transcortin in normal
    subjects, In:Proceedings, 12th International
    Conference of the International Society for
    Chronobiology, Hayes, D, L Scheving and F Halberg
    (eds.), Milano, Publishing House Il Ponte, 197-204,
    1977

12. Hiroshige, T, M Sakakura and S Itoh, Diurnal variation
    of corticotropin-releasing activity in the hypo-
    thalamus of normal and adrenalectomized rats.
    Endocrinol Jap 16:465-467, 1969

13. Krieger, DT, Factors influencing the circadian perio-
    dicity of plasma corticosteroid level. Chronobio-
    logia 1:195-216, 1974

14. Krieger, DT, Circadian rhythm of ACTH and adrenal
    corticosteroids : treatment of ACTH hypersecretion
    in Cushing's disease, In:The endocrine function of
    the human adrenal cortex, Serono Symposia 18,
    London and New York, Academic Press, 193-206, 1978

15. Di Raimondo, VC and PH Forsham, Some clinical impli-
    cation of spontaneous diurnal variation in adrenal
    cortical secretion activity. Amer J Med 21:321-
    323, 1956

16. Grant, SH, PH Forsham and VC Di Raimondo, Suppression
    of 17-hydroxycorticosteroids in plasma and urine
    by single and divided doses of triamcinolone. New
    Engl J Med 273:1115-1118, 1965

17. Nichols, T, CA Nugent and FH Tyler, Diurnal variation
    in suppression of adrenal function by glucocorti-
    coids. J Clin Endocrinol Metab 25:343-349, 1965

18. Ceresa, F, A Angeli, G Boccuzzi and G Molino, Once-a-day neurally stimulated and basal ACTH secretion phases in man and their response to corticoid inhibition. J Clin Endocrinol Metab 29:1074-1089, 1969

19. Ceresa, F, A Angeli, G Boccuzzi and L Perotti, Impulsive and basal ACTH secretion phases in normal subjects, in obese subjects with signs of adrenocortical hyperfunction and in hyperthyroid patients. J Clin Endocrinol Metab 31:491-501, 1970

20. Ceresa, F, A Angeli and G Boccuzzi, Nuovi concetti sui meccanismi di regolazione a livello ipotalamico del ritmo circadiano corticotropinico, In:Fisiologia e fisiopatologia ipotalamo-ipofisaria. Atti del 14° Congresso della Società Italiana di Endocrinologia, Roma, Il Pensiero Scientifico, 20-65, 1972

21. Krieger, DT, Neurotransmitter regulation of ACTH release. Mt Sinai J Med 40:302-314, 1973

22. Scapagnini, U and P Preziosi, Role of brain norepinephrine and serotonin in the tonic and phasic regulation of hypothalamic-hypophyseal-adrenal axis. Archs Int Pharmacodyn Ther 196:205-220, 1972

23. Agrimonti, F, D Boggio-Bertinet, L Merighi, R Frairia and A Angeli, Profilo circadiano del cortisolo e dell'aldosterone plasmatici in craniolesi politraumatizzati in trattamento con alte dosi di desametazone, In: Giornate Endocrinologiche Pisane, Pisa, 23-24 November 1979, in press, 1980.

24. Halberg, F, YL Tong and EA Johnson, Circadian system phase, an aspect of temporal morphology : procedures and illustrative examples, In:The cellular aspects of biorhythms. Symposium on Biorhythms, Von Mayersbach, H (ed.), Berlin, Springer-Verlag, 20-48, 1967

25. Carroll, BJ and J Mendels, Neuroendocrine regulation in affective disorders, In:Hormones, Behavior and Psychopathology, Sachar, EJ (ed.), New York, Raven Press, 193-224, 1976

26. Ceresa, F, E Strumia, A Angeli and M Dellepiane,
    Behaviour of the feed-back mechanism controlling
    ACTH secretion in normal subjects and under diffe-
    rent endocrine conditions, and relative clinical
    implications. Excerpta Med Intern Congr Series
    83:1027-1040, 1965
27. Martin, MM and DE Hellman, Temporal variation in SU-
    4885 responsiveness in man : evidence in support of
    circadian variation in ACTH secretion. J Clin
    Endocrinol Metab 24:253-260, 1964
28. Takebe, K, Temporal variation in the response of uri-
    nary 17-OHCS to metopirone in Cushing's syndrome
    due to bilateral adrenal hyperplasia. J Clin
    Endocrinol Metab 36:433-438, 1973
29. Angeli, A, D Fonzo, P Bertello, G Gaidano and F
    Ceresa, Circadian rhythm of urinary 17-hydroxycor-
    ticosteroids during metyrapone-induced ACTH release
    Chronobiologia 2:133-144, 1975
30. Angeli, A, D Fonzo, R Frairia, D Bertello and F
    Ceresa, Circadian variations in metyrapone-induced
    ACTH release in normal subjects and in patients
    with anorexia nervosa, In:Rhythmische Funktionen
    in Biologischen Systemen, Ihre Bedentung für
    Theorie un Klinik, Lassman, G, and F Seitelberger
    (eds.), Wien, Facultas-Verlag, 32-43 (Teil II),
    1977
31. Ceresa, F, C Cravetto and L Dughera, Le métabolisme
    des hormones corticosurrénales au cours des ano-
    rexies mentales. Actual Endocrinol (Paris) 1:145-
    163, 1960
32. Angeli, A and R Frairia, Some physiological aspects of
    ACTH rhythmicities in man, In:Neuroendocrinology :
    biological and clinical aspects, Polleri, A and
    RM McLeod (eds.), London and New York, Academic
    Press, 145-154, 1979
33. Angeli, A, D Fonzo, R Frairia, D Bertello, G Gaidano
    and F Ceresa, Independence of the circadian rhythm
    in metyrapone-induced ACTH release from variations

in adrenal 11-beta-hydroxylase inhibition, In:
Proceedings, 12th International Conference of the
International Society for Chronobiology, Hayes, D,
L Scheving and F Halberg (eds.), Milano, Publishing
House Il Ponte, 189-196, 1977

34. Telegdy, G and I Vermes, Effect of adrenocortical
hormones on activity of the serotoninergic system
in limbic structures in rats. Neuroendocrinology
18:16-26, 1975

35. Balfour, DJK and MEM Benwell, Betamethasone-induced
pituitary-adrenocortical suppression and brain 5-
hydroxytryptamine in the rat. Psychoneuroendocrinology 4:83-86, 1979

36. Cavagnini, F, AE Panerai, F Valentini, P Bultheroni,
M Peracchi and M Pinto, Inhibition of ACTH response
to oral and intravenous metyrapone by antiseroto-
ninergic treatment in man. J Clin Endocrinol Metab
41:143-148, 1975

37. Woolf, PD and L Lee, Effect of the serotonin precursor, tryptophan on pituitary hormone secretion.
J Clin Endocrinol Metab 45:123-133, 1977

38. Modlinger, RS, JM Schonmuller and SP Arora, Stimulation
of aldosterone, renin and cortisol by tryptophan.
J Clin Endocrinol Metab 48:599-606, 1979

39. Hyyppä, MT, T Jolma, J Liira, V-A Långvik and O
Kytömäki, L-tryptophan treatment and the episodic
secretion of pituitary hormones and cortisol.
Psychoneuroendocrinology 4:29-35, 1979

40. Krieger, DT and F Rizzo, Circadian periodicity of
plasma 17-OHCS : mediation by serotonin dependent
pathways. Amer J Physiol 217:1703-1707, 1969

41. Scapagnini, U, GP Moberg, GR Van Loon and WF Ganong,
Relation of brain 5-hydroxytryptamine content to
the diurnal variation in plasma corticosterone in
the rat. Neuroendocrinology 7:90-96, 1971

DISCUSSION

REINBERG: My first question is related to comatose patients. A study by Assenmacher in Montpellier in patients with coma resulting from vascular disease included a spectral analysis of longitudinal records of cortisol levels and demonstrated that the cortisol rhythm was free-running. Thus, the period was different from 24 hours. You observe a small change in acrophase in such patients. Did you check the period length?

CERESA: No.

REINBERG: What type of coma did you study?

CERESA: Type III, IV. "Coma dépassé" mainly resulting from car crashes.

REINBERG: In patients with toxic coma admitted in an anti-poison center, we found that the rhythm of urinary excretion of potassium persists but with a different acrophase. We were not able to find out whether the period length was different or whether there was a real acrophase change.

CERESA: In our study, the change in acrophase is very slight. There could be a difference in the nature of coma.

REINBERG: The age of the subjects could also play a role.

CERESA: Of course. But in all of the 6 patients we studied, the cortisol rhythm persisted.

REINBERG: Which results did you obtain in comatose patients, Dr. Krieger?

KRIEGER: The patients I referred to in my presentation were taken from the literature. Thus, I cannot comment on these results. With regard to the comparison between the comatose patients and the depressed patients that

Dr. Ceresa made concerning the abnormality of the dexamethasone suppressibility, there are actually some differences and some similarities. In depressed patients, it has been reported that there is an altered circadian periodicity. What is actually observed is not that the circadian periodicity is altered, because the amplitude and the acrophase remain normal, but that the number and magnitude of secretory episodes are much greater than in normals. Most of the studies in comatose patients reported in the literature have not been conducted in great detail as far as estimation of the episodic secretion is concerned.

CERESA: The depressed patients we mentioned in our presentation were taken from Carroll and Mendels. We made this comparison between depressed and comatose patients only with regard to the lack of suppressibility by very high doses of dexamethasone (12 mg/day).

MENDLEWICZ: Concerning these data of Carroll and Mendels on the cortisol escape from dexamethasone suppression in depression, a recent study by Langer in Vienna showed that if diazepam is given I.M. before the dexamethasone test, a normal cortisol suppression is observed. What is your interpretation of these data?

REINBERG: The interpretation of these data has to take into account the exact time at which the drugs are administered. You deal with a pharmacological phenomenon involving two drugs.

MENDLEWICZ: As far as I remember, dexamethasone was given at midnight and diazepam was given in the early morning hours.

REINBERG: The pattern of the response could be different if different timing was used.

QUABBE: We have studied 4 comatose patients with a frequent blood sampling technique over 24 hours and have observed dissociations in the responses of the different hormones, cortisol, PRL and GH, to the comatose state. In one of these patients, we performed a brain autopsy and we were surprised by the degree of damage in different areas of the brain, including the hypothalamus, which was not predicted by clinical signs. All 4 patients had a different pattern of alteration of cortisol, PRL and GH secretion. Therefore, studies in comatose patients will be of interest regarding the control of the rhythms only if there is a very detailed clinical description, preferably confirmed by autopsy.

REINBERG: If there is a free-running rhythm in coma, it will depend on the timing at which you perform the circadian rhythm analysis with regard to the beginning of the coma.

WEITZMAN: One has to be careful as to what one means with "coma". The true coma implies absolutely no responsiveness with a flat and very low EEG.   These patients almost always die if they don't recover within 24 to 48 hours, depending on the cause of the coma. In "coma dépassé", another form of vegetative coma state, there is a changing EEG pattern, especially after head injury or vascular disease. Part of these changes is the development of a type of sleep-waking cycle, even though the patient does not achieve consciousness. Thus, there is a problem of defining waking without consciousness. We followed such a patient and observed the reestablishment of the rhythm of cortisol as the sleep-waking process developed even prior to true consciousness, that is interactive relationship. Dr. Quabbe made a very important point by stressing that a very detailed clinical picture of the coma is needed.

REINBERG: Including the type of treatment of the coma.

Unidentified Discussant: You have shown that whatever the time of the day when metyrapone is given, an effect on the enzyme system converting 11-deoxycortisol to cortisol is observed.

CERESA: Yes, but there is a diurnal variation in the capacity of inhibition.

Unidentified Discussant: OK. Now, the adrenal cortex secretory response to metyrapone administered at midnight and 04.00 consists of an increased secretion but no response is observed at other times. Do you think that, at the times when there is no secretory response to metyrapone, ACTH fails to influence the gland or do you think that there is no ACTH secretion?

CERESA: ACTH secretion is always present. In my opinion, the gland is not sensitive to ACTH at these times.

Unidentified Discussant: Would you be led from these data to think that there is also a periodicity in the feedback system relating ACTH and cortisol secretion?

CERESA: We feel that the feedback mechanism acts mostly on the passive vagal secretion of ACTH, not on the active secretion which seems to be less sensitive to the inhibition. This is of course a working hypothesis.

Unidentified Discussant: You suggest that the hypothalamo-pituitary system might fail to sense the inhibitory signal.

CERESA: Yes.

REINBERG: When you administer metyrapone continuously for 36 hours, you still maintain the rhythmicity in 11-deoxycortisol and its tetra-hydro-derivative in the urine and these rhythms are in phase with the cortisol secretory rhythm.

HORMONAL RHYTHMS IN PITUITARY TUMORS

P. Jaquet[*], M. Guibout[*], E. Castanas[*], E. Goldstein[*],
C. Jaquet[*], F. Grisoli[**], P. Bert[***]

[*]Laboratoire des Hormones Protéiques - Faculté de Médecine
et Clinique Endocrinologique CHU Timone, Marseille, France;
[**]Clinique Neurochirurgicale, CHU Timone, [***]Clinique de
Neurophysiologie, CHU Timone.

INTRODUCTION

Anterior pituitary hormones are characterized by their episodic secretion patterns during the 24-hour period. Each
hormone displays periodic variations on an ultradian, circadian or monthly basis. This periodic hormone release is
dependent on neuroendocrine control mechanisms. In cases
of secreting pituitary tumors circadian variations of the
hypersecreted hormone are absent. This loss of rhythm has
been observed on GH profiles in acromegaly (1, 2), PRL
profiles in prolactinoma (3, 4) and on ACTH patterns in
Cushing's disease (5, 6).

The aim of this study was to analyse the 24-hour secretion
patterns of GH and PRL in patients with acromegaly, prolactinoma and mixed (GH and PRL) secreting adenoma. Studies
were performed in three distinct cases : 1° prior to treatment, 2° after tumorectomy and presumed cure, 3° after
long-term suppression of hypersecretion by bromocriptine.
Modifications of GH and PRL secretory rhythm in these studies furnished data allowing a better understanding of the
hormonal anomalies in these pituitary adenomas.

PATIENTS AND METHODS

Patients
Circadian studies were performed in 4 groups of subjects.

1. Normal_subjects
24-hour GH and PRL profiles were examined in a control group
of 10 healthy adult volunteers (7 women not on oral contra-

ceptives and 3 men), 21 to 35 years old.

2. Untreated patients with pituitary adenoma

Circadian patterns of GH and PRL plasma levels were studied
prior to all therapy in 12 acromegalics, 13 women with prolactinoma and in 4 patients with a mixed GH and PRL secreting adenoma. The acromegalic group was composed of 6 women and 6 men with a mean age of 49 years (range : 25-69
years). The mean 24-hour GH plasma value varied from
7.8 ± 2 to 98 ± 17 ng/ml (m ± SD). Each patient's mean GH
value is shown in Fig. 1. The 13 women with a PRL secreting adenoma were 16 to 37 years old (mean age : 24 years).
Their mean 24-hour PRL plasma level varied from 39 ± 7 to
3440 ± 600 ng/ml (Fig. 1). Four patients, 32 to 57 years
old, presented a syndrome of acromegaly associated with
hypersecretion of PRL. The mean 24-hour GH and PRL plasma
values varied from 9 ± 2 to 37 ± 18 ng/ml and 18 ± 5 to
61 ± 6 ng/ml, respectively.

3. After transsphenoidal surgery

This group only consists of patients (8 acromegalics, 9
women with a PRL secreting adenoma and 1 patient with mixed
GH + PRL hypersecretion) in whom normalization of hormone
hypersecretion (baseline GH level < 10 ng/ml; baseline PRL
level < 15 ng/ml) was evidenced immediately after surgery
and persisted during 1 to 5 years follow-up. Clinical data
and pre- and post-operative endocrine status in these patients have been reported in a previous study (7).

In the 8 acromegalics, the 24-hour mean GH plasma values
were 1.1 ± 0.9 to 10.8 ± 4.9 ng/ml, 1 to 4 years post-operatively. Dynamic studies of GH regulation (oral glucose,
intravenous TRH and oral bromocriptine) led to identify
2 sub-groups. Cases 1 to 5 (group 1) responded normally
to all 3 tests, whereas a paradoxical GH response to at
least one of the 3 stimuli was evidenced in cases 6 to 8
(group 2).

The 9 women, 16 to 41 years old, who underwent surgery for
a PRL secreting adenoma displayed 24-hour mean PRL plasma
levels from 4.7 ± 0.7 to 32.1 ± 15.6 ng/ml, 1 to 5 years
post-operatively. Post-operative pharmacodynamic tests

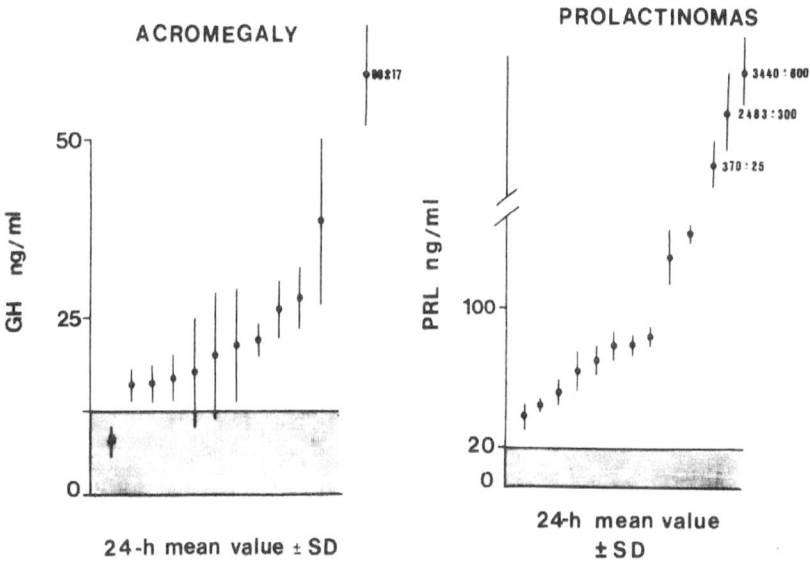

Figure 1 : Mean (± SD) 24-h plasma GH and PRL values in untreated acromegaly and prolactinoma. The stippled areas represent range of values in normals.

showed a return to normal PRL regulation (8) which was confirmed by the resumption of ovulation in all cases. Finally, in one 30 year old patient with hypersecretion of GH
and PRL, mean 24-h plasma levels of both hormones returned
to normal after surgery, i.e. GH : 2.5 ± 4 ng/ml, PRL :
2.6 ± 1.4 ng/ml.

4. Acromegalics treated by bromocriptine

In 5 acromegalics, administration of bromocriptine resulted
in reduction of residual GH hypersecretion which was evi-

denced after surgery. Prior to bromocriptine, but after surgery the baseline GH plasma levels ranged from 4.6 ± 1.0 to 77 ± 9 ng/ml. In 2 patients whose baseline GH plasma values were less than 10 ng/ml, bromocriptine therapy was started due to the persistence of a paradoxical GH rise after TRH and the existence of a fall in GH plasma levels after bromocriptine.

METHODS
24-hour studies
Two types of circadian studies were performed. The following study was made in the group of acromegalics after surgery, in 3 of the 5 acromegalics on postoperative bromocriptine and in one untreated patient with acromegaly. Before blood sampling the patients spent two nights in an air conditioned soundproof room. Lights were turned off between 2200 and 0600 h and during this time period sleep was continuously monitored by nucchal electromyography, electroencephalography (EEG) and eye movement recording. On the third day, an indwelling catheter was inserted in the antecubital vein and GH and PRL 24-h profiles were determined from blood samples withdrawn every 20 minutes. Meals were given at 0800, 1300 and 2000 h. During the daytime patients were free to move about. During the lights-off period blood samples were taken remotely and the timing of sampling was recorded on the EEG tracing. The EEG recordings were analyzed by 15 second sequences according to established criteria for defining sleep stages (9) and results were computer-processed to obtain hypnograms.

Circadian studies in all other patients were performed by the same technique, except that blood samples were withdrawn hourly and EEG sleep recordings were not made.

Hormone assays
RIAs of GH and PRL plasma levels were performed using commercial reagent kits (IRE, CEA, SORIN, Gif sur Yvette, France). In conditions used in this study, the normal baseline GH plasma level was 2.4 ± 1.2 ng/ml (mean ± SE) and that of PRL was 7.3 ± 1.1 ng/ml based on a control group of

32 women and 18 men, 18-52 years old. Intra- and inter-
assay variabilities did not exceed 7.5 % and 10 %, respectively. During 24-h studies, plasma levels were measured in
duplicate at appropriate dilutions. Measurements were performed as a single series in order to eliminate between
assay variability. RIA data were computed as described previously (8).

Statistical analysis

Analysis of GH and PRL circadian profiles was performed after dividing the 24-hour period into three equal intervals,
i.e. morning (0600-1340 h), afternoon (1400-2140 h) and
night (2205-0540 h). Analysis was performed on log transformed data in order to achieve homogeneity of variance.
Two-way analysis of variance followed by the Student's t
test was used to evaluate the statistical significance of
differences between patients and time periods. The residual variance was used as a common estimation of the standard deviation.

To evaluate differences between daytime (morning plus afternoon) and nighttime secretion, the method of linear contrast focused on comparisons between group means was used,
followed by one-way analysis of variance (10).

RESULTS

24-h secretory patterns in normal subjects

The mean 24-h GH plasma levels (mean of the 24 blood samples) showed a large dispersion in this group, the mean
value ranging from 1.3 ± 1.2 to 11.8 ± 13.9 ng/ml. Each
patient's circadian profile demonstrated the presence of
pulsatile bursts of GH secretion (defined as at least a
two-fold increase over the preceding plasma value). These
secretory spikes varied, in number (3-6 during the 24-h
period), amplitude and duration. Low level GH secretory
activity (GH < 1 ng/ml) occurred between the bursts. In
all cases a rise in GH plasma levels was detected around
the time of sleep onset.

The mean 24-h PRL levels were more homogeneous in this
group, ranging from 8.1 ± 6.2 to 18.3 ± 10.3 ng/ml. Analysis

of the overall 24-hour secretory patterns showed that minimum PRL secretion (nadir) occurred between 1000 and 1200 h
and that maximum plasma levels (zenith) were reached between
0100 and 0400 h. After dividing the 24-h period into 3
intervals (I : morning; 0700-1400 h; II : afternoon : 1500-
2200 h; III : night, 2300-0600 h), the lowest mean PRL
plasma level was found during the morning, whereas the
highest mean level occurred at night. In all cases, the
mean nightime PRL levels were significantly greater than
those observed during each of the daytime periods ($P < 0.05$)

24-hour GH and PRL secretory patterns in untreated patients
with pituitary adenoma

In 10 of the 12 acromegalics, the mean 24-h GH values (GH
< 30 ng/ml) showed the presence of moderate hypersecretion.
The circadian GH profile varied from case to case. Secretory bursts were sometimes observed, especially in the cases with high GH plasma levels. In most of the remaining
cases, the amplitude of GH fluctuations was small. None of
the patients displayed low level secretory activity. A
rise in GH levels was not found at the onset of sleep, as
illustrated in one patient presenting a low level of GH
hypersecretion (Fig. 2).

In 11 of the acromegalics, PRL plasma levels were analyzed
during the 24-h period and demonstrated the presence of an
abnormal circadian rhythm. In 8/11 cases, the mean 24-h
PRL plasma levels (1.1 ± 0.3 to 4.9 ± 0.7 ng/ml) were less
than the mean value in normal adults (Fig. 3). In 8 patients, the mean nightime PRL values did not differ significantly from those measured during the daytime periods.

Among the 13 cases of prolactinoma, 10 patients displayed
a mean 24-h PRL level ranging from 39 ± 7 to 141 ± 5 ng/ml,
with slight fluctuations occurring during the 24-h period.
In the remaining 3 patients who displayed higher secretion
levels, PRL variations were more pronounced. The 24-h
profiles consistently showed the absence of both the PRL
secretion zenith and nadir (Fig. 4). In 11/13 cases, a
normal GH plasma profile persisted with 2-5 pulsatile
bursts of GH secretion occurring during the 24-h period. In

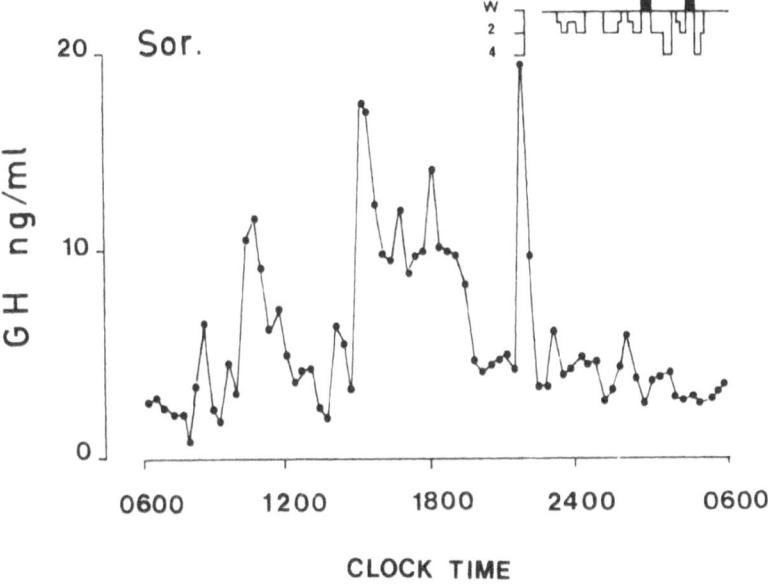

	Glucose		TRH		Bromocriptine	
	basal	test	basal	test	basal	test
GH ng/ml	4.0	22.0	3.2	14.5	6.5	10

Figure 2 : Circadian GH variations in acromegalic with the lowest level of GH secretion. Sleep histograms are shown at top. Rapid eye movement, waking, stage 2 and 4 sleep. Table at bottom of figure shows the paradoxical responses to dynamic tests.

10 of the 11 cases a sleep-related GH rise was observed. However, in three of these cases the mean GH plasma level was very low and although diurnal and nocturnal bursts of GH secretion were present, their amplitude was very small.

In the cases of mixed GH and PRL secreting tumors, the circadian profiles of both hormones showed the loss of normal secretory rhythm. The secretion level and circadian fluctuations of each hormone varied independently.

24-hour GH and PRL profiles after surgery

In the 9 cases of prolactinoma, the mean PRL plasma level for the entire group was 12.8 ± 10.1 ng/ml 1 to 4 years after surgery, and thus was very similar to the mean value in the normal group (13.1 ± 8.9 ng/ml). In 8 cases, the mean

214

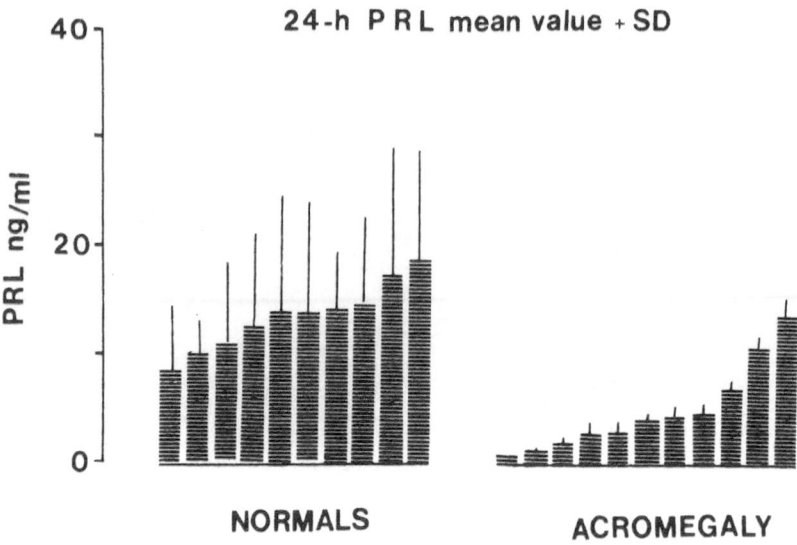

Figure 3 : Histogram showing mean (± SD) 24-hour PRL levels in untreated acromegalics compared to normal subjects.

nighttime PRL levels were significantly higher than those
detected during the daytime periods (P < 0.01). The lowest
level of PRL secretion was found in the morning in 7 of the
8 cases (Fig. 5a). In one patient (Mil.), 24-hour studies
were performed on several occasions 1 month to four years
after surgery (Fig. 5b). One month postoperatively, the
24-hour plasma profile showed that PRL values ranged from
1 to 4 ng/ml without significant circadian variations. On
the other hand, one year after surgery a physiological
rhythm of PRL secretion was observed and persisted throughout the 4 year follow-up period. In all 9 cases, the normal circadian GH pattern present preoperatively persisted
after surgery.

PROLACTINOMAS

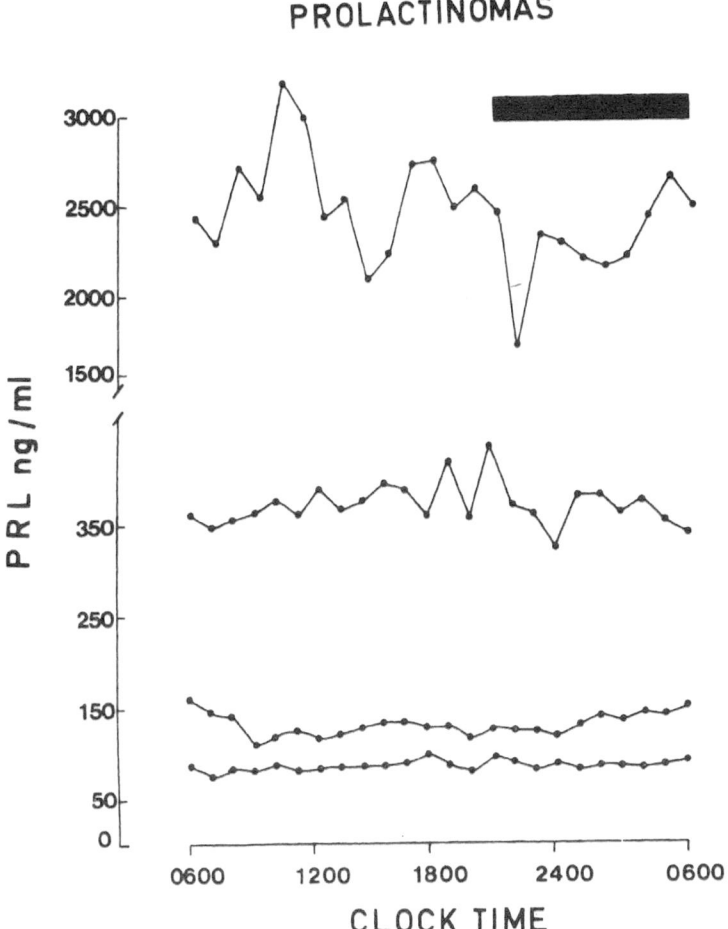

Figure 4 : 24-hour PRL profiles in 4 untreated cases of prolactinoma. Heavy bar at top indicates night.

In acromegaly : Group I patients (cases 1 to 5) were studied 1 to 4 years after surgical cure (Fig. 6). Analysis of GH plasma levels in each patient evidenced 1 to 4 GH bursts during the day. Plasma levels of GH remained at low levels (about 1 ng/ml) between the bursts. During sleep a

PROLACTINOMAS

Post Surgery

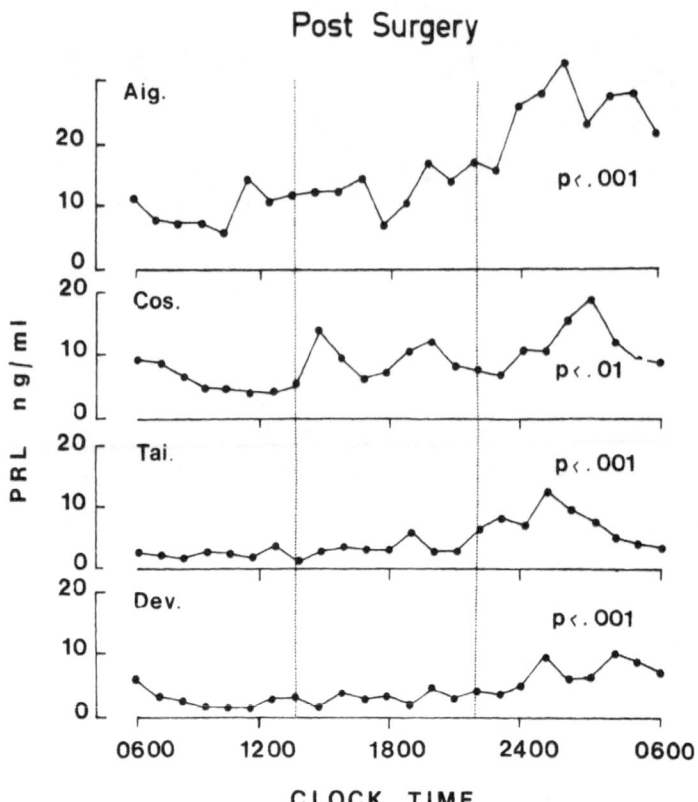

Figure 5a : Postoperative 24-h PRL profiles in 4 of 9 patients, 1 to 4 yrs after surgery. Dotted vertical lines divide the 24-h period into 3 intervals, morning, afternoon and night. Nocturnal values are significantly higher than during the 2 daytime periods.

GH rise was observed in strict correlation to deep sleep (stages 3-4) in cases 1 and 2. In the other 3 patients, a GH rise occurred around the onset of sleep but did not coincide with the stages of deep sleep. In all group I patients 24-h studies showed that PRL plasma values were significant-

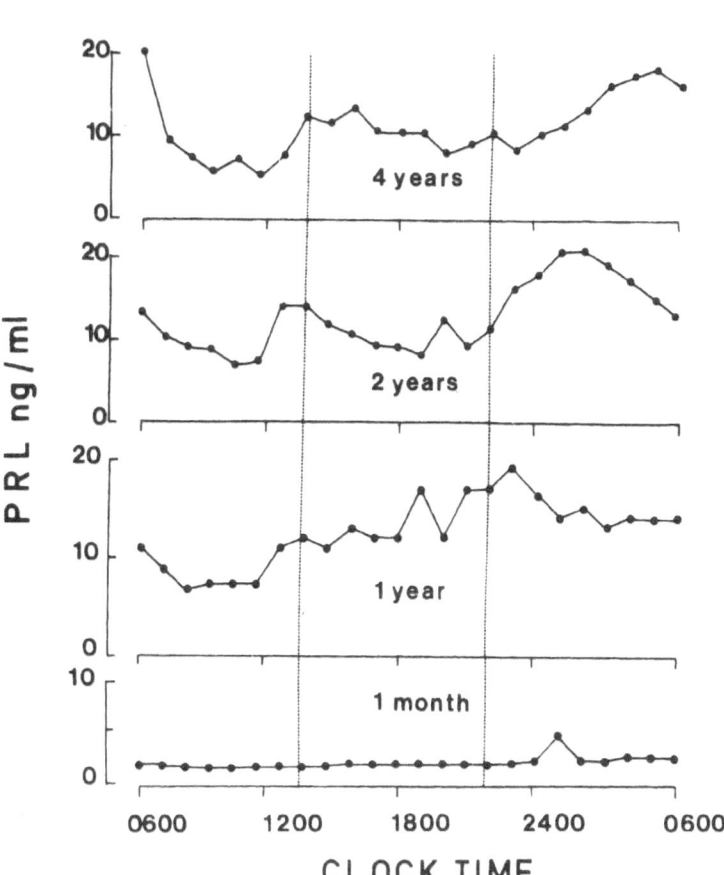

Figure 5b : 24-h PRL secretion pattern in one patient, 1 mo to 4 years after removal of prolactinoma.

ly higher during the night (P < 0.001). The mean 24-hour PRL value was at the lower limit of the normal range (2.5 ± 1.3 to 8.4 ± 4.8 ng/ml).

In case 5, as in the previously described cases of prolactinoma, a normal GH rhythm did not resume immediately after surgery. In this patient studied 3, 12 and 18 months

218

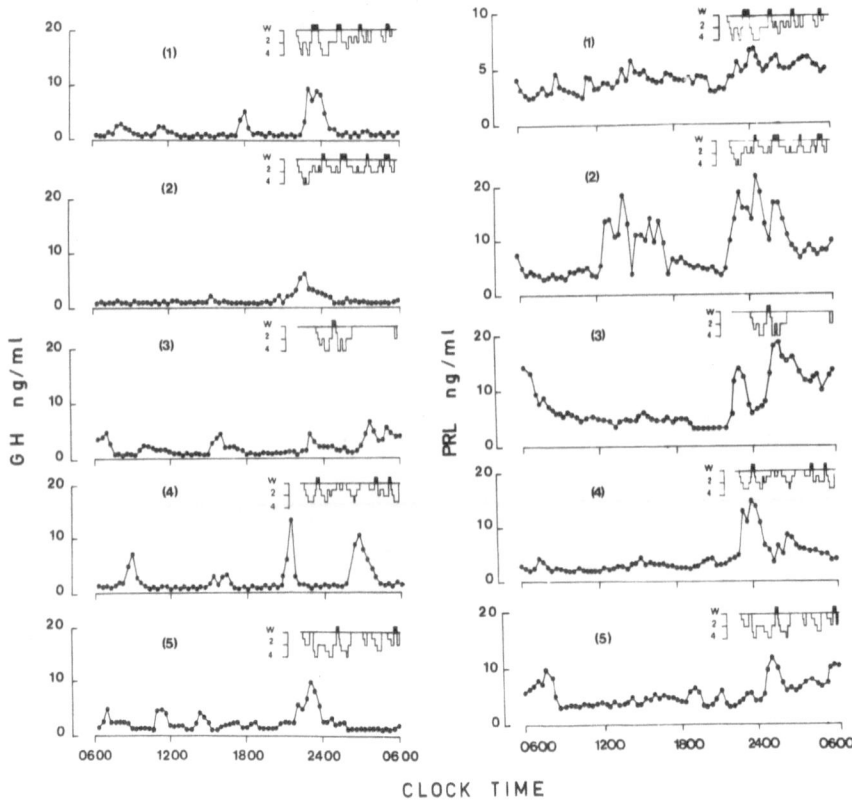

CLOCK TIME

Figure 6 : 24-h GH and PRL secretion patterns in group I acromegalics, 1-4 yr after surgery. Sleep histograms as in Fig. 2. Case nb is shown in brackets.

postoperatively, diurnal GH pulsatility and a clear nocturnal rise were found only 12 and 18 months after surgery. At 3 months postoperative follow-up GH levels were less than 2 ng/ml throughout the 24-h period. Details of the data in this case are presented elsewhere (11).

In the group II patients (cases 6 to 8) GH secretory patterns were consistently abnormal 1 to 4 years after surgery (Fig. 7). Periods of low secretory activity were not detected and the 24-h profiles in cases 7 and 8 displayed bursts of GH secretion occurring at random times without a sleep-related nocturnal rise. 24-hour secretion profiles demonstrated that plasma PRL levels were consistently less than 5 ng/ml. In cases 6 and 8, a significant nocturnal

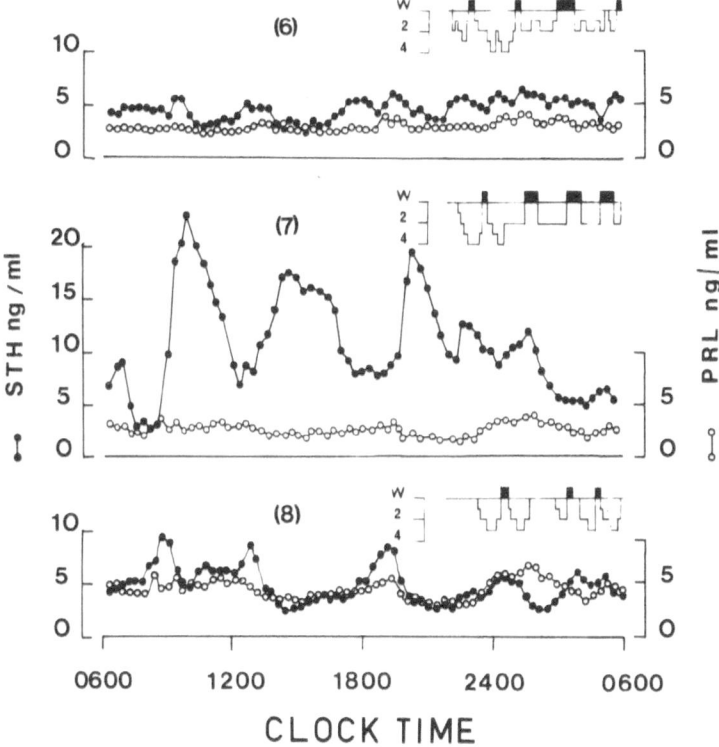

Figure 7 : 24-h GH and PRL profiles in group II acromegalics 1-4 yr after surgery. Case nb is shown in brackets.

PRL rise was observed despite the fact that PRL levels were low.

Circadian variations in GH and PRL levels were also measured before and after surgery in one patient with a mixed GH and PRL secreting adenoma. Plasma levels of both hormones returned to normal values postoperatively. Resumption of a normal GH secretory pattern occurred postoperatively, as in the previously presented cases.

24-hour GH profiles in acromegalics on bromocriptine
In 2 patients, the mean GH plasma level was 77 and 14 ng/ml prior to therapy. After 6 months of bromocriptine (5 mg t.i.d.) 24-hour studies were performed (Fig. 8). In the first patient, a fall in GH plasma levels of at least 50 % was observed 1 to 3 hours after each dose of bromocriptine,

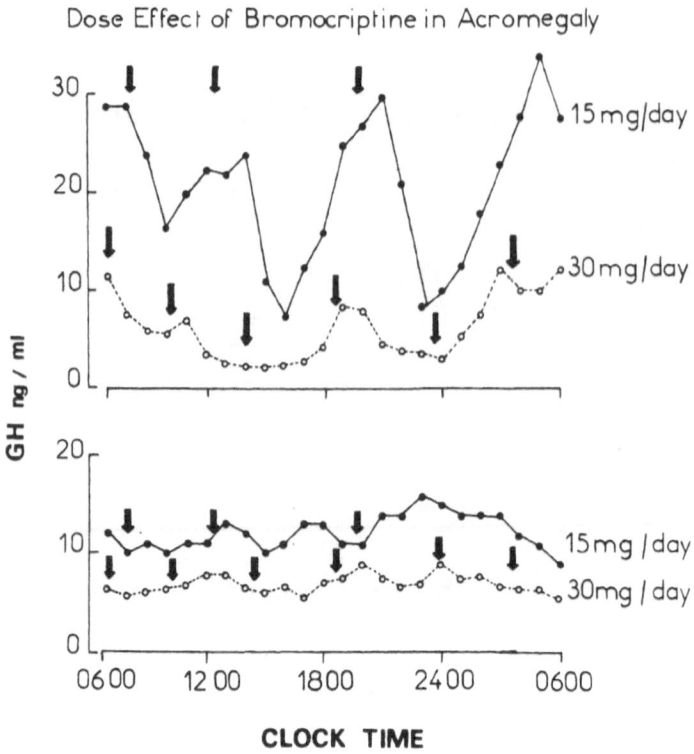

Figure 8 : 24-hour GH profiles in 2 acromegalics on bromocriptine therapy. Arrows indicate timing of each 5 mg oral dose.

followed by a rebound. The mean 24-h GH plasma value was 20.7 ± 7.5 ng/ml. In the second patient, the 24-hour mean GH plasma value (12.2 ± 1.8 ng/ml) did not differ from the pretherapeutic level and circadian GH variations were not observed. Studies of 24-h patterns were done again in both cases after administration of 30 mg bromocriptine per day. Each patient's GH profile was similar to that observed after 15 mg bromocriptine. In the first patient, 30 mg bromocriptine yielded a more pronounced GH suppressive effect and in the second case GH values were lowered after the higher dose of bromocriptine.

In three other patients presenting moderate postoperative levels of residual GH hypersecretion, the mean circadian GH value was significantly lower after 15 mg bromocriptine

therapy. No nocturnal rise at the onset of sleep was detected. However, in one patient a clear GH rise occurred in
the second half of the night (Fig. 9).

DISCUSSION

Hypersecretion of GH and PRL in acromegaly (1, 2) and in
patients with a PRL secreting adenoma (3, 4) is characterized by loss of 24-hour secretory rhythm of the hormones. In
these pathological states the loss of the normal secretory
pattern is independent of the level of hypersecretion since
such a loss is found even in cases of slightly active acromegaly where baseline plasma levels of GH are less than 10
ng/ml (12). Disrupted circadian regulation was found prior
to all treatment in one of our acromegalic patients (Fig. 4)
who presented pronounced diurnal fluctuations of GH levels,
ranging from 2 to 17 ng/ml, without daytime periods of low
secretory activity nor a nocturnal GH rise. These anomalies
of GH and PRL secretory rhythm are apparently a specific
feature of secreting pituitary tumors. Indeed, in the
hyperprolactinemic states of pregnancy (13) or during longstanding estrogen therapy (14) a normal 24-hour PRL profile
is maintained, despite the presence of PRL hypersecretion.
Likewise, in cases of high level pituitary stimulation due
to peripheral hormone deficiency, secretory rhythms persist.
This has been demonstrated in cases of ACTH hypersecretion
with cortisol deficiency in Addison's disease (15) or in
congenital adrenal hyperplasia (16). In these pathological
conditions, the reactional hypersecretion of ACTH consistently displays a 24-hour profile featuring a clear rise at
the end of the night.

Regarding the pathological interpretation of secreting pituitary tumors, the origin of the disrupted circadian profiles is currently open to debate. The loss of 24-hour GH
and PRL patterns could be related to a primary anomaly involving the regulation of hypothalamic catecholamines or
neuropeptides controlling the secretion of anterior pituitary
hormones. For example, in the rat bilateral lesions of the
ventromedial hypothalamic nuclei or administration of

222

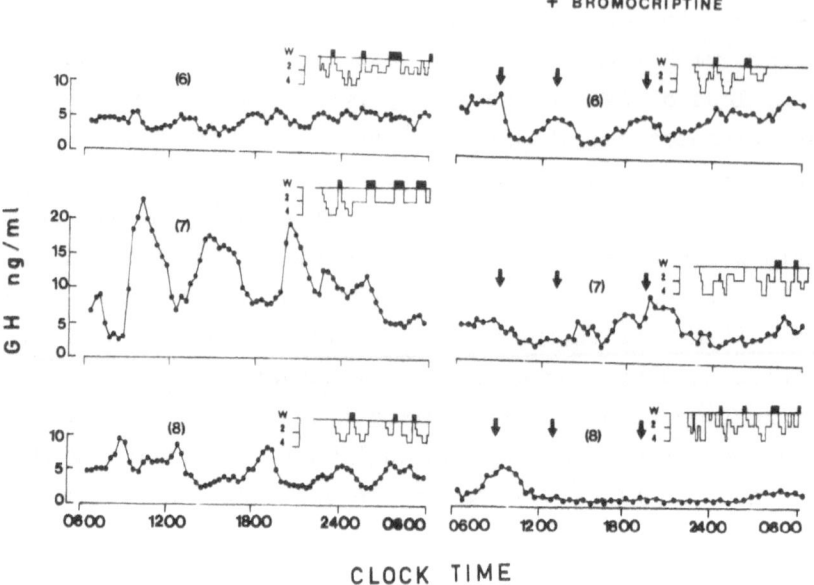

Figure 9 : Group II acromegalics : 24-h GH secretion patterns before
(left) and during (right) the third month of 15 mg daily bromocriptine
therapy. Timing of 5 mg oral doses is shown by arrows. Sleep histograms as in Fig. 2.

somatostatin significantly decrease the pulsatile pattern
of GH secretion (17). In certain cases of human pituitary
tumors this view is further supported by the loss of periodic regulation involving not only the hypersecreted hormone
but also other anterior pituitary hormone functions. In
Cushing's disease, the loss of circadian ACTH rhythm is
sometimes accompanied by abnormal 24-hour profiles of plasma GH and PRL (18). Conversely, the loss of secretory
rhythm may reflect the autonomous behavior of the pituitary
adenoma which no longer responds to physiologic stimuli. In
acromegaly, abnormal GH responses to TRH (19) and to dopaminergic drugs (20) have been observed in more than 50 % of
cases. These paradoxical responses to pharmacodynamic
stimuli are related to dedifferentiation of the tumor cells,

as recently shown in studies of such tumors in vitro (21).
Accordingly, if the loss of hormonal secretory rhythms
results from the primary autonomy of these pituitary adenomas, then total selective adenomectomy allowing conser-
vation of both healthy pituitary tissue and the hypothalamo
pituitary connections should lead to full cure accompanied
by a return to normal circadian rhythm of the involved hormone. The resumption of physiological GH and PRL secretory patterns after tumor removal in our cases of acromegaly
and prolactinoma lends support to the latter hypothesis.
Similar observations have been reported in one case of
acromegaly (22) and in Cushing's disease (23, 24).

In the majority of our cases of untreated acromegaly circadian studies demonstrated the existence of inappropriate
PRL regulation. The mean 24-hour PRL values were at the
lower limit of the normal range and the secretory rhythms
were characterized by the consistent loss of the nocturnal
PRL rise. Excess growth hormone in rats (25) with subcutaneous implants of GH_3 pituitary tumor cells or intra-
peritoneal injection of GH is able to suppress pituitary
production of PRL and to reduce TSH secretion. In our
cases, the return to normal PRL regulation when GH plasma
values fell to normal levels also suggests that the GH
hypersecretion may have altered the synthesis or turnover
of hypothalamic neuromediators involved in PRL regulation,
thus leading to abnormally low PRL plasma levels.

Repeated evaluations of 24-hour GH and PRL plasma profiles
demonstrated a delayed resumption of physiological regulation of the two hormones. During the 1-3 month period
following interruption of pathological hypersecretion, PRL
and GH levels were characterized by low amplitude plasma
profiles and the absence of periodic secretion. Similar
transient deficiencies have also been described after surgical removal of corticotropic adenomas (26). This transient disruption of regulation is not only found in pituitary tumors. A similar situation involving reversible
corticotropin deficiency has been described in subjects
after interruption of longstanding corticosteroid therapy

(27) or after surgical removal of adrenal adenoma (28). The delayed return to normal PRL or GH regulation after adenomectomy is currently poorly understood. In our patients, stimulation of GH by arginine or hypoglycemia (data not shown) showed weak responses when tested 3 months postoperatively, after which normal responsiveness resumed. Recent studies in rats bearing ectopic PRL and GH secreting pituitary tumors (29) showed that the excess PRL induces a selective increase of dopamine synthesis in the hypothalamus. Increased dopamine release into the portal pituitary circulation has also been demonstrated in pregnant rats (30). It is thus conceivable that the tumoral hormone excess, acting through short loop feedback, is able to modify the activity of hypothalamic structures which, after

tumor removal would require a certain delay before returning to normal activity. The existence of such anomalies is suggested by the inappropriate variations in plasma catecholamine levels occurring after pharmacological stimulations by bromocriptine and LHRH in acromegaly and prolactinoma (31, 32).

Comparison of 24-h GH profiles before and after bromocriptine therapy shows that the drug produced a variable GH-suppressive response in the 5 patients receiving 15 or 30 mg daily. This variable responsiveness is directly related to the tumor cells, as previously shown in adenomas studied in vitro using a cell culture system (33). In our patients (cases 6-8), despite the return to normal GH plasma values, resumption of physiological GH secretion rhythm was not found. Particularly, none of the patients displayed a nocturnal GH rise at the onset of sleep. In another study (34), a nocturnal GH rise was reported in 6 acromegalics on bromocriptine therapy. The authors pointed out that this nocturnal rise did not follow a physiological pattern since the GH plasma values increased gradually, reaching maximum levels during the second half of the night and did not correlate to the stages of sleep. It should be noted that in these patients the mean GH plasma levels under bromocriptine therapy were around 20 ng/ml. Because of the partial blocking of GH hypersecretion in these cases, the rise occurring in the second part of the night may have been due to the escape of tumoral secretion some time after the last dose of bromocriptine.

In conclusion, analysis of GH and PRL 24-hour profiles after total selective adenoma removal shows that plasma levels of these hormones return to normal and physiological secretory rhythms resume after a postoperative refractory period. In acromegaly, the abnormally low levels of PRL secretion also regress after tumorectomy. During the 1 to 5 years follow-up in this study, modifications of the normal GH and PRL secretory patterns were not observed. Our results argue in favor of a solely pituitary origin of the disturbed hormone rhythms encountered in these tumors.

ACKNOWLEDGEMENTS

The authors express their gratitude to the technicians of the Laboratoire des Hormones Protéiques who performed the RIA measurements. The expert secretarial assistance of Mrs. N. Hastert was greatly appreciated. This work was supported by INSERM grant 78.5.034.4

REFERENCES

1. Cryer, PE, WH Daughaday, Regulation of growth hormone secretion in acromegaly. J Clin Endocrinol Metab 29:1102, 1969

2. Carlson, HE, JC Gillin, P Gorden and F Snyder, Absence of sleep related growth hormone peaks in aged normal subjects and in acromegaly. J Clin Endocrinol Metab 34:1102, 1972

3. Jacobs, LS and WH Daughaday, Pathophysiology and control of prolactin secretion in patients with pituitary and hypothalamic disease, In: Human Prolactin , Pasteels, JL, C Robyn (eds.),Excerpta Medica, 189, 1973

4. Boyar, RM, S Kapen, JW Finkelstein, M Perlow, JF Sassin, DK Fukushima, ED Weitzman and L Hellman, Hypothalamic-pituitary function in diverse hyperprolactinemic states. J Clin Invest 53:1588, 1974

5. Krieger, DT, Factors influencing the circadian periodicity of plasma corticosteroids levels. Chronobiologia 1:195, 1974

6. Krieger, DT and SM Glick, Growth hormone and cortisol responsiveness in Cushing's syndrome. Am J Med 52:25, 1972

7. Guibout, M, P Jaquet, JC Lissitzky, F Grisoli and F Vincentelli, Résultats de l'exérèse transsphénoïdale des adénomes hypophysaires sécrétants. Ann Endocr (Paris) 39:95,1978

8. Jaquet, P, F Grisoli, M Guibout, JC Lissitzky and P Carayon, Prolactin secreting tumours. Endocrine status before and after surgery in 33 women. J Clin Endocrinol Metab 46:459, 1978

9. Rechtsaffen, A and A Kales, A manual of standardized terminology, techniques and scoring system for sleep stages of human subjects. National Institute of Neurological Disease and Blindness, Neurological Information Network, Bethesda, Md, 1968

10. Armitage, P, Statistical methods in medical research. Blackwell, Oxford, 217, 1971

11. Jaquet, P, M Guibout, C Jaquet, F Grisoli, B Conte-Devolx, D Dumas and J Bert, Circadian regulation of GH secretion after treatment in acromegaly. J Clin Endocrinol Metab 50:322, 1980

12. Mims, R and J Bethune, Acromegaly with normal fasting growth hormone regulation. Ann Int Med 81:781, 1974

13. Boyar, RM, JW Finkelstein and S Kapen, 24 hr prolactin secretory patterns during pregnancy. J Clin Endocrinol Metab 40:1117, 1975

14. Vekemans, M and C Robyn, The influence of exogenous estrogen on the circadian periodicity of circulating prolactin in women. J Clin Endocrinol Metab 40:886, 1975

15. Graber, AL, JR Givens, WE Nicholson, DP Island and GW Liddle, Persistence of diurnal rhythmicity in plasma ACTH concentrations in cortisol-deficient patients. J Clin Endocrinol Metab 25:11, 1965

16. West, DC, JB Stanchfield, JB Atcheson, ML Rallison and FH Tyler, Circadian variation in plasma ACTH and cortisol and its precursor in congenital adrenal hyperplasia. Clinical Research 21:190 (Abs), 1973

17. Martin, JB, LP Renaud and P Brazeau, Pulsatile growth hormone secretion : suppression by hypothalamic ventromedial lesions and by long-acting somatostatin. Science 186:538, 1974

18. Krieger, DT, PJ Howanitz and AG Frantz, Absence of nocturnal elevation of plasma prolactin concentrations in Cushing's disease. J Clin Endocrinol Metab 42:260, 1976

19. Irie, M and T Tsushima, Increase of serum growth hormone concentration following thyrotropin-releasing hormone injection in patients with acromegaly or gigantism. J Clin Endocrinol Metab 38:200, 1974

20. Chiodini, PG, A Liuzzi, L Botalla, G Gremascoli and F Silvestrini, Inhibitory effect of dopaminergic stimulation on GH release in acromegaly. J Clin Endocrinol Metab 38:200, 1974

21. Ishibashi, M and T Yamaji, Effect of thyrotropin-releasing hormone and bromoergocriptine on growth hormone and prolactin secretion in perfused pituitary adenoma tissues of acromegaly. J Clin Endocrinol Metab 47:1251, 1978

22. Bachelot, J, JM Muller, H Millet, H De Rougemont and J Tourniaire, Régulation normale de la sécrétion d'hormone de croissance chez un patient guéri par exérèse d'une tumeur hypophysaire. Ann Endocr (Paris) 34:398, 1973

23. Lagerquist, LG, AW Meikle, CA West and FH Tyler, Cushing's disease with cure by resection of a pituitary adenoma. Amer J Med 57:826, 1974

24. Boyar, RM, M Witkin, A Carruth and J Ramsey, Circadian cortisol secretory rhythms in Cushing's disease. J Clin Endocrinol Metab 48:760, 1979

25. Seo, H, S Refetoff and VS Fang, Induction of hypothyroidism and hypoprolactinemia by growth hormone producing rat pituitary tumors. Endocrinology 100: 216, 1977

26. Tyrrel, JB, RM Brooks, PA Fitzgerald, PH Cofoid, PH Forsham and CB Wilson, Cushing's disease selective transsphenoidal resection of pituitary microadenomas. New Engl J Med 298:753, 1978

27. Liddle, GW, Endocrine and other physiological derangements following long term glucocorticoid therapy. Chronobiological Aspects of Endocrinology, Symposia Medica Hoechst, 401, 1974

28. Krieger, DT and G Gewirtz, Recovery of pituitary adrenal function, growth hormone responsiveness and sleep EEG pattern in a patient following removal of an adrenal cortical adenoma. J Clin Endocrinol 38:1075, 1974

29. Perkins, NA, TC Westfall, CV Paul, R Mac Leod and AD Rogol, Effect of prolactin on dopamine synthesis in medical basal hypothalamus : evidence for a short loop feedback. Brain Research 160:431, 1979

30. Ben-Jonathan, N, C Oliver, HJ Weiner, RS Mical and JC Porter, Dopamine in hypophysial portal plasma of

the rat during the estrous cycle and throughout pregnancy. Endocrinology 100:452, 1977

31. Van Loon, GR, Abnormal catecholamine responses in
acromegalics. J Clin Endocrinol Metab 48:784, 1979

32. Van Loon, GR, A defect in catecholamine neurons in
patients with prolactin-secreting pituitary adeno-
mata. Lancet 2:868, 1978

33. Guibout, M, P Jaquet, E Goldstein, C Lucas and F
Grisoli, Effects of TRH and bromocriptine in acromegaly in vivo and in vitro studies. In: Synthesis
and Release of Adenohypophyseal Hormones : cellular
and molecular mechanism, Mc Kerns, KW (ed.). Plenum,
New York, 753, 1979

34. Chihara, K, Y Kato, H Abe, M Furumoto, K Maeda and H
Imura, Sleep-related growth hormone release following
2-bromo-ergocriptine treatment in acromegalic patients. J Clin Endocrinol Metab 44:78, 1977

DISCUSSION

BARDIN: I was interested in your patients showing a refractory period after the removal of the adenoma. How many patients did you have who were acromegalic but also had suppressed prolactin even after surgery? Also, do you feel that you have evidence showing that GH from the tumor can suppress GH from the normal cells and that PRL from the tumor can suppress PRL secretion from the remainder of the pituitary, etc?

JAQUET: We had 8 patients who resumed 24 hour PRL patterns at normal levels with the sleep increase. Regarding the second point, one should remember the work of Nancy Perkins in rats. After injecting GH_3 cells, she was able to demonstrate that an acceleration of the synthesis of dopamine occurred in the hypothalamus. Thus, the explanation could be that GH excess stimulates dopaminergic neurons which in turn block prolactin secretion.

BARDIN: Don't those tumors also make prolactin?

JAQUET: We have studied them in vitro in primary cell culture. The 24-hour release of one million cells in a Petri dish is low. We search for contamination or mixed secretion. Compared to normal cells, very little PRL is produced.

L'HERMITE: Concerning the possible regulation of PRL secretion by GH, we have observed a similar effect in hypopituitary children treated with GH for one year. PRL levels were in the normal range but, at the end of this 1-year treatment with GH, PRL levels were significantly lower than before treatment. Regarding PRL rhythms in patients with prolactinomas, in such patients treated for a long time with bromoergocryptine without surgery, there has been, in some instances, normalization of PRL secretion after interruption of bromoergocryptine treatment and even possibly disappearance of an adenoma. We have a case treated with bromoergocryptine by Dr. Copinschi for about 9 years. When

bromoergocryptine was interrupted, PRL levels remained
low for about 5 months and then increased. One month
after the interruption of the bromoergocrytpine, a 24-
hour study was performed and no PRL elevation associated
with sleep was observed. We would thus suggest that the
restoration of the rhythm would be the best indicator of
a real cure. Do you have any experience of such cases
supposedly cured after bromoergocryptine treatment only?
Finally, did you have any hyperprolactinemic patients
who underwent surgery and in whom no microadenoma was found
but had instead for example hyperplasia of PRL secreting
cells? How was the PRL rhythm? In some of our hyperprolactinemic patients, for example in patients with primary
myxedema in which we suppose there is hyperplasia of PRL
cells and no PRL microadenoma, we found a normal PRL rhythm.

JAQUET: We have not seen any medical cure of adenoma.
We have no 24-hour study of PRL in these conditions. Are
there hyperplastic forms of pituitary tumors secreting
PRL? Certainly. We have 5 or 6 cases in which an adenoma
was tentatively diagnosed but no tumor was found at surgery.
Indeed, neuropathological data revealed hyperplasia of
both cell lines controlling PRL and LH. The involvement
of LH has been evidenced using an anti β-LH antiserum.
Curiously, in those patients, we observed that the PRL 24-
hour pattern could be normal or abnormal with or without
a nocturnal rise but that the LH pattern was very similar
to what is generally observed in patients with polycystic
ovaries syndrome, that is, high LH levels and low FSH
levels. I think that, in this specific case, there is
hyperplasia of PRL cells but the pathological interpretation may differ from what might be observed in patients
with adenomas.

L'HERMITE: I wonder whether one could use the blunt-
ing of the nocturnal surge of PRL as a diagnostic predic-
tive test of the existence of an adenoma.

JAQUET: Certainly not. Indeed, in various conditions such as pregnancy or under treatment with neuroleptics, the nocturnal surge is not clearly present.

HANSEN: We and several others infused somatostatin in acromegalic patients and generally found that the GH levels can be suppressed to a certain extent but not beyond a certain point, even if the amount of somatostatin infused is increased to near toxic doses. One interpretation is that one can only suppress one fraction or one type of GH. Is it your impression that a similar effect on GH level is observed in the studies where bromoergocryptine is infused in acromegalic patients?

JAQUET: There seems to be a critical time period in the treatment with bromoergocryptine. In one patient whom we studied after one year of treatment and after two years of treatment, we observed once lowering of the 24-hour mean GH level and once an escape from bromoergocryptine inhibition. Moreover, it seems difficult, from our limited experience, to lower the GH level very substantially. The decrease is always partial, even with high doses of bromoergocryptine.

CIRCADIAN VARIATION OF PLASMA GROWTH HORMONE IN NORMAL SUBJECTS AND DIABETIC PATIENTS. EFFECTS OF SOMATOSTATIN INFUSION, AGE AND BODY WEIGHT

Aage Prange Hansen and Stig Engkjaer Christensen

First and Second University Clinic of Internal Medicine, Kommunehospitalet, 8000 Aarhus C, Denmark

INTRODUCTION

When these studies were initiated late in 1968 the 24-h plasma growth hormone pattern in normal subjects was just discovered. Hunter and Rigal (1) had reported raised plasma growth hormone values during night in children. Quabbe and coworkers (2) had found in adults low day time plasma growth hormone values, intermittent bursts during night with high peaks occurring during times of deeper sleep. Glick and Goldsmith (3) had shown an effect of various feeding procedures on the 24-h plasma growth hormone level. Takahashi et al. (4) and Honda et al. (5) had demonstrated that the release of growth hormone during night coincides with the onset of electroencephalographically determined deep sleep. Experiments in which they had delayed or interrupted sleep provided evidence that the nocturnal growth hormone secretion was related to the onset of sleep and did not reflect a true endogenous circadian rhythm in growth hormone secretion. Extensive studies by Parker and coworkers (6, 7) have amply confirmed and extended these findings

24-H GROWTH HORMONE SECRETION IN NORMALS AND DIABETICS

We were interested in studying the 24-hour growth hormone secretion in diabetic patients. This was because we knew that pituitary ablation followed by hormonal substitution

234

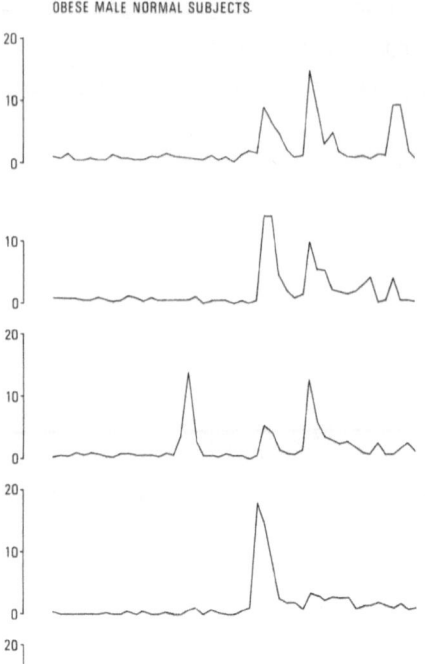

24-hr. GROWTH HORMONE LEVELS (ng/ml) IN 5 YOUNG NON-OBESE MALE NORMAL SUBJECTS.

Figure 1.

not as high as in the young juvenile diabetics (11). The values in the old obese maturity-onset diabetics (Fig. 6) are very low without distinct peaks during day or at sleep onset (11). Fig. 7 gives the mean 24-h growth hormone levels in the three groups of diabetic patients studied and their matched controls. As was clear already from the individual curves, the 24-h growth hormone level is 2-4 times higher in the young juvenile diabetics and in the old lean was able to inhibit the further development of retinopathy in juvenile diabetic patients (8). We therefore believed that the growth hormone secretion in one way or the other was abnormally elevated in these patients.

All experiments started in the morning with overnight fasted subjects. Blood was collected half-hourly or hourly from indwelling venous catheters. Heparin was not used. During the study the subjects were at leisure, sitting, talking, listening to the radio and moving quietly around in the rooms. They slept only during night where great precautions were taken in order to prevent sleep disruptions. No electroencephalographic monitoring of sleep was performed.

In order to clarify this presentation we have decided not to include results from studies in females. It is well known that the growth hormone secretion in females is increased, especially around ovulation (9).

Fig. 1 shows the growth hormone level in 5 young non-obese normals. The pattern is identical to that found earlier by others, with low day time values, some postprandial peaks and sleep-onset peaks (10). Fig. 2 shows the growth hormone levels in 7 old non-obese normals. "Old" indicate in this and all following studies ages between 40 and 70 years. The basal line level during day-time is a bit more fluctuating with less discernible postprandial peaks. The sleep- onset peaks are lower and more inconsistent, although these subjects slept as well and as deep as the younger ones, estimated clinically (11). Fig. 3 shows the growth hormone values in 9 old obese normals. All growth hormone peaks are clearly suppressed in this group (11).

Three age and body weight matched groups of diabetic patients were now studied. Fig. 4 shows the growth hormone levels in young juvenile diabetics. The pattern is wildly fluctuating without distinct postprandial peaks, but discernible and high sleep-onset peaks (10). The pattern of wild fluctuation is also seen in a group of old lean maturity-onset diabetics (Fig. 5), although the peak values are

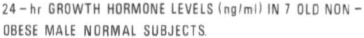

24 – hr GROWTH HORMONE LEVELS (ng/ml) IN 7 OLD NON – OBESE MALE NORMAL SUBJECTS.

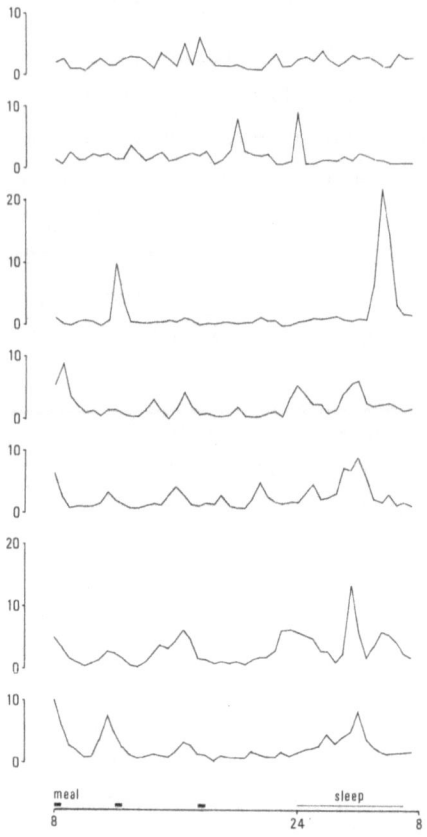

Figure 2.

maturity-onset diabetics than in their controls. The mean level however, was equally suppressed in the obese maturity-onset diabetics and the obese normals.

Although it has been shown that the metabolic clearance rate of growth hormone is somewhat reduced in diabetic patients, the many sudden and high growth hormone peaks observed in these patients indicate an increased secretion

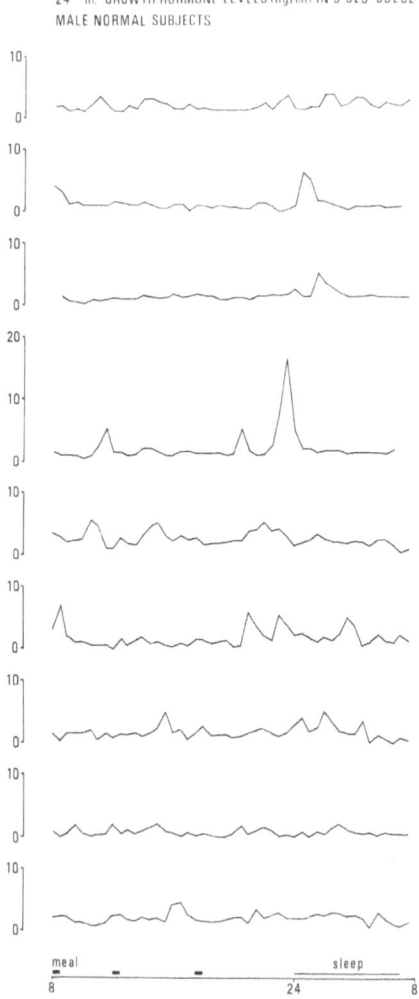

Figure 3.

rate as the major factor in the growth hormone abnormality.

It has been possible to show that the growth hormone hypersecretion in diabetes is due to the deranged metabolism and
not to a primary factor characterizing diabetes mellitus.
This conclusion was drawn because it could be shown that

238

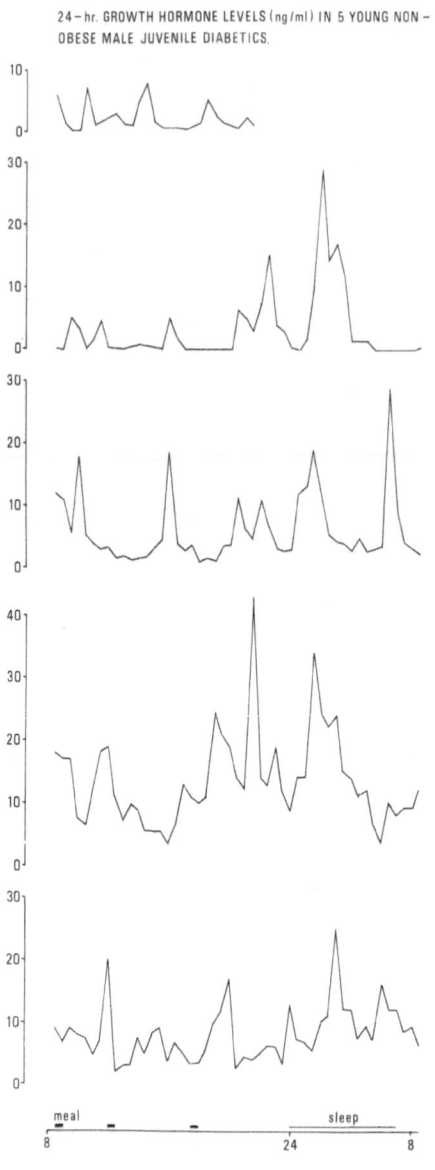

24-hr. GROWTH HORMONE LEVELS (ng/ml) IN 5 YOUNG NON-OBESE MALE JUVENILE DIABETICS.

Figure 4.

very strict diabetes control over prolonged periods of time
could normalize the growth hormone hypersecretion (12, 13).
Also, prediabetics and juvenile diabetics in complete

24 – hr GROWTH HORMONE LEVELS (ng/ml) IN 10 OLD NON –
OBESE MALE MATURITY–ONSET DIABETICS.

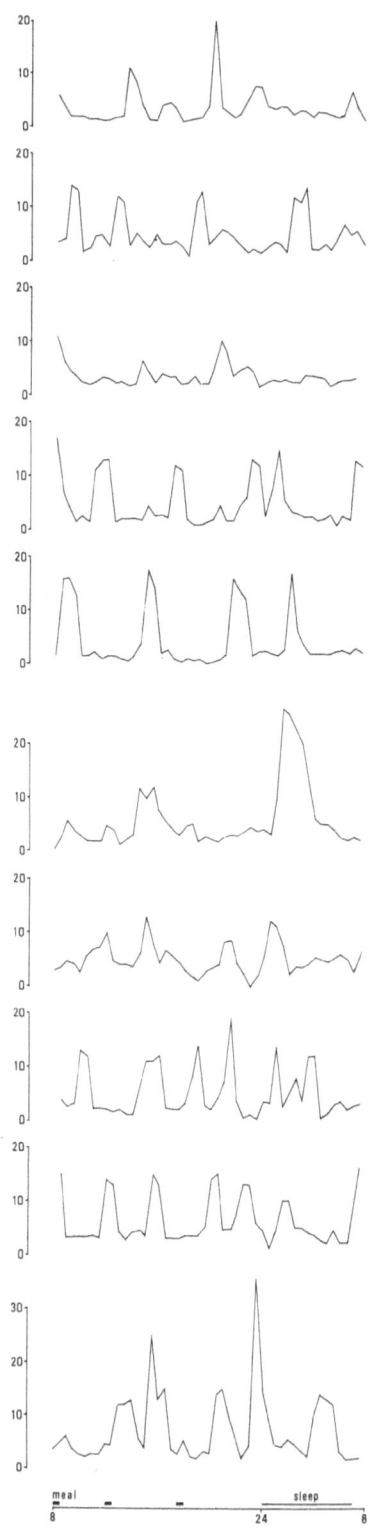

Figure 5.

240

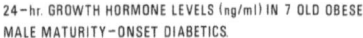

24-hr. GROWTH HORMONE LEVELS (ng/ml) IN 7 OLD OBESE
MALE MATURITY-ONSET DIABETICS.

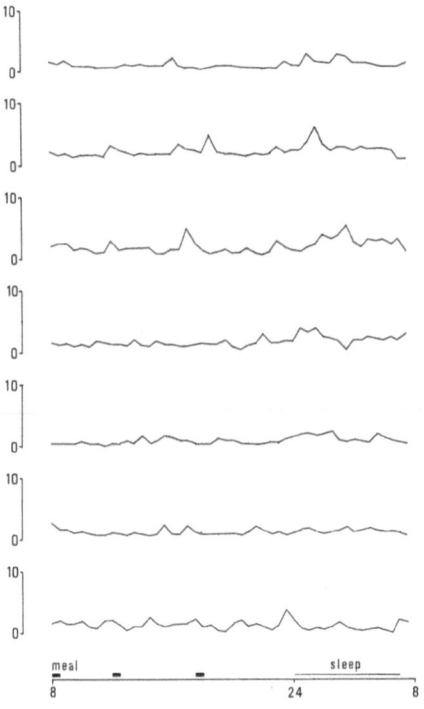

Figure 6 :

remission have normal 24-h growth hormone patterns, and
finally patients with secondary diabetes have highly fluctuating 24-h plasma growth hormone levels as have patients
with juvenile diabetes (14). It has not been possible,
however, to characterize the factor or metabolite responsible for the growth hormone hypersecretion, although we
know by now that the factor can be removed by hemodialysis
(15).

In order to study the growth hormone release during the
night in more detail in normal subjects, Parker et al. (16,
17) induced acute hyperglycemia by glucose infusion and
found that the sleep-onset growth hormone peak remained unchanged. The same finding was obtained by others (18). The

24-hr. GROWTH HORMONE LEVELS (ng/ml)

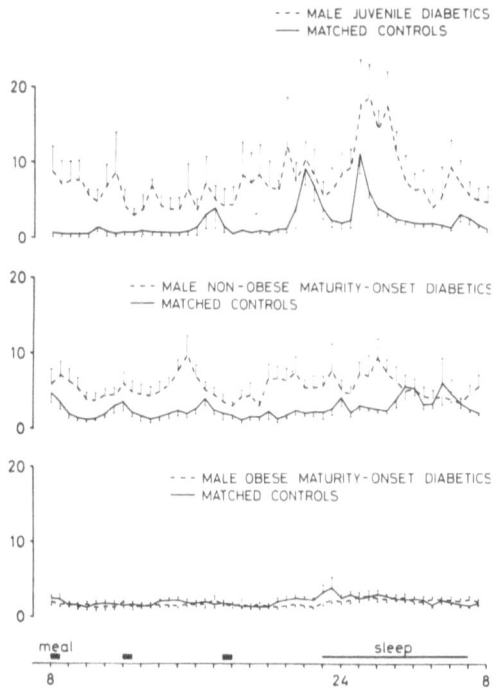

Figure 7 :

infusion of alpha and beta-adrenergic blockers was also
unable to modify the sleep-onset growth hormone peak (19).
On the other hand Lucke et al. (20) and Lipman et al. (21)
found that the infusion of lipids and heparin resulting
in a 2-4 times increase in plasma free fatty acids was able
to suppress the growth hormone release during deep sleep.
These results may indicate a regulatory role of free fatty
acids in modulating growth hormone secretion. Many questions are still to be answered, however, before this simple
negative feed-back mechanism between plasma free fatty acids
and growth hormone, already discussed by Hunter and Rigal
(1) and Quabbe et al. (2), can be demonstrated. We were not
able to inhibit the growth hormone hypersecretion in diabetic patients by infusions of glucose or lipids plus heparin
(22, 23).

24-H SOMATOSTATIN INFUSION

Parker et al. (24) demonstrated early that infusion of the growth hormone release inhibiting hormone, somatostatin, was able to inhibit the sleep-onset growth hormone peak in normal subjects without interfering with the electroencephalographic recorded sleep patterns. We tested somatostatin in normal subjects for its ability to suppress the postprandial and the sleep-onset growth hormone peaks and in diabetics for its ability to suppress the growth hormone hypersecretion. Fig. 8 shows the effect of somatostatin infusion (4 mg/24 h) in 5 young non-obese normal subjects. All spontaneous, postprandial and sleep-onset growth hormone peaks are completely blocked. Cessation of somatostatin infusion results sometimes in a large rebound secretion (25). Fig. 9 shows the effect of somatostatin infusion (2 mg/24 h) on the growth hormone hypersecretion in 4 young juvenile diabetics. In most cases somatostatin inhibits the spontaneous and sleep-onset peaks, but occasionally a peak breaks through (25). Fig. 10 shows the effect of a large somatostatin dose (6 mg/24 h) on the growth hormone hypersecretion in 4 young juvenile diabetics. As before, somatostatin infusion results in a clearcut suppression of the many growth hormone peaks, but a few peaks break through. Cessation of somatostatin infusion sometimes results, as in normals, in rebound secretion (25). Old maturity-onset diabetics, non-obese as well as obese, react to somatostatin infusion as do young normals and young juvenile diabetics (Figs. 11, 12) (26).

SIGNIFICANCE OF AGE AND BODY WEIGHT

The preceding results gave the impression that the circadian growth hormone secretion, especially the number and height of growth hormone peaks, decreased with increasing age and body weight in both normal subjects and diabetics. In order to verify statistically this impression, two parameters representative of the circadian growth hormone secretion were selected, namely the mean 24-h plasma growth hormone level and the highest plasma growth hormone peak

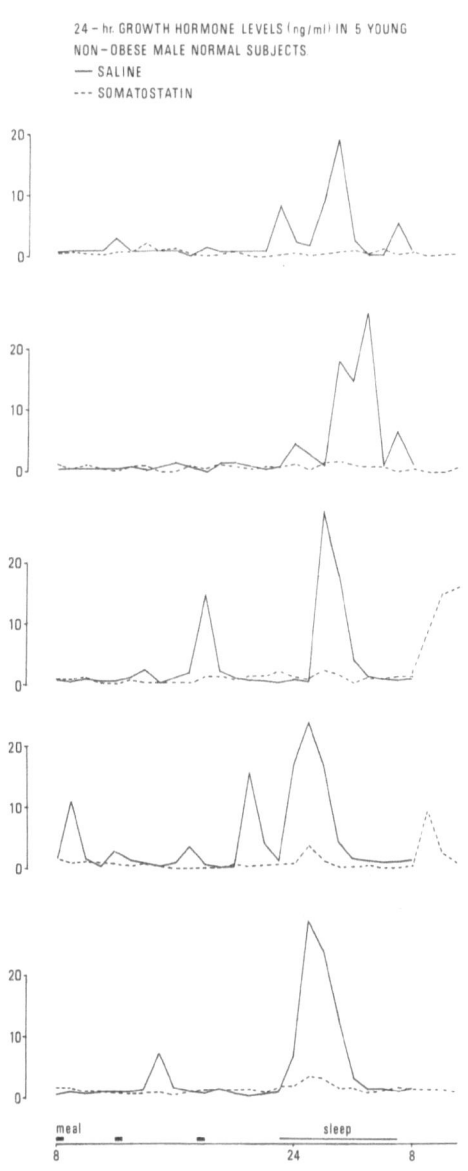

24 - hr. GROWTH HORMONE LEVELS (ng/ml) IN 5 YOUNG
NON-OBESE MALE NORMAL SUBJECTS.
— SALINE
--- SOMATOSTATIN

Figure 8.

during the night.

When the effects of age were examined,only non-obese subjects
could be included in the calculations because the studies
did not comprise groups of young obese normals and,for

244

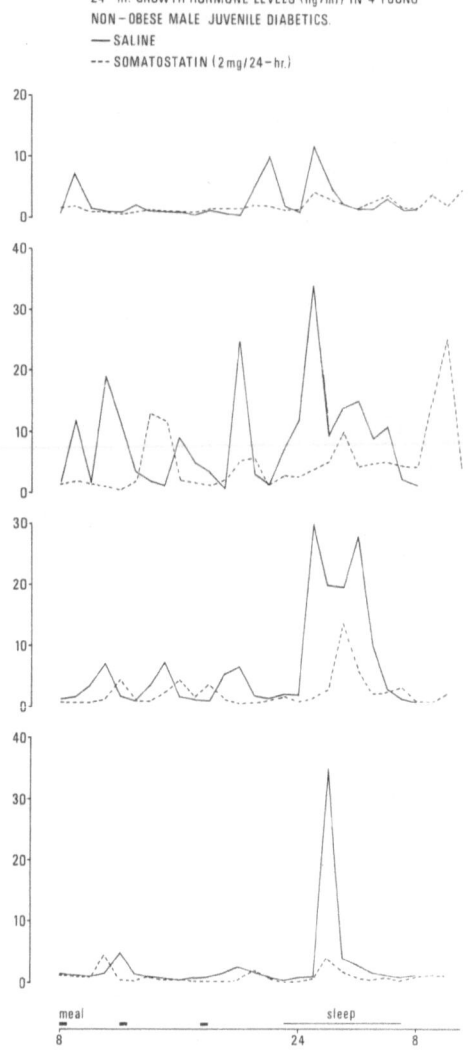

24- hr. GROWTH HORMONE LEVELS (ng/ml) IN 4 YOUNG
NON-OBESE MALE JUVENILE DIABETICS.
—SALINE
--- SOMATOSTATIN (2mg/24-hr.)

Figure 9.

obvious reasons, young obese juvenile diabetics.

In the diabetics (n = 38), a significant negative correlation was demonstrated between the mean 24-h plasma growth hormone level and age (r = - 0.48; p < 0.005) (Fig. 13); and between the night peak plasma growth hormone value and age (r = - 0.65; p < 0.0001) (Fig. 14).

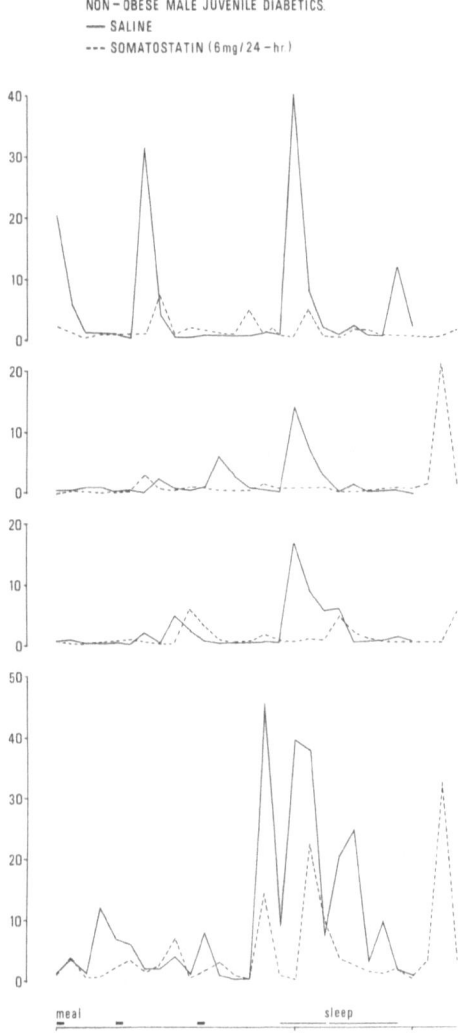

24 - hr. GROWTH HORMONE LEVELS (ng/ml) IN 4 YOUNG
NON - OBESE MALE JUVENILE DIABETICS.
— SALINE
--- SOMATOSTATIN (6 mg / 24 - hr.)

Figure 10.

In the normal subjects (n = 17), a significant negative correlation was demonstrated only between the night peak plasma
growth hormone value and age (r = - 0.82; p < 0.0001) (Fig.
15). The mean 24-h plasma growth hormone level could not
be correlated to age, probably because plasma growth hormo-

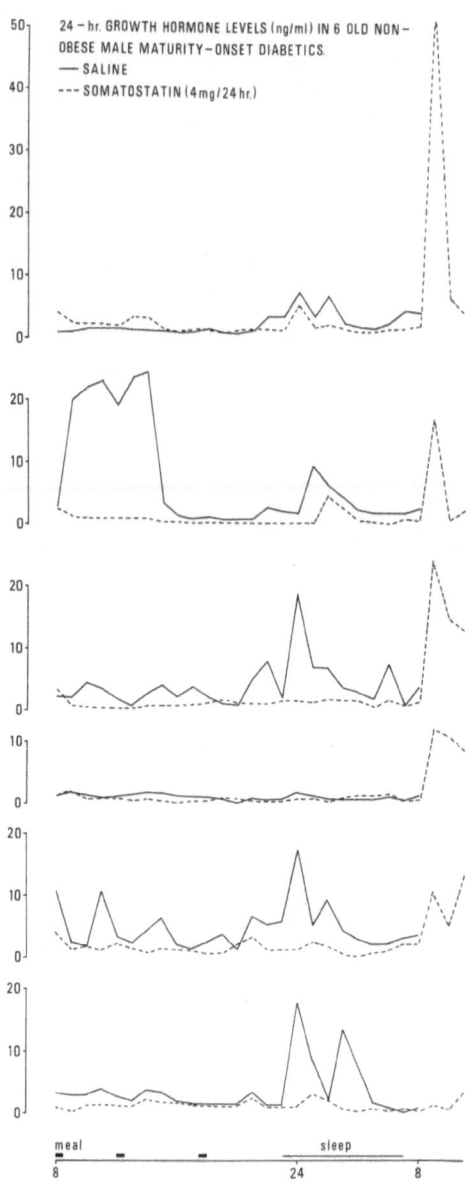

Figure 11.

ne in normal subjects is very low throughout day and night except for the physiological peaks occurring postprandially, after heavy exercise and at sleep-onset.

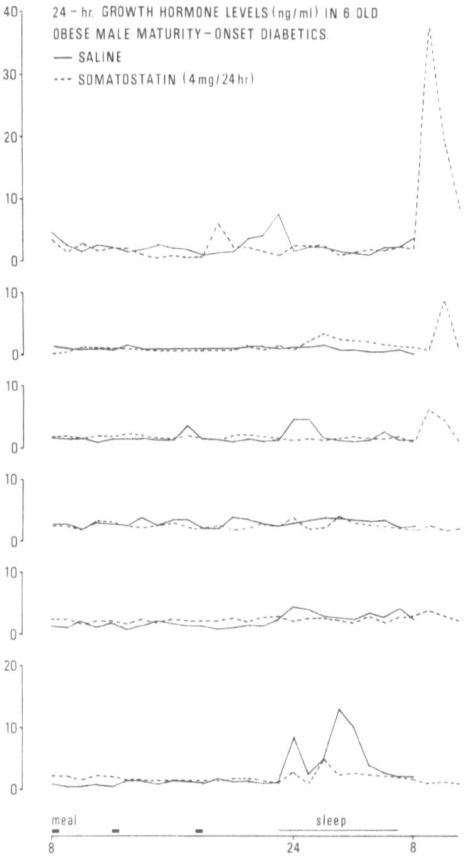

Figure 12.

The negative correlation between growth hormone secretion and age demonstrated here is compatible with the finding of Carlson et al. (27) of absent sleep-onset growth hormone peaks in 4 out of 6 normal subjects studied over the age of 50 years. Three of the 4 non-responders developed electro-encephalographically determined deep sleep.

When the effects of body weight were examined, only the old group of subjects could be included in the calculation, again, because the studies did not comprise groups of young obese normals and diabetics.

248

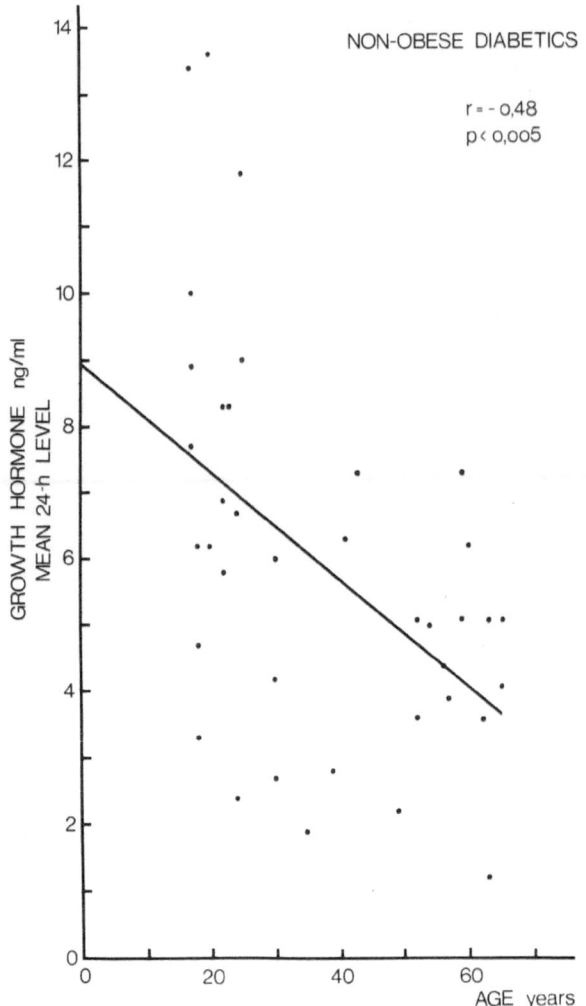

Figure 13.

In the diabetics (n = 29), a significant negative correlation
was demonstrated between the mean 24-h plasma growth hormone level and body weight (r = - 0.64; p < 0.001) (Fig.
16); and between the night peak plasma growth hormone value
and body weight (r = - 0.56; p < 0.01) (Fig. 17).

In the normal subjects (n = 16), a significant negative correlation was demonstrated only between the mean 24-h plasma

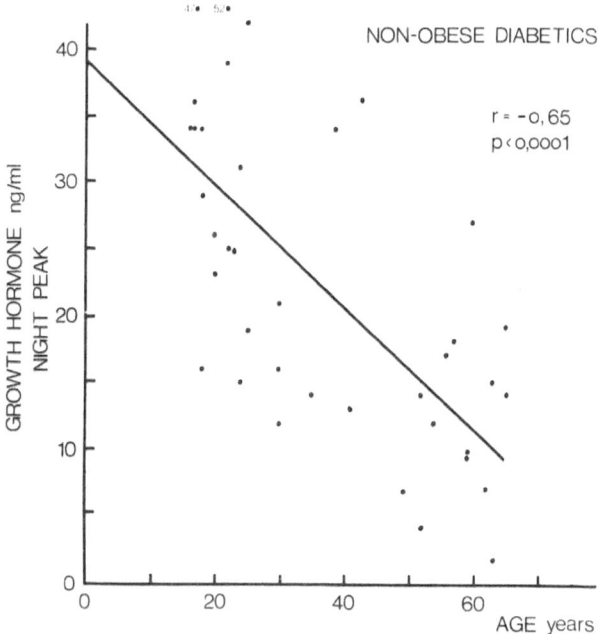

Figure 14.

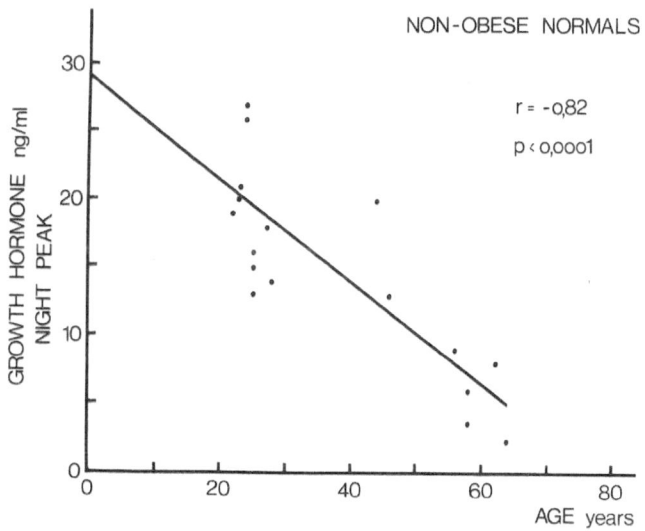

Figure 15.

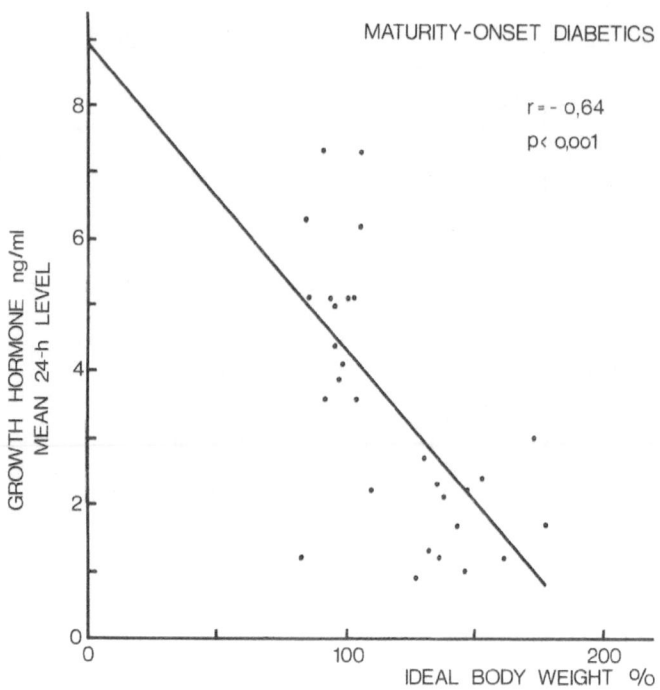

Figure 16.

growth hormone level and body weight (r = - 0.61; p < 0.05) (Fig. 18).

The negative correlation between the circadian growth hormone secretion and body weight demonstrated here is in accordance with the finding of Quabbe et al. (28) of fewer and smaller night-time plasma growth hormone peaks in obese children and with the finding of Copinschi et al. (29) that the difference between integrated day-time and night-time plasma growth hormone values were abolished in obese adults, but became normal at the end of a 12-day fast.

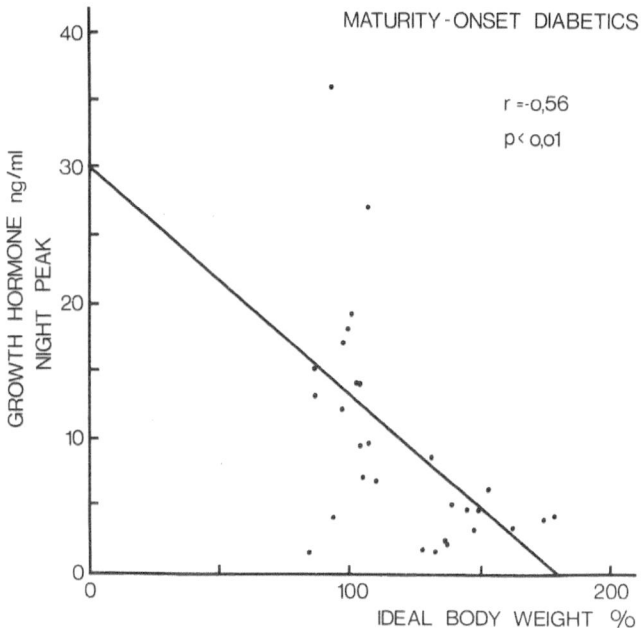

Figure 17.

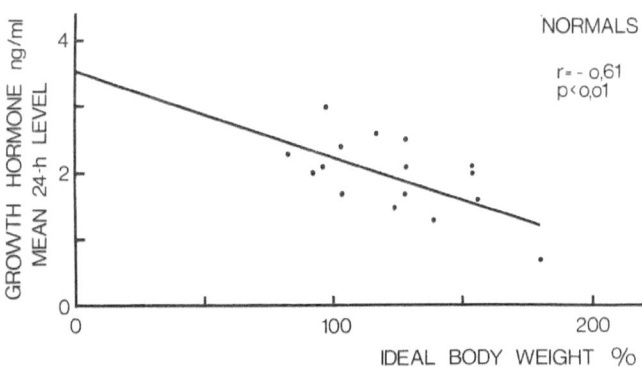

Figure 18.

SUMMARY

1. The circadian growth hormone secretion in normal subjects is characterized by low day-time values, postprandial peaks and sleep-onset peaks or deep-sleep
   peaks.

2. The circadian growth hormone secretion in diabetic subjects is wildly fluctuating without distinct postprandial peaks, but distinct   and high sleep-related
   peaks.

3. The circadian growth hormone secretion is 2-4 times
   higher in juvenile and lean maturity-onset diabetics
   than in matched controls. The secretion is equally
   suppressed in obese diabetics and normals.

4. Somatostatin infusion inhibits the postprandial and
   sleep-related growth hormone peaks in normals and the
   many spontaneous peaks in diabetics, but a few peaks
   break through.

5. A negative correlation can be demonstrated between the
   circadian growth hormone secretion and age in normals
   and diabetics.

6. A negative correlation can also be demonstrated between
   the circadian growth hormone secretion and body weight
   in normals and diabetics.

ACKNOWLEDGEMENTS

Professor Knud Lundbaek is thanked for his indefatigable
inspiration and help through this study. We are also
grateful to Inga Bisgaard and Joan Hansen for their excellent technical assistance. The Danish Medical Research
Council and P. Carl Petersen's Foundation have supported
the studies.

REFERENCES

1. Hunter, WM, and WM Rigal, The diurnal pattern of plasma growth hormone concentration in children and adolescents. J Endocrinol 34:147-153, 1966

2. Quabbe, HJ, E Schilling, and H Helde, Pattern of growth hormone secretion during a 24-hour fast in normal adults. J Clin Endocrinol Metab 26:1173-1177, 1966

3. Glick, SM, and SG Goldsmith, The physiology of growth hormone secretion, In: Growth Hormone, Pecile, A, and EE Müller (eds.). Proceedings of the First International Symposium, Milan, Italy, September 11-13, Amsterdam, Excerpta Medica Foundation, 1968, pp 84-88

4. Takahashi, Y, DM Kipnis, and WH Daughaday, Growth hormone secretion during sleep. J Clin Invest 47:2079-2090, 1968

5. Honda, Y, K Takahashi, S Takahashi, K Azumi, M Irie, M Sakuma, T Tsushima, and K Shizume, Growth hormone secretion during nocturnal sleep in normal subjects. J Clin Endocrinol Metab 29:20-29, 1969

6. Parker, DC, JF Sassin, JW Mace, RW Gotlin, and LG Rossman, Human growth hormone release during sleep Electroecenphalographic correlation. J Clin Endocrinol Metab 29:871-874, 1969

7. Sassin, JF, DC Parker, JW Mace, RW Gotlin, LC Johnson, and LG Rossman, Human growth hormone release : relation to slow-wave sleep and sleep-waking cycles. Science 165:513-515,1969

8. Lundbaek, K, R Malmros, HC Andersen, JH Rasmussen, E Bruntse, PH Madsen, and VA Jensen, Hypophysectomy for diabetic angiopathy. A controlled clinical trial, In:Supplement to the Proceedings of the Sixth Congress of the International Diabetes Federation, Stockholm, 1967, Östman, J, and RDG Molner (eds.). Amsterdam, Excerpta Medica Foundation, 1969, p 127-139

9. Hansen, AaP, and J Weeke, Fasting serum growth hormone levels and growth hormone responses to exercise during normal menstrual cycles and cycles of oral contraceptives. Scand J Clin Lab Invest 34:199-205, 1974

10. Hansen, AaP, and K Johansen, Diurnal patterns of blood glucose, serum free fatty acids, insulin, glucagon and growth hormone in normals and juvenile diabetics. Diabetologia 6:27-33, 1970

11. Kjeldsen, H, AaP Hansen, and K Lundbaek, Twenty-four hour serum growth hormone levels in maturity-onset diabetics. Diabetes 24:977-982, 1975

12. Johansen, K, and AaP Hansen, Diurnal serum growth hormone levels in poorly and well-controlled juvenile diabetics. Diabetes 20:239-245, 1971

13. Hansen, AaP, Abnormal serum growth hormone response to exercise in juvenile diabetics. J Clin Invest 49: 1467-1478, 1970

14. Hansen, AaP, T Ledet, and K Lundbaek, Growth hormone and diabetes, In:Handbook of Diabetes Mellitus, Brownleed, M (ed.). New York, Garland STPM Press, 1980, in press

15. Hansen, AaP, HE Hansen, H Ørskov, R Nosadini, G Noy, and KGMM Alberti, Normalization of growth hormone hypersecretion in uremic diabetics and non-diabetics. Studies with artificial pancreas and artificial kidney, In: Proceedings of the XVIth Congress of the European Dialysis and Transplant Association. Amsterdam, June 1979, in press

16. Parker, DC, and LG Rossman, Human growth hormone release in sleep : nonsuppression by acute hyperglycemia. J Clin Endocrinol Metab 32:65-76, 1971

17. Parker, DC, and LG Rossman, Sleep release of human growth hormone in treated juvenile diabetics. Similarity to normal subjects and nonsuppression by hyperglycemia. Diabetes 20:691-695, 1971

18. Schnure, JJ, P Raskin, and RL Lipman, Growth hormone secretion during sleep : impairment in glucose tolerance and nonsuppressibility by hyperglycemia. J

Clin Endocrinol Metab 33:234-241, 1971

19. Lucke, C, and SM Glick, Experimental modification of the sleep-induced peak of growth hormone secretion. J Clin Endocrinol Metab 32:729-736, 1971

20. Lucke, C, Adelman, N, and SM Glick, The effect of elevated free fatty acids (FFA) on the sleep-induced human growth hormone (hGH) peak. J Clin Endocrinol Metab 35:407-412, 1972

21. Lipman, RL, AL Taylor, A Schenk, and DH Mintz, Inhibition of sleep-related growth hormone release by elevated free fatty acids. J Clin Endocrinol Metab 35:592-594, 1972

22. Hansen, AaP, The effect of intravenous glucose infusion on the exercise-induced serum growth hormone rise in normals and juvenile diabetics. Scand J Clin Lab Invest 28:195-205, 1971

23. Hansen, AaP, The effects of intravenous infusion of lipids on the exercise-induced serum growth hormone rise in normals and juvenile diabetics. Scand J Clin Lab Invest 28:207-212, 1971

24. Parker, DC, LG Rossman, TM Siler, J Rivier, SSC Yen, and R Guillemin, Inhibition of the sleep-related peak in physiologic human growth hormone release by somatostatin. J Clin Endocrinol Metab 38:496-499, 1974

25. Christensen, SE, AaP Hansen, J Weeke, and K Lundbaek, 24-hour studies of the effects of somatostatin on the levels of plasma growth hormone, glucagon and glucose in normal subjects and juvenile diabetics. Diabetes 27:300-306, 1978

26. Christensen, SE, AaP Hansen, and K Lundbaek, Somatostatin in maturity-onset diabetes. Diabetes 27:1013-1019, 1978

27. Carlson, HE, JC Gillin, P Gorden, and F Snyder, Absence of sleep-related growth hormone peaks in aged normal subjects and in acromegaly. J Clin Endocrinol Metab 34:1102-1105, 1972

28. Quabbe, HJ, H Helge, and S Kubichi, Nocturnal growth hormone secretion : correlation with sleep   EEG

in adults and pattern in children and adolescents
with non-pituitary dwarfism, overgrowth and with
obesity. Acta Endocrinol (Kbh) 67:767-783, 1971

29. Copinschi, G, MH Delaet, JP Brion, R Leclercq, M
L'Hermite, C Robyn, E Virasoro, and E Van Cauter,
Simultaneous study of cortisol, growth hormone and
prolactin nyctohemeral variations in normal and
obese subjects. Influence of prolonged fasting in
obesity. Clin Endocrinol (Oxf) 9:15-26, 1978

DISCUSSION

DESIR: You gave no quantitative information regarding the degree of control of the blood glucose levels in your subjects. What was the effect of somatostatin on blood glucose levels? Somatostatin has very complex effects in diabetes and can induce marked hyperglycemia, particularly if infused at such doses during 24 hours. Do you have any idea regarding the correlation between the control of the blood glucose levels and the degree of abnormality of the GH pattern?

HANSEN: Our studies were performed in juvenile diabetes and adult onset diabetes under poor diabetes control with blood glucose levels between 200 mg/dl and 400 mg/dl. Some of the subjects were slightly ketotic but most of them were not. In other studies we have shown that, by controlling the diabetes better, such as by giving insulin several times a day, or over a prolonged period, the GH level can be normalized but first the glucose levels have to be totally normalized for several days. The patient has to be hospitalized.

DESIR: Do you have recordings of the blood glucose fluctuations? What do you call "normal" blood glucose? In juvenile diabetes, it is very exceptional to be able to normalize the blood glucose levels by means of subcutaneous injections of insulin.

HANSEN: This is why I said that the patient has to be hospitalized. What we have been most concerned with is the normalization of the GH response after exercise. It is possible, but very difficult, to normalize this response. Regarding the question of how somatostatin influences GH secretion in normals and in diabetics, it depends on the insulin levels. Indeed, somatostatin has also other effects than suppression of GH, it also suppresses insulin and other hormones. In case there is an insulin secretion in normals or in maturity onset diabetics whether lean or obese, this secretion is suppressed and the blood glucose levels in-

crease over control or saline study levels. In juvenile
diabetics, however, who have no insulin secretion at least
postprandially, the insulin levels will not be suppressed
further and therefore the effect of somatostatin will be
to decrease glucose levels, though not to hypoglycemic
levels, for example, from 200 mg/dl to 100 mg/dl. This
is an effect that many of us would like to use in the
treatment of diabetic angiopathy because insulin alone
cannot normalize blood glucose levels but insulin plus
somatostatin can.

VIGNERI: We published similar data on the normalization of GH levels in diabetic patients under strict control. Referring to Dr. Desir's question, strict control
means blood glucose levels constantly below 150 mg/dl. Do
you have data about the lag time required to observe normalization of GH levels after reaching normalization of
blood glucose levels?

HANSEN: A few years ago, we studied newly diagnosed
but not yet insulin treated diabetics and performed exercise tests. Then we started insulin treatment very effectively and after about 20 days, blood glucose levels were
normal, and, much before that, free fatty acid levels were
normal. Still the GH secretion was elevated. Approximately 10 days after the blood glucose levels returned to
normal, GH levels were totally normalized. However, many
juvenile onset diabetics coming in the clinic have normal
GH secretion.

QUABBE: Your GH patterns in diabetic patients resem-
ble strikingly patterns in monkeys, with regular occurrence of peaks, suggesting that the development of suppression of GH may be one of the important differences
between the non-human primate and the primate. If a
patient has at the same time adult onset diabetes and
obesity, the effect of obesity seems to override the effect of diabetes. Could this be related to elevated free

fatty acid levels?

HANSEN: It is tempting to simply speculate that there is a disturbed relationship between free fatty acids and GH in such patients. We did studies where lipids and heparin were infused in order to elevate free fatty acids and we did not see suppression of the GH levels in these patients. The night peak would be suppressed in normals under these conditions. Thus, it might be a question of fasting.

QUABBE: Concerning the dialysis in diabetic patients, my interpretation of your data was that the lack of intra-cellular glucose was probably responsible for the elevation of GH. Now, you seem to look for a dialysable effector other than glucose responsible for the GH elevation. What was the glucose level after dialysis? Why can it not be the glucose normalization after dialysis that is respon-sible for the clearance in GH secretion?

HANSEN: When juvenile diabetics are dialyzed with fluid containing no glucose, which is most common, the blood glucose levels fall rapidly during dialysis. They can reach values of 10 mg/dl but, curiously, most of these patients do not develop signs of hypoglycemia. If glucose is included in the dialysis fluid, or if you in-fuse glucose, or if you use the artificial pancreas to stabilize blood glucose during the procedure, you will see that the GH secretion is totally abolished during the first hour. This may be observed in juvenile diabetics as well as in uremic patients who do not have diabetes and who just present, as diabetics do, highly fluctuating GH levels. Thus, glucose is certainly not responsible for the GH suppression.

JAQUET: Do you have data on the pattern of GH shortly after the start of insulin treatment in your patients with juvenile onset diabetes? When you block rapidly the catabolic state, do the abnormalities you observe disappear rapidly?

HANSEN: Insulin treatment does not change the GH secretion dramatically in juvenile onset diabetics. After a few days, GH levels are lower but the effect is not acute.

CIRCADIAN AND CIRCANNUAL CHANGES OF PITUITARY AND
OTHER HORMONES IN HEALTHY HUMAN MALES : THEIR RELATIONSHIP
WITH GONADAL ACTIVITY

Michel Lagoguey and Alain Reinberg

Laboratoire de Physiologie
Equipe de Recherches de Chronobiologie Humaine CNRS n° 105
Fondation A. de Rothschild 29, rue Manin 75940 Paris Cedex
Service de Biochimie Médicale
Faculté de Médecine Pitié-Salpétrière
91, bld de l'Hôpital 75634 Paris cedex

INTRODUCTION

Circadian and circannual rhythms must be investigated in
the same experiment since the bioperiodicity of a given
physiologic variable can be expressed, among others, in these two frequency domains. Moreover, not only the 24 h mean
level M, but also the circadian crest time $\emptyset$ of a physiologic variable can be the subject of circannual changes.

SUBJECTS, MATERIAL AND METHODS

During 14 months, five mature, apparently healthy (routine
clinical examinations and biological tests) young males (medical student and biochemists) living in Paris, volunteered
to document circadian changes. At the beginning of the study
they were 26, 26, 28, 29 and 31 years old. Their respective
height and weight were : 168 cm, 64 kg; 183 cm, 70 kg;
180 cm, 78 kg; 178 cm, 63 kg; 171 cm, 64 kg.
At the time of the 28-h tests (every other month for plasma
sampling; monthly for urine sampling) the subjects were taking no medication and had no sexual activity. Food and water intakes were not controlled, and meals were taken at
about 07.00, 13.00 and 20.00. The subjects' circadian periodicity was synchronized with light-on at 07.00 (7 a.m.) $\pm$
1 h and light-off at 23.00 (11 p.m.) $\pm$ 1.5 h during the
year.
Circadian rhythms in levels of plasma hormone were explored
simultaneously in the five subjects during the same two days
in January,March,May,July,September,November 1973 and again

in February 1974. On test days, venous blood samples were
withdrawn in a EDTA vacutainer (Becton and Dickinson) at
fixed 4-h intervals for 28 h, starting at 08.00 on day 1.
Plasma (after centrifugation) and urine samples were stored
at -25°C, ten tubes per sample to facilitate control and
multiple determination, each tube being thawed only once.
Determinations were performed in large series at the end of
the entire study. Radioimmunoassay procedures were used for
plasma variables and urinary aldosterone determinations.
Specificity, sensitivity, and precision were tested according to the best current methodology.
Both conventional and single cosinor (Halberg et al, 1) methods were used for the statistical analysis of time series
thus obtained. In a first step, data were plotted as a function of time (mean $\bar{X} \pm 1$ SE). Rhythmic changes can be visua-
lized when the curve is roughly sinusoidal and associated
with a statistically significant crest-trough difference.
Thereafter, detection and quantification of rhythms were
achieved by fitting a sine curve of either 24 hours or 365
days, by the method of least squares, to each time series
of respectively one day or one year in duration. With this
cosinor method a rhythm is validated when its amplitude differs from zero with $p < 0.05$. The rhythm, when detected,
can be characterized by several parameters : the acrophase,
$\emptyset$, circadian or circannual crest time (more precisely,
crest-time - clock hour of day, or day of a specified month
- of the sine function approximating all data); the amplitude, A, equal to 1/2 the within daily or yearly rhythmic
variability; and the mesor, M, or rhythm-adjusted mean. $\emptyset$
and A are given as mean values with their 95% confidence
limits and M as mean ± 1 SE.

RESULTS

Circadian and circannual rhythms in plasma testosterone,FSH,
and LH were first analyzed in 1975, 1976 (2,3,5). We want
to report here the obtained results giving more details
than in our previous papers.

Plasma LH and FSH

FSH circadian rhythm was detected neither in any monthly

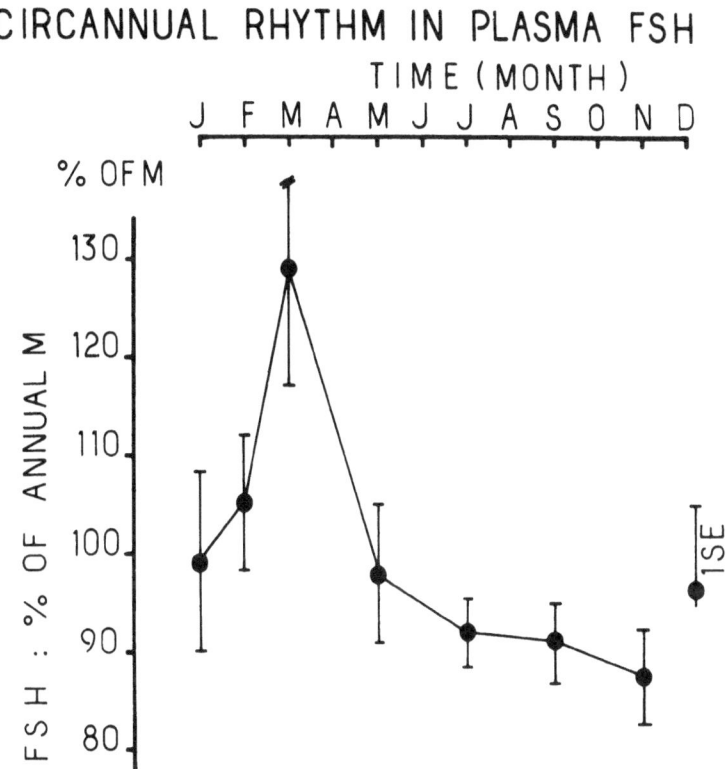

CIRCANNUAL RHYTHM IN PLASMA FSH

NO DETECTION OF CIRCADIAN RHYTHMS
ANNUAL M = 7.63 mu/ml ± 0.27 (1SE)

Figure 1 : Circannual rhythm in plasma FSH. Data for all figures were gathered during a 14 month span and are displayed in a 12 month plexogram. Annual changes are expressed as per cent of the annual monthly M in order to minimize interindividual differences. M is the circadian mesor or the 24-hour adjusted mean with reference to a given month.

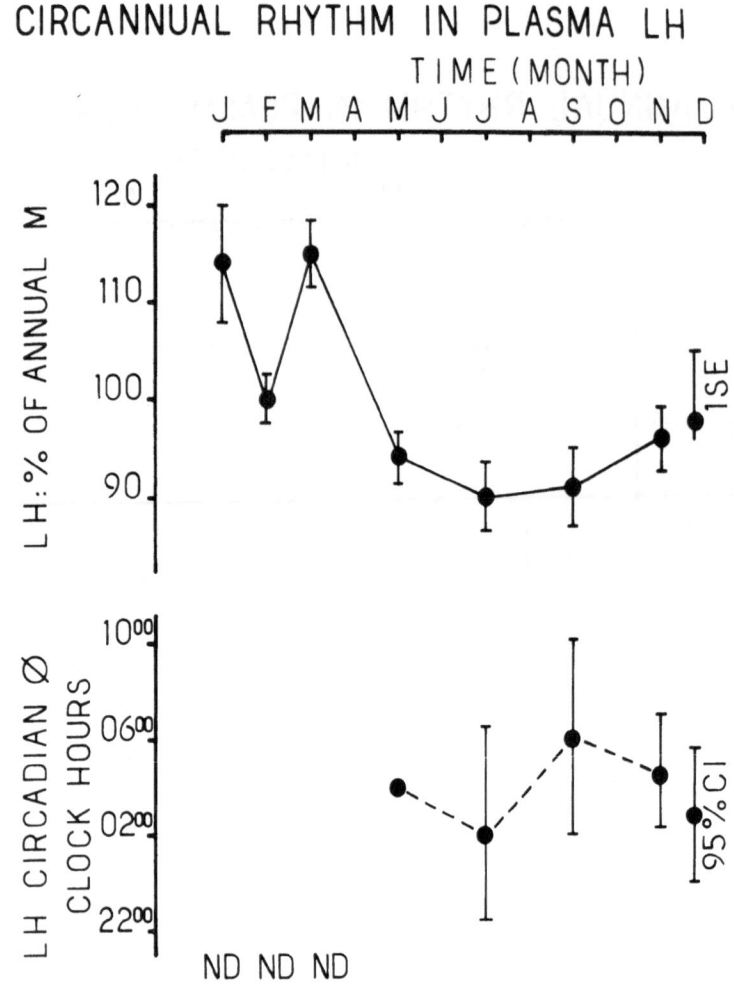

CIRCANNUAL RHYTHM IN PLASMA LH

ND = NO DETECTION OF THE CIRCADIAN RHYTHM
ANNUAL M = 8.91 mu/ml ± 0.29 (1SE)

Figure 2 : Circannual rhythm in plasma LH.
Top : Annual changes expressed as per cent of the annual monthly M.
Bottom : Location of the circadian crest time Ø when the circadian
rhythm was detected (p < 0.05). Ø is given with its 95 % confidence
limits. Circadian rhythm of LH with a nocturnal Ø was detected only
in July, September and November. In May Ø is only estimated since
p < 0.10.

time series nor in pooled data. LH circadian rhythm was
detected only in July, September, November and in pooled
data (with a relatively small amplitude for this latter and
   a nocturnal acrophase (Figs. 1 and 2).
Statistically significant circannual rhythms in plasma FSH
and LH were detected with both the conventional and cosinor methods. This latter shows (Fig. 7) that the circannual acrophase was located in February for FSH (from December 1 to April 10) and in March for LH (from January 18 to
April 26).

Plasma testosterone

Statistically significant (p < 0.05) circadian rhythms were
detected in January, February, May, July, September, and
November but not in March (Fig. 3). The plasma testosterone circadian acrophase varied as a function of time of
year; it occurred in the early morning in May and in the
early afternoon in November, the difference of 6 h and 22
min between extreme Øs being statistically significant. The
circannual Mesor showed a statistically significant annual
change validated by both conventional. and cosinor methods.
With this latter the detected rhythm (p < 0.025) had its
annual acrophase located in October (from July 16 to December 20 with 95% confidence limits) (Fig.   7).

Plasma cortisol

A statistically significant circadian rhythm was detected
for each of the documented months. The crest time occurred
in February while the trough time was located in September
(Figs. 4 and 7).
A small but statistically significant change in the circadian acrophase location was observed between February and
September.

OTHER PLASMA AND URINARY VARIABLES

Plasma prolactin

In the 5 male subjects here studied a circannual rhythm
was detected neither for the circadian M nor for the circadian Ø (Fig. 5). In other words, both the circadian mean
level and the nocturnal crest time Ø of the plasma prolactin
   did not vary as a function of the time ot the year.

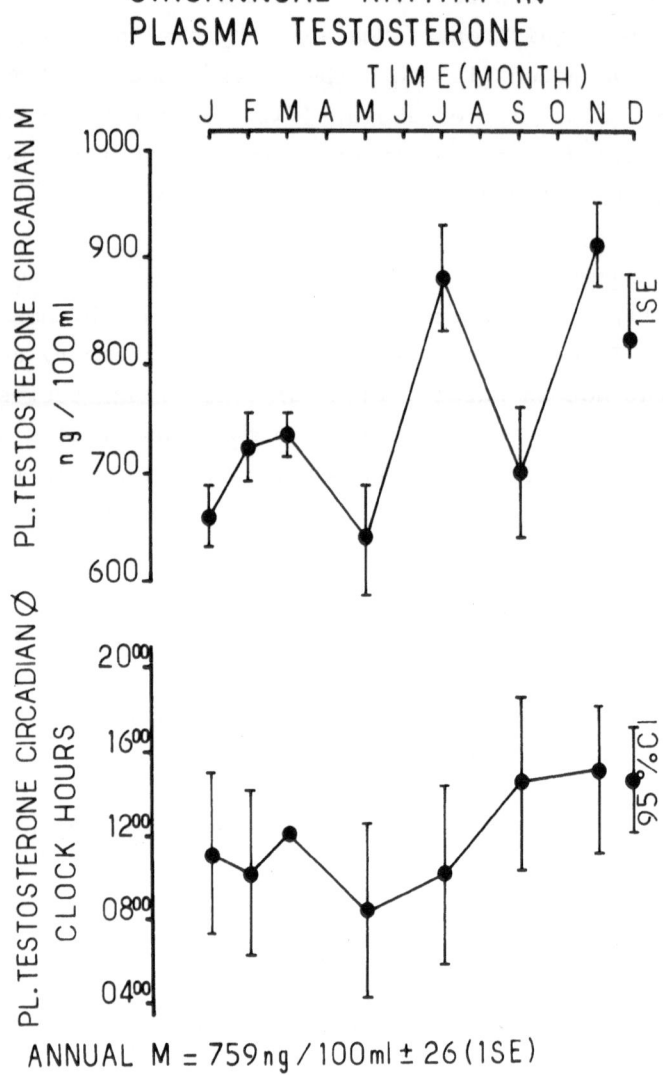

Figure 3 : Circannual rhythm in plasma testosterone.
Top : Annual changes of the 24-h adjusted mean in ng/100 ml.
Bottom : Location of the circadian acrophase ∅.

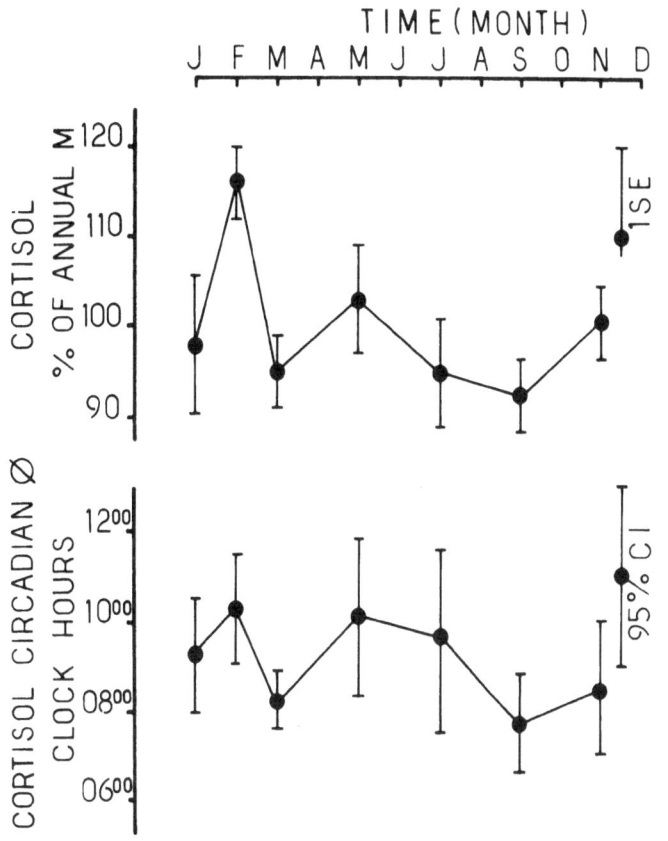

CIRCANNUAL RHYTHM IN PLASMA CORTISOL

Figure 4 : Circannual rhythm in plasma cortisol.
Top : Annual changes expressed as per cent of the annual monthly M.
Bottom : Location of the circadian crest time Ø.

Plasma thyroxine

An annual change in the mean level was observed with a peak
time in September and a trough time in March (Fig. 6). The
circadian acrophase varied as well and was located in the
evening in February and the early afternoon in March.

Other variables

Circannual changes of all the documented variables are summarized in   Fig. 7. The single cosinor method was used to
re-analyze circannual changes of circadian M. Results thus
obtained showed the annual acrophase location as well as
the circannual amplitude when the rhythm was detected. Both
circannual ∅ and A are given with their 95% confidence limits. This figure confirms the detection of circannual rhythms for plasma FSH, LH, thyroxine, cortisol, testosterone
but not for prolactin.

In addition, statistically significant circannual rhythms
were detected for plasma HGH and plasma TSH with regard to
pituitary hormones.

Other circannual rhythms were also validated, such as :
plasma renin activity, urinary excretion of 17-OHCS, aldosterone, potassium, catecholamines (VMA) and para mandelic
acid as well as sexual activity and body weight.

COMPLEMENT OF INVESTIGATION

The difference of about 6 months between peak times of plasma FSH and LH on the one hand, and plasma testosterone on
the other hand, is intriguing and remains to be explained.
One of the hypotheses to be considered is the existence of
an annual change in the gonadal sensitivity to gonadotro-
phic hormones (5). Such a change has been demonstrated in
the male duck (6). Another hypothesis which does not exclude the first one takes into consideration chronopharmacolo-
gic phenomena (7, 8). The effectiveness of an agent
(including hormones) varies as a function of the timing of
its circadian changes in plasma concentration.
Therefore we explored the testicular response (with plasma
testosterone as index) to the specific stimulation of HCG
as a function of both time of day (07.00, 14.00, 20.00) and

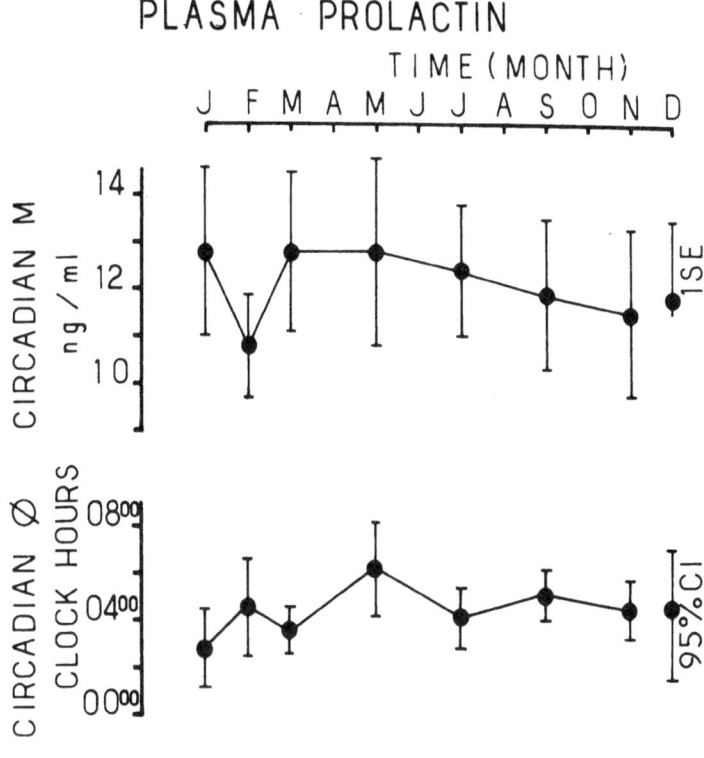

Figure 5 : Plasma prolactin.
Top : Circadian M in ng/mℓ. No circannual change.
Bottom : Circadian ∅ location. No circannual change.

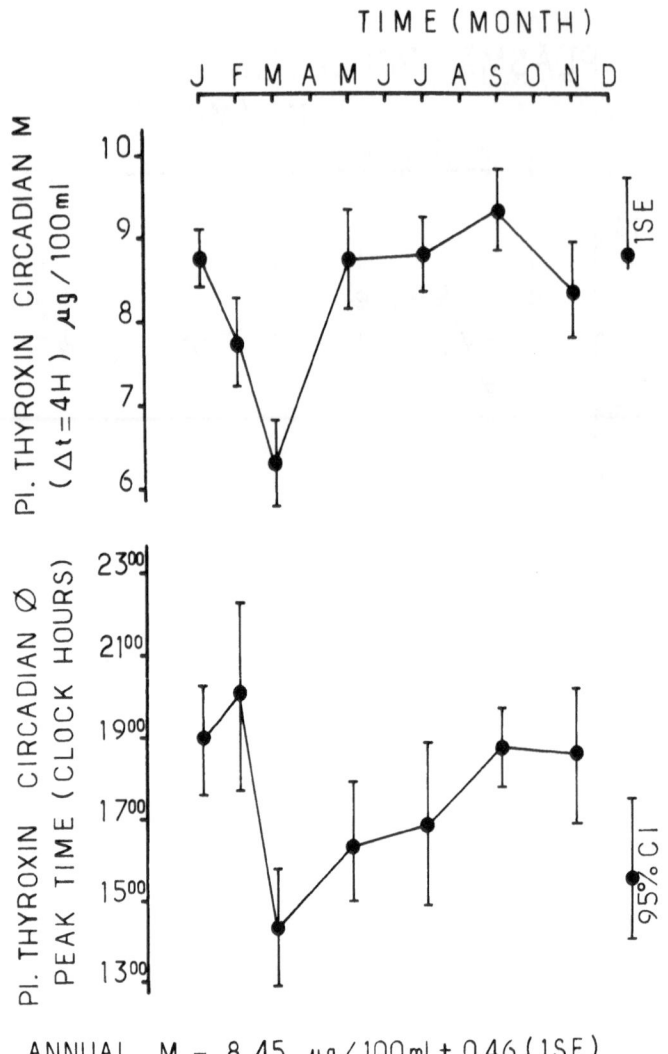

CIRCANNUAL RHYTHM IN PLASMA THYROXINE

TIME (MONTH)

Figure 6 : Circannual rhythm in plasma thyroxine.
Top : Annual changes in the circadian M expressed in µg/100 mℓ.
Bottom : Annual changes in the circadian Ø.

time of year (May-June and October-November) in four (out
of five) of the subjects who volunteered for the studies
reported above. This complementary investigation was done 4
years later. Each subject was studied twice in a year for
his responses to 6 different tests. 2500 IU/0,5 ml HCG
(Organon) intra-muscular injections were done one week apart
at 07.00, 14.00 and 20.00 as well as control injections of
saline. Days and order of fixed clock hours of the 6 tests
were randomized. Venous blood was sampled immediately before and 30, 60, 90, 150 and 240 minutes after each injection
of either saline or HCG.

Changes occurring after the IM administration of HCG in any
individual and for any stimulation (both for time of day
and time of year) are referred to plasma testosterone control values (T control) corresponding to the five determinations expressed as X $\pm$ 1 SE. Plasma testosterone changes
resulting from the HCG injection were estimated according
to several parameters : (1) plasma testosterone mean value
recorded after the HCG stimulation (HCG stimulated T) resulting from 5 determinations ($\overline{X} \pm 1$ SE); (2) HCG stimulated T/T
control ratio; (3) The highest value of plasma testosterone
resulting from the stimulation expressed as T peak height/T
control ratio; (4) The span of time to reach the testosterone peak. Each parameter was determined for each subject/
time of day/time of year.

Plasma testosterone mean value recorded after the HCG stimulation

Plasma testosterone control levels were higher both in the
morning than in the evening and in the autumn rather than
in the spring.

For all subjects and times of year, there was no rise of
testosterone level when HCG was injected at 07.00. To the
contrary a statistically significant rise of testosterone
level ($p < 0.01$ to < 0.0005) was observed when HCG was
injected at 20.00. The HCG stimulation at 14.00 resulted
in an intermediate response with regard to data obtained at
the other considered time points (Tables 1 and 2).

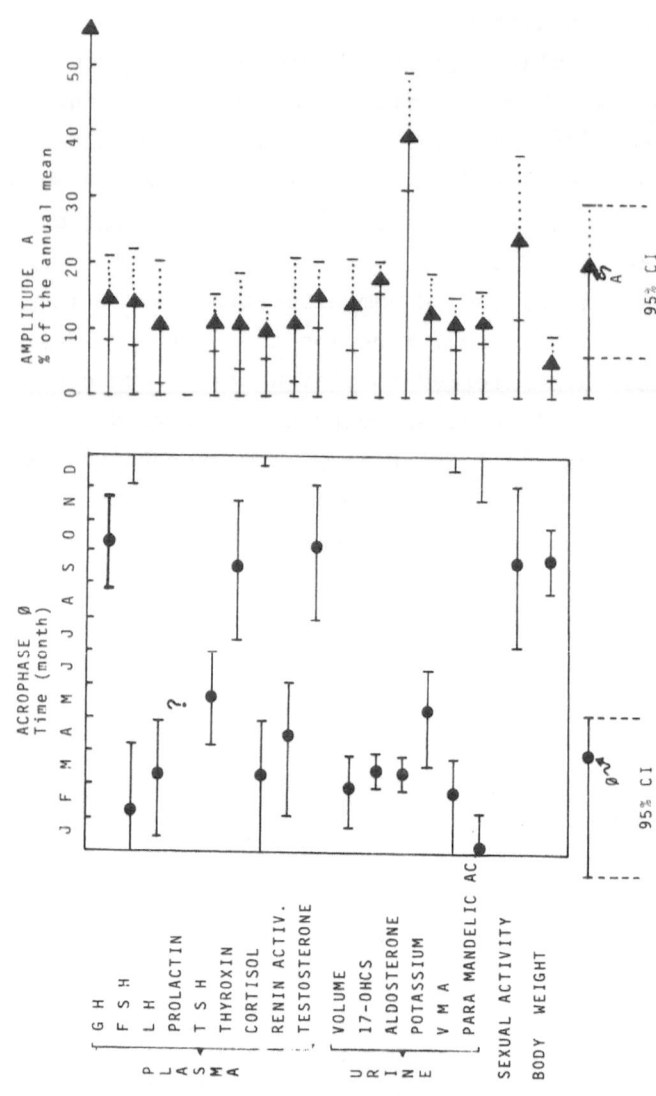

Figure 7 . Single cosinor summary of circannual changes in 5 healthy young males.

Left : circannual acrophase Ø location.

Right : circannual amplitude A.

Table 1 . Test time of year : May-June. Individual changes in plasma testosterone levels (5 determinations) after IM injections of HCG (HCG-stimulated) and saline (control) at 07.00, 14.00 and 20.00 (test time of day).

Subject n°	Test time clock hour	Control	HCG stimulated	t	P
		plasma testosterone in ng/100 ml ± 1 SE			
1	07.00	342+37	245+26	no stimulation	
	14.00	320+12	450+40	5.26	<0.0005
	20.00	100+19	626+44	10.97	<0.0005
2	07.00	99+10	112+2	1.17	N.S.
	14.00	117+12	664+241	2.05	<0.05
	20.00	104+14	1054+100	9.40	<0.0005
3	07.00	320+108	180+22	no stimulation	
	14.00	160+45	156+6	no stimulation	
	20.00	82+2	230+35	2.22	<0.05
4	07.00	206+24	192+30	no stimulation	
	14.00	88+18	141+26	1.58	N.S.
	20.00	63+3	319+30	7.13	<0.0005

Table 2 . Test time of year : October-November.

Subject n°	Test time clock hour	Control	HCG stimulated	t	P
		plasma testosterone in ng/100 ml ± 1 SE			
1	07.00	453+33	332+10	no stimulation	
	14.00	230+18	355+18	4.91	<0.0025
	20.00	260+19	404+38	3.38	<0.005
2	07.00	638+9	537+37	no stimulation	
	14.00	788+109	601+52	no stimulation	
	20.00	303+25	525+51	3.90	<0.0025
3	07.00	425+43	358+18	no stimulation	
	14.00	285+21	369+26	2.51	<0.0025
	20.00	243+11	323+14	4.49	<0.0025
4	07.00	574+74	731+88	1.36	N.S.
	14.00	343+31	360+33	0.37	N.S.
	20.00	364+31	515+33	3.33	<0.01

N.S. : not statistically significant.

Testosterone peak height/testosterone control ratio

The highest peak of T occurred when HCG was injected at
20.00 rather than at 14.00 or 07.00, the response being more pronounced in May-June than in October-November.
When data were analyzed as a group phenomenon, testosterone
peak height/testosterone control ratio in May-June was
1.15 $\pm$ 0.30 (1 SE) at 07.00 and 8.21 $\pm$ 1.94 at 20.00
(p < 0.01). In October-November this ratio was 1.08 $\pm$ 0.19
at 07.00 and 2.02 $\pm$ 0.16 at 20.00 (p < 0.005).

Span of time to reach the testosterone peak after the HCG
injection

The inspection of individual data and the statistical analysis for the group indicated that in May-June the span of
time to reach the peak was shorter when the HCG test was
done at 20.00 than at other time points. Such a difference
did not appear in October-November.

HCG stimulated testosterone (mean)/testosterone control
ratio

In May-June the ratio was 0.84 $\pm$ 0.12 (1 SE) at 07.00 and
6.07 $\pm$ 1.53 at 20.00, the difference being statistically
significant (p < 0.01).
Finally the HCG-induced rise of plasma testosterone levels
was not only 8 times greater but also more than twice as
fast at 20.00 than at 07.00 in May-June. In October-Nevem-
ber the ratio was 0.91 $\pm$ 0.12 at 07.00 and 2.02 $\pm$ 0.16 at
20.00, again with a statistically significant difference
(p < 0.005).

DISCUSSION

It is likely that with regard to the timing of HCG injection the lower the plasma testosterone level, the stronger
the response of the testes. Such findings can be compared
to the circadian stage related response of the mouse corti-
coadrenal (in vitro) to a fixed dose of ACTH : the increased release of corticosterone resulting from the ACTH induced secretion corresponds to the time point of the lower
(non-stimulated) level of plasma corticosterone (9).

If we consider circadian and circannual changes of plasma
testosterone, the obtained results suggest that we must take into consideration :

a) circadian and circannual changes in LH secretion (as
reflected presumably by LH plasma levels).

b) circadian and circannual changes in the susceptibility
of the testes to LH (chronesthesy of a target organ (8)).
In the reported experiments we were dealing with a "single
pulse" administration rather than a cyclic (e.g. circadian)
stimulation.

As suggested by Weitzman (10), it could well be that the
circadian rhythmicity with a nocturnal crest time of plasma
LH plays a major role in stimulating the gonads in peribu-
beral children, both girls and boys. As shown in Fig.2
the same male subjects had a plasma LH circadian rhythm
detected only in July, September and November with a nocturnal acrophase $\emptyset$ = 03.02 (from 00.07 to 05.57) while this
latter circadian rhythm was not detected in January, February, March and May. The existence of a circadian rhythm of
LH roughly from mid-summer to mid-winter may lead to a more
effective stimulation of the human testes even if the 24
hour mean level of plasma LH is lower at this time of year.
In addition, the plasma LH circadian crest in the 24 hour
scale at this time of year corresponds roughly to the circadian trough of testosterone : 02.14 (from 22.24 to 07.04).
One has also to consider the circannual rhythm of thyroxine
as a possible "modulator". Thyroid hormones play an important role in the circannual change of the gonadal activity
of other species such as the duck (6). In the drake thyroxine
has an inhibitory effect on the gonad while in some mammals
(including man) thyroxine is likely to have a permissive effect on the testicular activity. From this point of view it
is interesting to see (Fig. 7) that plasma thyroxine and
plasma testosterone are in phase with regard to their circannual rhythmicity.

In conclusion both circadian and circannual endocrinological rhythms in man need to be considered as a function of
hormone secretions as well as a sensitivity of the target
organs to these hormones.

REFERENCES

1. Halberg,F., Johnson, E.A., Nelson, W., and Sothern, R., Autorhythmometry-procedures for physiologic self-measurements and their analysis. Physiology Teacher 1, 1-7, 1972.

2. Reinberg,A., Lagoguey, M., Chauffournier, J.M., Cesselin, F., Circannual and circadian rhythms in plasma testosterone in five healthy young Parisian males. Acta Endocrinol. 80, 732-743, 1975.

3. Lagoguey, M. and Reinberg, A., Circannual rhythms in plasma LH, FSH and testosterone and in the sexual activity of healthy young Parisian males. J. Physiol., 257, 19-20 P, 1976.

4. Smals, A.G.H., Kloppenborg, P.W.C. and Benraad, T., Circannual cycle in plasma testosterone levels in man. J.Clin. Endocrinol. Metab. 42, 979-982, 1976.

5. Reinberg, A., Lagoguey, M., Cesselin, F., Touitou, Y., Legrand, J.C., Delasalle, A., Antreassian, J. and Lagoguey, A., Circadian and circannual rhythms in plasma hormones and other variables of five healthy young human males. Acta Endocrinol. 88-417-427, 1978.

6. Assenmacher, I., External and internal components of the mechanism controlling reproductive cycle in drakes. In : Circannual Clocks. Pengelley, E.T. (Ed), New York : Academic Press, 1974.

7. Reinberg, A., Halberg, F., Circadian chronopharmacology, Ann. Rev. 11, 455-492, 1971.

8. Reinberg, A., Advances in human chronopharmacology. Chronobiologia, 3, 151-166, 1976.

9. Ungar, F. and Halberg, F., Circadian rhythm in the in vitro response of mouse adrenal to adrenocorticotropic hormones. Science, 137, 1058-1060, 1962.

10. Weitzman, E.D., Boyar, R.M., Kapen, S. and Hellman, L., The relationship of sleep and sleep stages to neuroendocrine secretion and biological rhythms in man. Recent Progress in Hormone Research. Academic Press, 31, 399-446, 1975.

DISCUSSION

QUABBE: Regarding your detection of a circadian rhythm of LH in the fall, was the rhythm related to sleep? Did you see the depressive effect of sleep that Weitzman reported in women in the early follicular phase of the menstrual cycle?

REINBERG: We cannot answer this question because in our study, plasma was collected at 4-hour intervals whereas, in Weitzman's study, the sampling interval was much shorter. Moreover, we did not make polygraphic recordings of sleep.

VAN CAUTER: Regarding circannual changes in sexual activity, we have analyzed data from the Institut Royal de Statistique de Belgique giving month by month the number of births and marriages of the Belgian population over the last 25 years. After 1950, a peak in the number of births develops in April and becomes very sharp in the seventies. It corresponds to conception in July and August, at the time of summer holidays. It seems thus that social schedule might be the most powerful zeitgeber of circannual changes in sexual activity.

REINBERG: Social schedule is usually provided as an explanation for any circannual changes in behaviour. Summer holidays may be involved but there is no demonstration for it so far. Circannual changes of hormones are another possible explanation. I do not think that the number of births is a good index of the sexual activity because they are not closely related. We are presently studying the incidence of rape in Paris and in Houston, with Dr. Smolensky. There is clear-cut circannual change in the number of rapes in both locations, with a peak concomitant with the peak of testosterone. Surprisingly, this observation was already reported at the end of the last century in England in a paper called "Violence Against Chastity". At that time, the social habits were very different from now.

It could be that social habits and vacation play a role but it is not a proven explanation. Moreover, there is an analogue of testosterone which competes with testosterone and reduces sexual activity in subjects prone to sexual violence. Finally, if you consider the transmission of veneral diseases, there is again an annual peak concomitant with the abnormal testosterone elevation.

VAN CAUTER: I did not mean to exclude the possibility of hormonal changes as a factor responsible for circannual changes in sexual activity. However, data on 9,000,000 Belgian subjects clearly show that the number of births in April and May is significantly larger than at all other times of the year. Dr. Aschoff mentioned yesterday that these preliminary data on such circannual changes indicate that the latitude of the country plays a role. This would maybe help discriminating the relative influences of social habits and of hormonal changes.

REINBERG: A similar study has been published by Batschelet in the Intern. Journal of Chronobiology. A clear-cut relationship between the incidence of births and the latitude was demonstrated and shown to be similar to what is observed in monkeys. One can hypothesize that man is a seasonal long-night breeder as the other primates.

QUABBE: Is there evidence to prove or to exclude that the frequency of sexual activity has an influence on the level of testosterone?

REINBERG: It seems that there is an immediate influence but there is probably no effect on the 24-hour mean. Moreover, other factors such as muscular activity and exposure to sun may play a role. All these factors have to be studied separately.

CLINICAL IMPLICATIONS OF GONADOTROPIN RHYTHMS

C. Wayne Bardin

The Population Council, The Rockefeller University
New York, New York 10021

When radioimmunoassays for LH and FSH were devised, a number of investigators looked for cyclic variations of gonadotropin levels in human plasma. The lack of sensitivity of these initial assays and the failure to obtain frequent samples prevented the detection of variable LH secretion. Nankin and Troen (1) were the first to show that LH and, to some extent, FSH were secreted in a pulsatile fashion. Since these initial studies, numerous laboratories have confirmed that LH secretion is highly variable (2-5). In view of these observations, it was important to determine whether variable gonadotropin secretion occurred in patients and what were the implications of this mode of secretion for the clinician.

A series of normal men were sampled every 10 or 20 min for 6-24 hrs. The pulsatile secretion of LH was found to be expressed in three major secretory peaks over a 6 hr period. The shape of most peaks suggested that LH was released into the blood during a sudden burst of secretion. The increase of LH was rapid, followed by a slower decline from which an apparent half-life of the hormone could be deduced. With every large peak of LH, there tended to be a smaller peak of FSH. More precisely, if a 200% rise in LH occurs, the probability that there will be a smaller concomitant FSH peak is approximately 90%. In order to perform a detailed analysis of the pulsatile pattern a computer program was developed for calculating the number of peaks over a given period of time, the duration of their ascending and declining portions, the corresponding increment in hormone level, the total area under the curve and the apparent half-life after each spike (5).

When a given individual was sampled every 20 min for 6 hr and the cumulative mean LH level for consecutive samples calculated, the 95% confidence interval was extremely large when only a few samples were included in the calculation (Fig. 1). The confidence interval decreased with consideration of additional samples being reduced to $\pm$ 12% of the mean after 6 hr of sampling. Thus, the measurement of a cumulative mean of samples obtained every 20 min for 6 hr provides an accurate estimation of the actual mean LH level of the individual. It was further shown that measuring a cumulative mean was equivalent to measuring integrated concentrations, provided LH changes were changing rapidly (5).

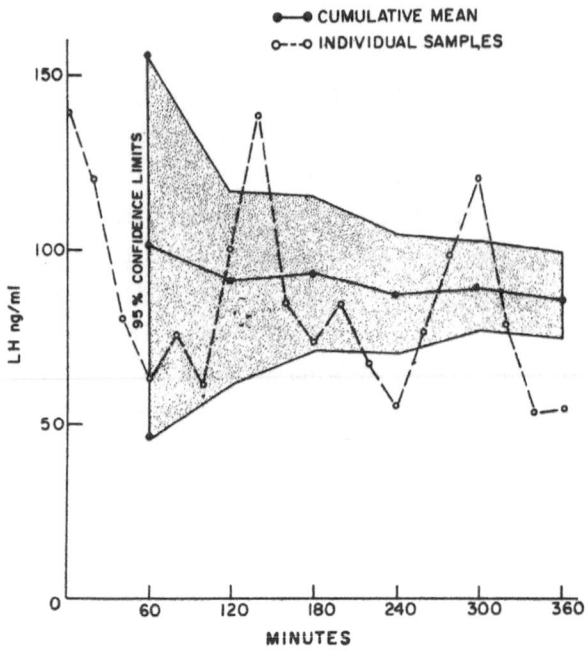

Figure 1: *The solid line and shaded area are the cumulative mean LH level and the 95% confidence limits of that mean at hourly intervals for 6 hr in a single normal man. For a comparison, the dotted line and open circles represent the actual estimate of serum LH in samples obtained from that subject at 20 min intervals (Santen and Bardin, 1973).*

In women, the pulsatile pattern of LH and FSH varies with the phase of the menstrual cycle. In subjects sampled every 30 min during the luteal and follicular phases it was observed that the height of the secretory spikes was larger and the apparent half-life of LH shorter in the luteal than in the follicular phase (Fig. 2). These observations suggested that the pattern of gonadotropin secretion was influenced by hormonal status. This suspicion was, in part, confirmed by an analysis of a large group of individuals with a variety of clinical disorders. The results indicated that, as a group, the pattern of LH secretion in patients with hirsutism and hypergonadotropic hypogonadism resembled that of women in the luteal phase, whereas the patterns in patients with hypogonadism were more similar to those in the follicular phase. However, with the exception of a few disease states such as anorexia nervosa and primary amenorrhea, a given individual could usually not be singled out only on the basis of the pulsatile properties of the LH pattern (5,6).

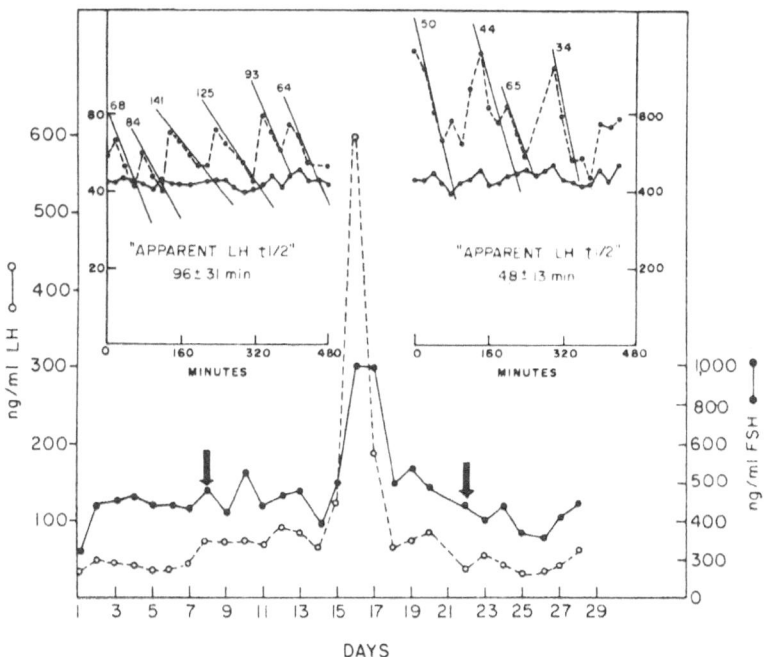

Figure 2: Pattern of LH and FSH (linear scale) and daily samples of blood collected from a normal woman during a menstrual cycle. The inserts represent the LH and FSH levels (log scale) in serum samples collected at 20 min intervals for 8 hr on days 8 and 22 (solid arrows) after the onset of menses. The solid lines represent the decrements of LH after secretory spikes which meet the criteria of linearity. The numbers above each solid line represent the apparent LH half-life calculated from that decrement (Santen and Bardin, 1973).

In an effort to understand the relation between various components of the LH pattern, many patients were sampled every 20 min for 6 hr. Analysis of these data indicated mean LH is linearly related to the mean height of the spikes. Thus, a postmenopausal woman with a very high basal LH level will have large secretory peaks whereas, in an individual with low basal LH level, the height of the spikes will be smaller. The individuals who did not obviously exhibit this linear relationship tended to be women in the luteal phase in whom fewer but higher spikes were observed (5).

The factors which determine the pattern of LH secretion were further investigated in a study focused on understanding the alterations in the apparent half-life. When patients with hypogonadotropic hypogonadism were given a large dose of non-radioactive LH, the disappearance curve of this gonadotropin from blood could be described by two exponentials. The half-life for the first exponential ranged from 32 to 65 min and, for the second exponential, from 90 to 145 min. If the apparent half-life which followed endogenous LH secretion was in the range of the first exponential, then it could be postulated that LH was secreted as a burst and that the secretion was then discontinued until the next burst. However, only about one-third of all observed spikes in both patients and normal individuals could be described in that way. Approximately another third of all observed spikes had apparent half-lives longer than the greatest half-time (145 min) of the second exponential. As a consequence, LH secretion is not always discontinuous. Continuous LH secretion may not be the only reason for long apparent half-life. In a study using the computer program to evaluate the parameters of a very large number of LH spikes, we found an inverse relationship between the apparent half-life and spike increment. Thus, the higher the secretory spike, the shorter the half-life (5). After a large spike, one was more likely to observe a disappearance rate which corresponds to the first exponential of the disappearance curve for exogenously administered LH. After a low spike the apparent half-life was longer, possibly because the disappearance curve which follows the spike blends into the previous secretory episode. Another possible reason for variations in apparent half-life includes secretion of LH with variable glycoscillation.

Prior to puberty, testosterone and LH plasma levels are low around the clock. However, when LH levels were measured in the urine, higher values were observed during sleep (7). The relationship between gonadotropin and testosterone secretory patterns during puberty was first studied by Boyar et al. (8,9). In stage II of puberty, these investigators observed an augmentation of LH spiking activity and of testosterone secretion with the onset of sleep. After awakening, the spiking activity decreased and LH and testosterone levels declined. In later stages of puberty, the sleep-associated increase in LH and testosterone was still observed. When group means for all pubertal boys were considered, the LH level was 4 mU/ml while awake and 5 mU/ml while asleep, and the testosterone level, 200 ng/dl while awake and 300 ng/dl while asleep. The sleep-awake difference in these hormone levels gradually decreased as the individual approached adulthood and no differences were found in adults. The many conflicting reports on a possible diurnal variation of LH and testosterone secretion may be related to the failure to understand this maturation process (6).

Since studies on patients with a variety of endocrine disorders suggested that sex steroids may influence the pattern of LH secretion it was pertinent to determine the effects of testosterone and estradiol on the frequency and configuration of the LH secretory spikes. In this regard, it had been suggested that testosterone controlled LH secretion by way of its conversion to estradiol. If this were the case, then similar effects of both hormones on LH spiking activity might have been expected. Normal men were studied for 30 hr. A blood sample was obtained every 20 min throughout the experiment. After 12 hr, a 6 hr infusion of either testosterone or estradiol was carried out followed by a 12 hr recovery period. The amount of steroid infused in either case was twice the 6 hr production rate for normal males. During testosterone infusion, testosterone and estradiol levels increased and then returned to normal when the infusion was discontinued. When cumulative means of LH levels were calculated over 6 hr periods, a significant decline of LH occurred during testosterone infusion with a recovery over the next 12 hr. This pattern of decline and recovery of LH was also observed during estradiol infusion, and there was no significant difference between the magnitude of the decline produced by either steroid. However, when the amplitudes of the LH spikes (expressed as percentage of base line) were compared, peak heights were increased during testosterone infusion and decreased during estradiol infusion. The two hormones thus had opposite effects on the amount of LH released at each secretory episode. When the frequency of spikes (the number of LH spikes per 6 hr) was considered, no significant change was found during estradiol infusion. By contrast, the frequency of LH spikes was decreased during testosterone infusion (10). This study demonstrated that estrogens and androgens suppress LH secretion by different mechanisms—estradiol by reducing the amount of LH released at each secretory episode and testosterone by reducing the number of episodes. In each instance, the net effect of both hormones was the same (10,11).

The above study also provided the first evidence in men that testosterone does not control the LH pulsatile secretion by way of its conversion to estradiol. Further support for this conclusion was provided by a study where LHRH was injected into subjects infused with either testosterone and estradiol. The LH response to LHRH injection was blunted when the injection took place during estradiol infusion but remained normal when the releasing hormone was injected during testosterone infusion. Thus, estradiol and testosterone differ in some of their effects on the hypothalamo-pituitary unit (10). The final demonstration that estradiol and testosterone exert independent effects on the hypothalamo-pituitary axis was provided by an experiment with the non-aromatizable androgen, dihydrotestosterone. Using the same 6 hr infusion protocol as described above, dihydrotestosterone suppressed mean LH levels in normal men (10).

Having established the pattern of gonadotropin release, it was necessary to consider the constraints that variable hormonal secretion poses for the clinician. The number and height of secretory spikes were estimated from 19 samples collected over a 6 hr period in patients with a large variety of disease states. In each subject a mean LH level was calculated from the serial samples as shown in Figure 1. As noted above, the mean LH is equivalent to the integrated LH over 6 hrs. In normal women and men, the mean LH level over a 6 hr sampling period was 20-80 ng/ml (Fig. 3A). However, if single individual samples rather than 6 hr means were considered, a large number fell out of the range for 6 hr means (Fig. 3B). These observations present the clinician with a problem. If single LH samples are used, there is a marked overlap between normal subjects and patients with gonadal disorders. However, if 6 hr mean LH levels are used, then disease states, such as anorexia nervosa and hypogonadotropism, are very well separated from the normal range (Fig. 3C) (5). In contrast to LH, estimates of FSH concentrations from single samples provide a more accurate appraisal of the secretion of this gonadotropin since the secretory spikes are not great.

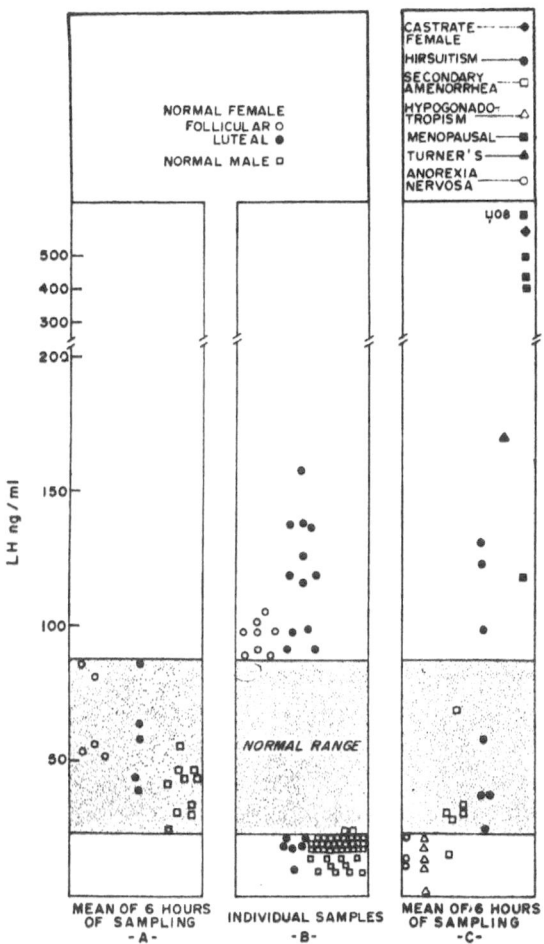

Figure 3: (A) *The normal range of 6 hr mean LH levels is represented by the shaded area. Each data point reflects the mean level of LH observed in blood samples collected at 10 or 20 min intervals for 6 hr. (B) Estimates of LH concentrations in individual samples which were above or below the normal range established by calculating 6 hr mean LH levels in these same normal subjects. (C) Six hr mean levels in patients with various abnormalities of the pituitary-gonadal axis (Santen and Bardin, 1973).*

In addition to the mean gonadotropin concentration, the pattern of secretion provides useful clinical information. Abnormal pulsatile patterns of LH were found in patients with primary amenorrhea (low LH level and no detectable secretory spikes), anorexia nervosa (very few secretory spikes of low amplitude) and liver disease (few secretory spikes in both hypo- and eugonadotropic patients). However, in

286

patients with hypogonadism due to pituitary disease, the spiking pattern was often preserved (6). If it is not possible to obtain frequent samples in a given individual, then the mean LH level may be approximated in a timed urinary sample. In this instance, information about the pattern of LH secretion is lost (7).

Another abnormality of gonadotropin secretion occurs in eugonadotropic women with secondary amenorrhea. In these women the normal pattern of LH secretion is preserved but the feedback control of LH and FSH release is markedly disturbed as demonstrated in a 10 day study (12). During the first 5 days, they received estradiol (10 µg/kg/day IM) in order to raise the levels of this steroid into a range where both negative and positive feedback effects on LH secretion were known to occur. In normal women, this treatment elicited negative feedback on day 3 (suppression of LH levels) followed by a positive feedback (elevation of LH levels) and complete recovery by day 10 (Fig. 4).

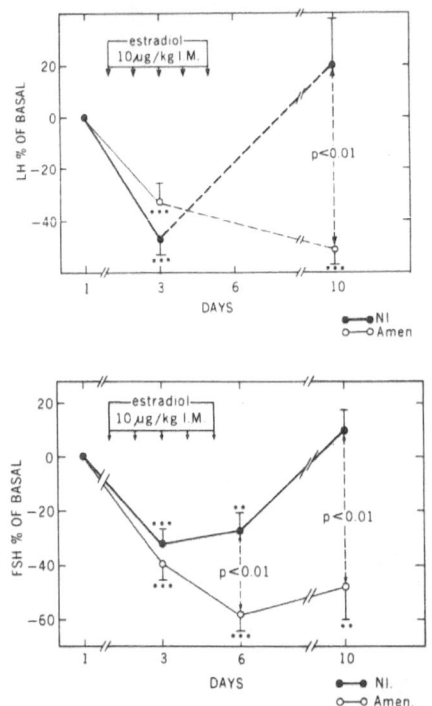

Figure 4: LH (top) and FSH (bottom) in normal and amenorrheic women in response to estradiol. The vertical dashed lines indicate the differences between groups. LH from days 4-6 are not plotted due to the asynchronous LH peaks resulting from positive feedback observed on these days. See Fig. 5, ref. 12 for positive feedback (from Santen et al., 1978).

In the eugonadotropic amenorrheic woman, a negative feedback effect on LH level occurred in all women but positive feedback was seen in only 3 of 11. LH and FSH remained suppressed even though no estradiol had been given for 5 days and the plasma levels of this hormone had returned to the normal range (Fig. 4). In another study these patients failed to recover from the negative feedback effects of estradiol in 16 days after the steroid was discontinued (Fig. 5).

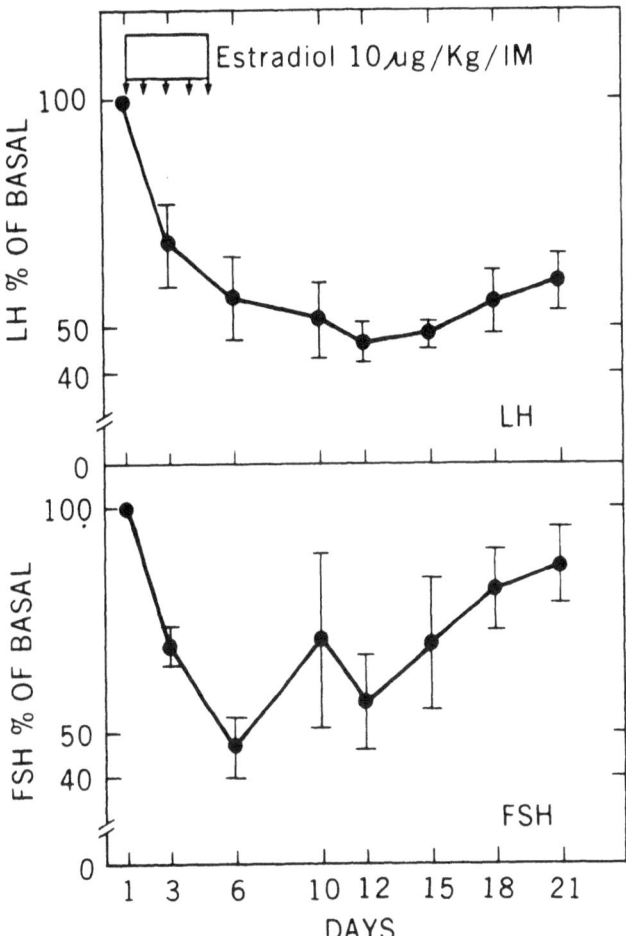

Figure 5: LH (top) and FSH (bottom) levels over a 21-day period after the start of estradiol injections observed in four women with secondary amenorrhea, mean ± S.E.M. (from Santen et al., 1978).

In these studies, FSH levels were also suppressed in both healthy and amenorrheic subjects. This gonadotropin recovered in the normal but not the amenorrheic group (12). These observations suggest that a defect in the recovery phase of negative feedback to estradiol rather than absent positive feedback may be the dominant physiological abnormality which causes secondary amenorrhea by preventing early follicular phase gonadotropin increments and follicular maturation.

Another alteration of the feedback control of LH in eugonadotropic women with secondary amenorrhea was evident with a LHRH test performed during the course of the daily estrogen treatment described above. When normal and amenorrheic women were injected with LHRH 3 times at 2 hr intervals, a low LH peak was produced by the first injection, followed by a larger peak after the second injection, and a still larger peak after the third injection. The series of LHRH injections was repeated after 3 days of estradiol treatment. The response was blunted in the normal women but unchanged in the amenorrheic woman. Five days after estradiol injections were discontinued, both normal and amenorrheic women had identical responses (12). These observations suggest that pituitaries of amenorrheic women are resistant to estradiol.

In summary, the pattern of LH secretion is influenced by the frequency, duration and amount of hormone in each secretory episode. In the child there is a day-night difference in the amount of LH secreted but this is only detected in urine. The day-night difference in LH secretion is markedly accentuated during puberty. In contrast to LH, the FSH secretion does not have a marked minute-to-minute variation. The pattern of gonadotropin secretion is altered in a variety of pathological states but, in some diseases, it remains remarkably normal even though feedback parameters can be strikingly altered.

Acknowledgements

This research was supported, in part, by NIH Grant No. HD-13541.

References

1. Nankin, H.R. and P. Troen. Repetitive luteinizing hormone elevations in serum of normal men. J. Clin. Endocrinol. Metab. 33:558, 1971.

2. Naftolin, F., S.S.C. Yen, and C.C. Tsai. Rapid cycling of plasma gonadotrophins in normal men as demonstrated by frequent sampling. Nat. New Biol. 236:92, 1972.

3. Rubin, R.T., A. Kales, R. Adler, T. Fagan, and W. Odell. Gonado-tropin secretion during sleep in normal adult men. Science 175:196, 1972.

4. Yen, S.S.C., C.C. Tsai, F. Naftolin, G. Vandenberg, and L. Aja-bor. Pulsatile patterns of gonadotropin release in subjects with and without ovarian function. J. Clin. Endocrinol. Metab. 34:671, 1972.

5. Santen, R.J. and C.W. Bardin. Episodic luteinizing hormone secretion in man: Pulse analysis, clinical interpretation, phy-siologic mechanisms. J. Clin. Invest. 52:2617, 1973.

6. Baker, H.W.G., R.J. Santen, H.G. Burger, D.M. DeKretser, B. Hud-son, R.J. Pepperell and C.W. Bardin. Rhythms in the secretion of gonadotropins and gonadal steroids. J. Steroid Biochem. 6:793, 1975.

7. Santen, R.J. and Kulin, H.E. The male reproductive system. In: Practice of Pediatrics, Kelly,V.C. (ed.), Vol. 1, Hagerstown, M.D., Harper & Row, Inc., pp. 1-44, 1976.

8. Boyar, R., J. Finkelstein, H. Roffwarg, S. Kapen, E. Weitzman, and L. Hellman. Synchronization of augmented luteinizing hormone secretion with sleep during puberty. N. Engl. J. Med. 287:582, 1972.

9. Boyar, R.M., R.S. Rosenfeld,, S. Kapen, J.W. Finkelstein, H.P. Roffwarg, E.D. Weitzman, and L. Hellman. Human Puberty: Simul-taneous augmented secretion of luteinizing hormone and testos-terone during sleep. J. Clin. Invest. 54:609, 1974.

10. Santen, R.J. Is aromatization of testosterone to estradiol required for inhibition of luteinizing hormone secretion in men? J. Clin. Invest. 56:1555, 1975.

11. Winters, S.J., R.J. Sherins, and D.L. Loriaux. Studies on the role of sex steroids in the feedback control of gonadotropin

concentrations in men. III. Androgen resistance in primary gonadal failure. J. Clin. Endocrinol. Metab. 48:553, 1979.

12. Santen, R.J., J.N. Friend, D. Trojanowski, B. Davis, E. Samojlik,
and C.W. Bardin. Prolonged negative feedback suppression after
estradiol administration: Proposed mechanism of eugonadal secondary amenorrhea. J. Clin. Endocrinol. Metab. 47:1220, 1978.

DISCUSSION

L'HERMITE: Did you check the half-life of LH in patients with thyroid disease?

BARDIN: No. We measured the half-life of LH in hypogonadotropic patients with very low endogenous LH levels.
We measured apparent half-lives from the backside of secretory spikes in patterns collected in over 200 patients.
These apparent half-lives did not relate to disease state
but instead to the height of the secretory spike.

L'HERMITE: Regarding the problem of the overlap of
normal and pathological LH values, should we go back to urinary determinations of gonadotrophins?

BARDIN: There are two simple ways for the clinician
to determine basal LH levels. One is to use a urinary
sample over a 3-hour or 6-hour period and the other is to
evaluate a mean LH level of plasma sampled every 20 minutes
over 6 hours. It is preferable to use urinary levels in
children prior to puberty.

L'HERMITE: Did you investigate the pulsatile pattern
of LH in hyperprolactinemic state?

BARDIN: No.

L'HERMITE: When you tested the lack of recovery of
the negative feedback effect of estrogens on gonadotrophins
in amenorrheic patients, were there any differences among
patients?

BARDIN: It is very hard to have an absolutely homogeneous group of amenorrheic patients since there is no
general agreement as to how to subdivide amenorrhea. As we
defined our patients, we selected patients with eugonadotropic hypogonadism, that is, with normal LH, FSH, oestradiol and prolactin levels. Thus, patients with tumors or
anorexia nervosa were excluded. The only non-homogeneity

was related to weight since about 50% of the patients were markedly obese but the recovery from estrogen suppression was uniformly abnormal. However, 3 of 11 patients had a positive feedback response to estrogens but then showed suppression and failed to recover. We found a positive feedback response to estrogen in only 11 of our 13 normal subjects.

JAQUET: I have two questions. First, is a 3-hour sampling period at 20-minute intervals sufficient to evaluate the secretory spikes of LH? Second, what is your interpretation of the differential effect of estradiol and testosterone on LH and FSH spikes? The question is related to the studies of the group of Dr. Labrie where pituitary cells were pre-incubated with estradiol and testosterone and the effects of LH, FSH and PRL following TRH or dopamine stimulation were investigated. In these *in vitro* studies, the pre-incubation time necessary to observe the effects of steroids was much longer (*i.e.*, 36 hours) than in your studies (6 hours).

BARDIN: 1) In a normal individual, there are 3 to 4 spikes per 6 hours. Thus, using a 3-hour sampling period, you would see 1-1/2 or 2 spikes. However, in an individual in the luteal phase of the menstrual cycle or in a patient with anorexia nervosa, you will most probably miss the spiking pattern. Six hours is probably a minimum time to look at a pulsatile pattern. With a 3-hour period, you will get a mean LH level with a confidence limit at a .95 probability level of 25% of the mean. 2) The second question refers to studies by Dr. Labrie showing that in pituitary cells incubated with sex steroids, the dose-response curve to GnRH is shifted either to the right or to the left depending on the incubation conditions. I would suspect that the difference in time of appearance of the effect between these *in vitro* experiments and our observation after 6 hours of injection has to do with the culture conditions and whether enough time was allowed for attachment of the cells.

JAQUET: In your experiments, you can appreciate the short effect of steroids on the release of preformed hormones. The necessity of incubating for a longer time in Dr. Labrie's experiments may be related to the fact that one can then observe not only the release of preformed hormone but also the synthesis.

BARDIN: Except that our studies have been repeated in another laboratory with a 96-hour instead of 6-hour infusion period, and the results were remarkably similar.

VAN CAUTER: In dealing with the statistical analysis of LH spikes data, we were faced with the problem of varying precision of the assay in different concentration ranges. How did you deal with that problem in your computer program?

BARDIN: In the middle of the concentration range of any RIA, the coefficient of variation is much smaller than at either extreme. One way to improve that is the use of weighing functions. We instead rejected samples which were not in the good portion of the assay curve even if the estimation was fairly good. The definition of a secretory spike was then based on the maximum coefficient of variation in that portion.

REINBERG: Did you try to inject testosterone, DHA and estradiol at different times of the day? In a recent study, we showed that the peak time of DHA was precisely in the middle of the day at the time when you injected DHA in your experiments but that the testosterone peak time was out of phase. On what basis did you select the injection time at the middle of the day? Did you use other time points of injection?

BARDIN: The middle of the day was selected only for convenience to laboratory personnel. All patients were studied at exactly the same time. We have not investigated different time points of injection.

L'HERMITE: Were your studies on the differential effects of estradiol and testosterone on the amplitude and frequency of LH pulses performed in males?

BARDIN: Yes.

L'HERMITE: Did you find a similar effect in females?

BARDIN: No, we limited these studies to males because we were primarily interested in the effect of testosterone on LH control. However, since there are differences in the pattern of LH secretion at different times of the menstrual cycle, studies in women would require several sub-groups. Finally, most of the women who volunteered for our studies were on the pill. It is difficult to find female controls nowadays.

PITUITARY AND PINEAL HORMONE RHYTHMS

IN MANIC-DEPRESSION

J. Mendlewicz, E. Van Cauter, J. Golstein, L. Vanhaelst,
P. Linkowski, M. L'Hermite and C. Robyn (1), U. Weinberg
and E.D. Weitzman   (2)
Universities of Brussels, Belgium (1) and Albert Einstein
  College of Medicine, New York, U.S.A. (2)

INTRODUCTION

Biological rhythms are an integral part of life. The day
and night 24-hour period is present in almost all biological systems, remaining constant in various environments.
This observation has led to the concept of endogenous
biological clocks. The exact synchronisation of the 24-
hour period also involves external synchronizers ("zeitgebers"). Besides circadian rhythms, living organisms also
present shorter ultradian rhythms such as the REM period of
sleep (paradoxical sleep) or longer infradian rhythms such
as the menstrual cycle in female.

The exact nature of biological clocks remains unclear, but
the hypothalamo-pituitary axis seems to play a role in the
maintenance of circadian rhythms both in animal and man (1).
It is by now clear that the pituitary gland constitutes a
major link in the neuroendocrine axis in man. Central neurotransmitters regulate the secretion of the hypothalamic
neurohormones which in turn may affect brain monoamine metabolism. These neuroendocrine parameters are subjected to
circadian variations both in animal and man and they may be
implicated in the pathogenesis of periodic psychoses. A
new approach called chronophysiology permits to study temporal changes in clinical and physiological symptoms in diseases such as cancer, endocrine disturbances, cardiovascu-
lar and psychiatric conditions. Furthermore, treatment
response may also show important temporal variations probably due to circadian variations in drug metabolism and receptor sensitivity (chronopharmacology).

Some affective disorders are characterized by an alternance
of depressive and manic episodes and by periodic as well as

diurnal disturbances in mood and biological functions such as sleep, energy, appetite and sex (evening improvement and morning worsening). These diurnal changes may be related to desynchronisation of day-night variation of the mood and drive system. According to this concept, desynchronisation may be an important pathophysiological aspect of depression with some biological rhythms following its non endogenous, or free running, circadian period, deviated from the normal 24 hour period (in general phase advanced).

Furthermore, experimental studies have shown jet lag and night shift (i.e. desynchronisation phenomenon) to modify energy level and concentration abilities while sleep deprivation has been reported to temporarily alleviate depression. It may be paradoxical to improve depression with sleep deprivation since this condition is usually associated with a reduction in sleep. The mechanism of sleep deprivation is unknown but it may be understood in light of the desynchronisation theory. During sleep deprivation, the previously desynchronised rhythm may come into plan with the free running cycle, and when this resynchronisation takes place, the depression may be relieved. As soon as the patient resumes its sleep pattern, desynchronisation occurs again, and the depression may return (chronotherapy).

The study of circadian and ultradian rhythms of biological functions are thus of great importance in psychopathology, in particular, manic-depression. According to this desynchronisation hypothesis, manic-depression may be conceptualized as a "biological clock" disorder.

Over several centuries, observations of remarkably predictable recurrences of periodic psychoses have stimulated interest and raised the hope that studies of these patients might help us understand important aspects of the pathophysiology of affective psychoses (2, 3). Despite the fact that precise periodicities of psychosis are rare, there is, nevertheless, a marked statistical tendency to approach a specific timetable in a large number of patients. Such phenomena are highly relevant to the structural changes in mood observed in affectively ill patients.

A minority of manic-depressive patients, called "rapid cyclers" show an unusually rapid shift from depression to mania and vice versa. These patients switch rapidly from the zenith of mania to the nadir of depression with little free normal intervals. This switch to mania offers a unique opportunity to monitor some biological variables in relation to sudden mood changes. Phase shifts in biochemical circadian rhythms in manic-depressive patients have also been suggested for steroids, electrolyte rhythms, neurochemical metabolites and body temperature. While these studies based on brief observations suggest that there are circadian disturbances in manic-depressives, longitudinal observations are essential to demonstrate consistent circadian patterns in affectively ill patients.

The existence of circadian variations in the release of several pituitary hormones, such as ACTH, TSH, PRL and adrenal hormones such as cortisol in man has been well documented. Moreover, for several of these hormones, such as ACTH, TSH, cortisol and melatonin, it has been shown that higher frequency non-periodic oscillations, corresponding to secretory episodes, were superimposed to the basal circadian rhythm. As a consequence of this hormonal variability, consistent studies of hormonal secretion imply repeated blood sampling over long periods of time (i.e. 24-hour periods). This approach has been used by Sachar and his colleagues (4) who have found that the normal 24-hour pattern of cortisol secretion was disrupted in some depressed patients. There was an increase in the number of secretory episodes, with active secretion during the normal non-secretory period, and with elevation of all peaks of plasma cortisol throughout the 24 hours. The pattern almost returned to normal after the patient recovered.

Other workers have previously shown that the effects of dexamethasone and of insulin-induced hypoglycemia on cortisol secretion were reduced in depressed patients (5), an observation relating to the same endocrine dysfunction. They postulated the existence of an "abnormal drive from limbic areas", i.e. there was a central limbic dysfunction in depression.

Other studies suggest that these disturbances cannot be explained entirely as a simple stress response, since these abnormalities are present in unanxious patients, during sleep, and are not corrected after the administration of large doses of sedative medications (6).

In light of the biogenic amine hypothesis of affective illness, recent studies have shown alterations in circadian and seasonal rhythms of various neurotransmitter substances in the plasma of depressed patients (7).

The above arguments led us to examine circadian variations of pituitary-pineal hormone levels in manic-depression.

METHOD

We have investigated pituitary activity in patients suffering from primary affective disorders. In this paper, we are now reporting preliminary results on the 24-hour secretion of prolactin, TSH and melatonin during the depressed phase of manic-depressive illness in subjects diagnosed as bipolar manic-depressives, i.e. patients experiencing both manic and depressive episodes and unipolar depressives, suffering from depression only.

Serum TSH (μU/ml) and prolactin (μU/ml) were measured by a double antibody radioimmunoassay (8, 9, 10). Plasma concentration of melatonin was determined by radioimmunoassay (11). Estimated amplitudes and phases (day and night) of TSH, prolactin and melatonin patterns observed in depressed patients were compared to the estimations obtained for control patterns recorded in healthy volunteers. All patients studied were free of medications for at least one week prior to the investigation and were hospitalized in an inpatient unit for a primary depressive episode severe enough to warrant hospitalization. Patients were diagnosed as bipolar and unipolar depression (12). Severity of the depressive illness was assessed by the Hamilton Rating Scale. Blood samples were drawn for 24 hours through a plastic indwelling catheter. Blood samples were collected every hour during day time and every thirty minutes during the night. All patients were confined to bed, had normal breakfast, lunch, supper and their nocturnal sleep was not interrupted. Day time sleep was prevented and sleep times were recorded by trained nurses. All patients and controls were investigated throughout the calendar year.

RESULTS

The prolactin patterns of all depressive patients as a group (n = 18) showed no significant difference with patterns observed in healthy subjects (n = 14). Nevertheless, the mean prolactin level over 24 hours was significantly lower in bipolar patients as compared to unipolars. This was mainly due to the absence of sleep related elevation of PRL in 6 out of 8 bipolar patients (75 %) in whom maximum PRL secretion occurred during wakefulness (phase advanced), whereas maximum PRL concentrations were observed during sleep in all unipolar patients as in normal controls.

24-HOUR PROLACTIN PROFILES IN UNIPOLARS AND BIPOLARS

	NORMALS N = 14	UNIPOLARS N = 10	BIPOLARS N = 8
24 HOUR MEAN (uU/ML)	283 ± 144	351 ± 156	165 ± 62
WAKE MEAN (uU/ML)	235 ± 136	321 ± 158	160 ± 59
DIFFERENCE BETWEEN SLEEP MEAN AND WAKE MEAN	+ IN 14/14	+ IN 8/10	+ IN 2/8
RATIO SLEEP MEAN/WAKE MEAN	1.77 ± .69	1.37 ± .46	1.06 ± .29

The diurnal patterns of TSH levels studied in unmedicated depressed female patients (n = 13) differed greatly from those exhibited by normal subjects previously investigated (n = 6 males, 10 females). The mean 24-hour TSH level was lower in all depressed patients when compared to normals. In these patients, the rhythm appears to be desynchronized, no early morning peak being evidenced. In some cases, a maximum occurred before midnight. Higher frequency variations of plasma TSH could also be observed in unipolar and bipolar patients. Furthermore, thyroid function was found to be normal in all patients and controls.

NYCTOHEMERAL PATTERN OF TSH IN DEPRESSION

UNIPOLAR DEPRESSION	BIPOLAR DEPRESSION
Normal thyroid function	Normal thyroid function
Normal basal TSH levels	Normal basal TSH levels
Abnormal circadian TSH rhythm :	Normal circadian TSH rhythm :
lower 24-hour TSH mean	normal 24-hour TSH mean
sleep-wake ratio of TSH is lower	normal sleep-wake ratio of TSH
absence of nocturnal rise of TSH	nocturnal rise of TSH

One interesting aspect of the desynchronization hypothesis could be related to the increased incidence of affective (manic and depressive) relapses in spring and autumn when day light is either longer or shorter. It is thus possible that in genetically predisposed subjects, some circadian physiological clock parameters may be desynchronized during these periods. In those susceptible individuals, circadian desynchronization may be triggered by infradian seasonal variations and then continue into a free running cycle. Melatonin is a pineal hormone particularly sensitive to day-night changes and exposure to light. It is also under central noradrenergic control. Melatonin is thus of great interest in studying cyclic manic-depressive patients. Preliminary data on 24-hour plasma melatonin concentrations are available for 2 female depressed patients before and after treatment and 5 normal controls (males). Secretory episodes are observed throughout the 24-hour span in all subjects but are of higher magnitude in depressed patients. Furthermore the circadian rhythm of melatonin is less apparent in depressed patients. The night/day ratio for

melatonin is 1.38 in depressed patients and 2.80 in normals.
The nocturnal rise of melatonin is practically absent in 3
of 4 depressed patients who show an elevation of the pituitary hormone during daytime. Finally, no significant changes in 24-hour melatonin patterns can be seen in depressed
patients after antidepressant treatment and following remission.

NYCTOHEMERAL PATTERN OF MELATONIN IN DEPRESSION	NYCTOHEMERAL PATTERN OF MELATONIN IN CONTROLS
Circadian rhythm : abnormal or absent	Circadian rhythm with noctur- nal rise of melatonin
Reduction or absence of nocturnal rise of melatonin	
Average night/day ratio = 1.38	Average night/day ratio = 2.80
Secretory episodes throughout the 24-hour span	Secretory episodes throughout the 24-hour span

No significant changes in 24-hour melatonin pattern
after recovery following antidepressant treatment

It seems thus that the altered circadian pattern of melatonin secretion in depression is not state dependent.

DISCUSSION

We have previously demonstrated striking alterations of the
24-hour profile of plasma dopamine-bêta-hydroxylase (DBH)
activity in the same depressed patients, with more episodic
variations during daytime and absence of the afternoon elevation of DBH in some depressed patients. These observations may provide an objective and quantitative biological
indicator of the alteration of circadian peripheral dopaminergic activity in affective illness (13). In the present
studies, several parameters could not be rigorously controlled. Among those are sex, age and ovarian status. Furthermore, the absence of polygraphic recordings of sleep does
not permit to disregard the possible influence of sleep disturbances on circadian hormonal rhythms, although the

abnormalities described in our depressed patients do not
seem to disappear after clinical remission (including norma-
lisation of sleep) following antidepressant treatment.
Alterations in circadian rhythms for plasma pituitary and
pineal hormones such as prolactin, TSH and melatonin are
present in some depressed patients and it is tempting to
hypothesize that these circadian disturbances may be related to desynchronization phenomena in manic-depressive
illness. This desynchronization may induce primary modifications of circadian rhythms of central catecholaminergic
and serotoninergic activity in affective illness, as suggested by the typical alterations in the 24-hour profile of
plasma DBH activity which we have previously described in
manic-depressive patients.

Moreover, it is possible that cholinergic-adrenergic inter-
actions are also of significance. Finally, there is no
reason to assume that groups of patients labelled as "depressive" are necessarily similar on genetic and biochemical grounds. As a matter of fact, we have previously
shown that it is possible to differentiate between several
genetic subgroups in depressive illness (14). It is thus
conceivable that some form of depressive illness may be
associated with an abnormality in serotonin metabolism
while catecholaminergic deficiencies may be present in
other forms of depression, and that there is a complex im-
balance between several neurotransmitters. The rapid changes in mood and the abruptness of the desynchronization observed in manic-depressive patients make it unlikely that
these phenomena be related to primary oscillations in
central neurotransmitter synthesis or turnover rate. More
fruitful hypotheses may be formulated in terms of infradian, ultradian or circadian variation in specific brain
receptor sensitivity or more complex behavioral modulation
through endogenous neuropeptide substances. This may be
more consistent with the concept of internal desynchronization of biological rhythms in some manic-depressive patients. As circadian clock frequency may be transmitted
on an X-chromosome gene as has been shown in animal studies
(15) (Drosophilia melanogaster) and may increase with age,

a circadian etiology is consistent with the genetics and age distribution of manic-depressive illness (as indicated by Kripke et al, 16). The brain distribution of other releasing factors and peptides has not yet been reported and when the brain effects of hypothalamic hormones and peptides will be further elucidated, the clinical conditions in which their actions are investigated may be better understood. Nevertheless, the chronobiological studies described above combining enzymatic and neuroendocrine evaluation over long periods of time in the study of abnormal behavior are most promising and may enable us to better understand cyclical alterations of hypothalamic and pituitary functions in man, although it is still premature to draw firm conclusions from the neuroendocrine abnormalities as to the specific nature of the underlying neurotransmitter or neuropeptide disturbances in psychopathology.

REFERENCES

1. RICHTER, C.P., Abnormal but Regular Cycles in Behavior and Metabolism in Rats and Catatonic-Schizophrenics. In : Psychoneuroendocrinology, M. Reiss, Ed. Grune & Stratton, New York : 168-181, 1958.

2. GJESSING, R, Beiträge zur Kenntniss der Pathophysiologie des Katatonen Stupors. Archiv. Fur Psychiatr. und Nervenkrank, 200 : 350-366, 1960.

3. JENNER, F.A. : Periodic Psychoses in the Light of Biological Rhythm Research. Intern. Rev. of Neurobiol., 11 : 129-169, 1968.

4. SACHAR, E.J., HELLMAN, L. and FUKUSHIMA, D.K. : Cortisol production in depressive illness. Arch. Gen. Psychiat., 23 : 289-298, 1970.

5. CARROLL, B.J., Hypothalamic-Pituitary Function in Depressive Illness : Insensivity to Hypoglycaemia. Brit. Med. Journ., 3 : 27-28, 1969.

6. STOKES, P.E., Studies on the Control of Adrenocortical Function in Depression. In : Recent Advances in the Psychobiology of Depressive Illnesses, Williams, Katz and Shiled, Washington D.C., U.S. Dehw Publ. : 199-220, 1972.

7. RIEDERER, P., BIRKMAYER, W., NEUMAYER, E., AMBROZI, L. and LINAUER, W., The Daily Rhythm of HVA, VMA, (VA) and 5HIAA in Depression Syndrome. J. Neural Transm., 35 : 23-45, 1974.

8. GOLSTEIN, J. and VANHAELST, L., Influence of Thyrotrophin Free Serum on the Radioimmunoassay of Human Thyrotropin. Clin. Chim. Acta, 49 : 141, 1973.

9. AUBERT, M.L., BECKER, R.L., SAXENA, B.B. and RAITI, S., Report of the National Pituitary Agency. Collaborative Study of the Radioimmunoassay of Human Prolactin. J. Clin. Endocr. Metab., 38 : 1115-1120, 1974.

10. BADAWI, M., BILA, S., L'HERMITE, M., PEREZ-LOPEZ, R.F. and ROBYN, C., Comparative Evaluation of Radioimmunoassay for Human Prolactin using Anti-ovine and Anti-human Prolactin Sera. In : Radioimmunoassays and Related Prodedures in Medicine. Vol 1. International Atomic Energy Agency, Vienna : 411-422, 1974.

11. WEINBERG, U., D'ELETTO, R.D., WEITZMAN, E.D., ERLICH, S and HOLLANDER, C.S., Circulating Melatonin in Man : Episodic Secretion throughout the Light-Dark Cycle. J. Clin. Endocrinol. Metab. , 48, 1 : 114-118, 1979.

12. MENDLEWICZ, J. and FLEISS, J.L., Linkage Studies with X-Chromosome Markers in Bipolar (Manic-Depressive) and Unipolar (Depressive) Illness. Biol. Psychiat., 2 : 1044, 1974.

13. VAN CAUTER E. and MENDLEWICZ, J, 24-Hour Dopamine-Bêta-Hydroxylase Pattern : A Possible Biological Index of Manic-Depression. Life Sciences, Vol. 22, 2 : 147-155, 1978.

14. MENDLEWICZ, J, Le Concept d'Hétérogénéité dans la Psychose Maniaco-Dépressive. L'Inf. Psychiat., 2 : 1044, 1974.

15. KONOPKA, R.J. and BENZER, S., Clock Mutants of Drosophilia Melanogaster. Proc. Natl. Acad. Scie. (U.S.), 68 : 21-22, 1971.

16. KRIPKE, D.F., MULLANCY, D.J., HATKINSON, M., WOLF, S., Circadian Rhythm Disorders in Manic-Depressives. Biol. Psychiat., 13, 3 : 335, 1978.

DISCUSSION

REINBERG: The hypothesis of beat has been proposed to explain the differences in period of several rhythms and is presently tested by various investigators, including D. Kripke. Did you perform a spectral analysis of your data in order to determine whether the period length was modified in your patients? Was it different from 24 hours?

MENDLEWICZ: The statistical analysis of the data was performed by E. Van Cauter. Does your question pertain to mood variations or hormonal variations?

REINBERG: It was shown that, in manic-depressive patients, the period of the body temperature rhythm is different from 24 hours. Lithium treatment acts on the length of the period. Thus, I wonder if in your patients the period length was altered.

VAN CAUTER: No patient was studied for longer than one 24-hour cycle. Since the alterations within a 24-hour cycle were considerable and different from one plasma constituent to another, we could not determine whether the period length was longer or shorter than in normal subjects.

KRIEGER: One other neuroendocrine abnormality which has been described in depressed patients concerns the response to TRH. Could you correlate the abnormalities you observed in the 24-hour profile of TSH with abnormal responses to TRH stimulation?

MENDLEWICZ: We studied the response to TRH in patients with manic-depression. We found abnormal responses of TSH in most of these patients.

KRIEGER: I was referring to the GH response to TRH which may be abnormal in manic-depression. Do these abnormalities correlate with alterations of the TSH periodicity?

MENDLEWICZ: In our patients, there was such a large interindividual variation in the GH response to TRH that it

is very difficult to draw conclusions. Some patients have
a clear abnormal response, sometimes the response is delayed but the interindividual variability is enormous.

QUABBE: Your patients had a higher mean 24-hour PRL
level. Were there any patients with mean 24-hour PRL
levels outside the normal range? Were the melatonin
studies conducted in unipolar or bipolar subjects?

MENDLEWICZ: Actually, bipolar patients had lower
mean PRL levels than normal controls while unipolar patients
had values higher than controls. However, basal PRL levels
were within the normal range for both groups. In our melatonin studies, we had 3 unipolar patients and 1 bipolar
patient.

JAQUET: A possible effect of lithium on TSH could
clearly be interpreted as resulting from altered T3 and
T4 levels. Do you have any data on the effect of lithium
on melatonin?

MENDLEWICZ: We have performed some studies but the
samples are still in Dr. Weitzman's laboratory.

L'HERMITE: The abnormalities of the 24-hour profile
of PRL on the one hand and of TSH on the other hand did
not occur in the same type of depression. Would you
interpret this finding in the light of inter-relation-
ships between these hormones and of the dopaminergic and,
perhaps also, the somatostatin effects on these secretions? Are there any data on the levels of somatostatin
in these patients?

MENDLEWICZ: Indeed, the abnormalities in the TSH pattern were only observed in unipolars whereas the abnormalities of PRL pattern were found in bipolars mostly.
There seems to be major neurochemical differences between
unipolar and bipolar patients. Which particular neurotransmitter is affected in either type of depression

remains unclear. My point of view is that, even within
unipolar patients, there are probably several different
specific neurochemical abnormalities involving dopamine
or serotonin or noradrenalin. There is a genetic and
biochemical heterogeneity within the unipolar and bipolar
groups. We do not have any data on somatostatin.

L'HERMITE: What is the relevance of this type of
studies to the management and therapy of patients?

MENDLEWICZ: I believe that psychiatry suffers from
the lack of biological tests providing objective basis
for diagnosis. If studies showing abnormalities in neurotransmitter metabolism and neuroendocrine tests are confirmed, reliable and sensitive biological tests for
the diagnosis of psychiatric diseases may be made available.

L'HERMITE: You showed alterations of melatonin secretion in depression. Are there any data on LH and FSH
secretion in these subjects? Because of the inter-rela-
tions between melatonin, LH and FSH, abnormalities in
gonadotrophin patterns might be expected.

MENDLEWICZ: There are indeed other studies showing
abnormalities in LH and FSH patterns in subtypes of depressive patients. LH-RH has been used as a potential
antidepressant treatment. It is however still controversial.

WEEKE: I would like to emphasize that, so far, no
assay is able to measure somatostatin levels in man.

JAQUET: If some differences in somatostatin levels
could be measured in psychiatric patients, they could
bring some support to the hypothesis of gastrointestinal
and pancreatic origin of psychiatric disorders. The
quantity of somatostatin which is exported by the gut
and the pancreas is enormous. It is thus very difficult

to assess differences.

WEEKE: It is possible to find a measure of somatostatin by studying the cerebrospinal fluid.

JAQUET: Only hemorragies have shown significant
differences in somatostatin. This has already been
studied unsuccessfully.

CIRCADIAN RHYTHM OF PLASMA GONADOTROPINS, PROLACTIN AND
GROWTH HORMONE LEVELS IN ANOREXIA NERVOSA : CORRELATIONS
WITH HYPOPHYSIAL TESTS

R. Roulier[1], B. Conte-Devolx[1,2], E. Castanas[3], J.
Bert[4] and J.L. Codaccioni[1]

(1) Service d'Endocrinologie et des Maladies Métaboliques,
Hôpital de la Conception, Marseille, (2) Laboratoire de
Physiologie, Faculté de Médecine, Marseille, (3) Laboratoire
des Hormones Protéiques, Faculté de Médecine, Marseille,
(4) Service de Neurophysiologie Clinique, Hôpital de la
Timone, Marseille.

Numerous hypothalamo -pituitary abnormalities have been
described in anorexia nervosa (for review see 1 and 2).

These abnormalities, especially those involving gonadotropin function, have been usually demonstrated by baseline
hormone levels and responses to dynamic tests.

The aim of the study was to examine 24-hour plasma profiles of PRL, GH, LH and FSH in anorexia nervosa and to compare the results to those obtained after dynamic testing.

PATIENTS AND METHODS

Patients

8 patients with anorexia nervosa defined according to the
criteria of Feighner et al. (3) were studied. The group
consisted of 7 girls with amenorrhea and 1 boy. At the
time of study, patient age ranged from 17 to 25 years and
body weight was 70 % to 94 % of ideal body weight as defined in the Metropolitan Life Insurance Tables (4). Initial
weight was less than 70 % in all the cases. None of the
patients received medication during the 3 months prior to
testing.

Methods

A. Sleep studies

Polygraph recordings (EEG, EMG and Eye movement tracings)
were made between 22.00 h and 06.00 h in three consecutive
nights. Recordings were done in a temperature controlled
(18°C) soundproof room. Lights were turned off from 22.00
h to 06.00 h. Sleep stages were analyzed as described in
(5). An indwelling cathether was placed in the antecubital
vein on the third night 3 hours prior to recording. Control
values were obtained in 20 age-matched healthy volunteers.
Ten subjects only underwent polygraphic recording as described above (group A) and the ten other controls (group B)
were tested by the full procedure (polygraph and catheter
on the third night).

B. Hormone studies

1° 24 h studies :

Blood samples for measurement of FSH, LH, PRL and GH were
taken remotely every 20 min for 24 h. The samples were
immediately centrifuged and stored at -20°C until measurement.

2° Dynamic tests :

FSH and LH plasma levels were measured after an I.V. bolus
of 100 µg LHRH (Roussel, France) and prolactin plasma values
were determined after a 250 µg I.V. bolus of TRH (Roche,
France). Blood samples were taken 15 min before and at the
time of injection and 20 min, 30 min, 60 min, 90 min, 120
min after. Both tests were performed shortly after the
sleep recordings. At this time, the patients' weight had not
changed significantly.

3° Hormone assays

Hormone determinations were made by radioimmunoassay with
the following reagents for FSH and LH : ^{125}I labelled hormones by the lactoperoxydase procedure, specific antibodies
(a generous gift of D. Reuter), MRC 68-39 LH Standard and
68-40 FSH Standard. Results are expressed in mIU/ml. Cold
and labelled hormones were incubated with the antibody at
4°C for 96 h, then separated by the double antibody technique (48 h incubation at 4°C). Using this method, the limit
of detectability of FSH and LH was 0.2 mIU/ml.

- PRL was assayed using a homologous human system as described by Reuter et al. (6); results are expressed in mIU/ml of the MRC 68-32 standard (40 mIU = 1 ng).
- GH was assayed using a commercial reagent kit (CEA - I.R.E., Sorin, GIF/S/Yvette, France); results are expressed in ng/ml.

4° Statistical analysis :

The different parameters studied (hormone plasma values, duration of sleep) were compared by Student's t test using the residual variance of the analysis of variance as a common estimator of the S.D. (7).

5° Analysis of hormonal results :

- A pulsatile GH burst is defined by at least a 100 % increase over the preceding value
- PRL values were analyzed every two hours during the night (22.00 h-06.00 h) and the mean prolactin level during each 2 h interval was compared to the mean daytime value (06.00 h-22.00 h); a prolactin rise is assumed to exist when at least one nocturnal value is statistically greater than the daytime mean
- The LH 24 h plasma profiles were analyzed according to Boyar et al. (8) with a few modifications.

The following criteria were used :

   infantile : no LH values greater than 1 mIU/ml throughout the 24 h period

   puberal : nocturnal LH values greater than 1 mIU/ml and statistically higher than daytime values (the latter may be less than 1 mIU/ml)

   adult : all values are greater than 1 mIU/ml and nocturnal LH levels do not differ from daytime values

- LHRH test : LH and FSH responses are expressed as cumulative response, i.e. the area circumscribed by the hormone response curve and the line passing through the mean baseline value

RESULTS

Sleep studies (Fig. 1)

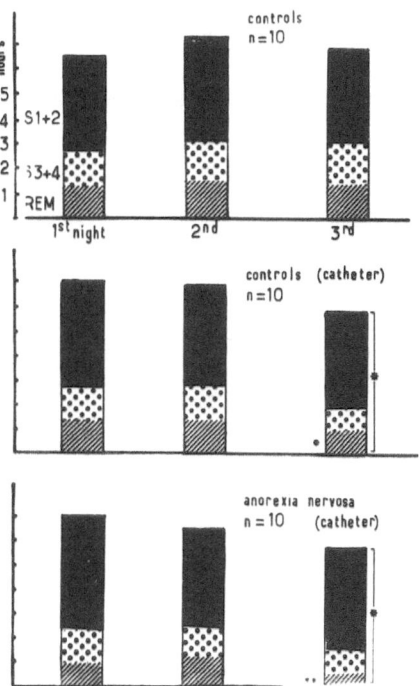

Figure 1 : *Total sleep time, duration of stages 1, 2, 3, 4 and REM sleep in control subject (without and with catheter) and in patients with anorexia nervosa.* ★ $P < 0.05$ - ★★ $P < 0.01$.

In the 3 groups studied (patients with anorexia nervosa, group A and group B controls), the polygraph recordings of the first two nights were not significantly different on the basis of total sleep time and duration of stages 1, 2, 3, 4 and REM sleep. In control group A (no catheter) sleep parameters were unchanged over the three nights period. Conversely, in control group B and in patients with anorexia nervosa, the positioning of the venous catheter coincided with a significant decrease in total sleep duration (group B : 386 ± 7 (SEM); anorexia nervosa : 326 ± 34 versus 410 ± 12 and 394 ± 20 minutes respectively on the second night) and in duration of REM sleep (group B : 64 ± 5; anorexia nervosa : 38 ± 8; versus 87 ± 2 and 71 ± 8 respectively on the second night).

Hormonal studies

1° GH (Table 1)

Table 1. Mean daytime and nighttime baseline GH (ng/ml)
plasma levels in patients with anorexia nervosa

CASE N°	SLEEP		WAKE	
	Mean	SEM	Mean	SEM
1	5.21	0.16	0.70	0.19
2	2.89	0.67	1.32	0.34
3	1.02	0.05	1.43	0.15
4	4.63	1.00	5.68	2.51
5	2.82	0.18	2.35	0.25
6	1.77	0.39	1.77	0.37
7	4.51	0.31	2.94	0.26
8	3.25	0.70	2.05	0.85

This table
Shows the mean daytime and nightime baseline GH plasma
levels in patients with anorexia nervosa. These values are
within the normal range in all cases. However, although at
least one nocturnal burst of GH is consistently observed in
normal subjects, 3/8 (cases 3, 5, 7) patients with anorexia
nervosa do not present such pulsatile secretion (Fig. 2).

2° PRL (Table II)

Table II. Mean diurnal and nocturnal prolactin (mIU/ml)
values observed in 8 patients with anorexia nervosa.

6 H	→	22 H	350 ± 87
22 H	→	24 H	453 ± 147
24 H	→	2 H	633 ± 212
2 H	→	4 H	504 ± 143
4 H	→	6 H	526 ± 119

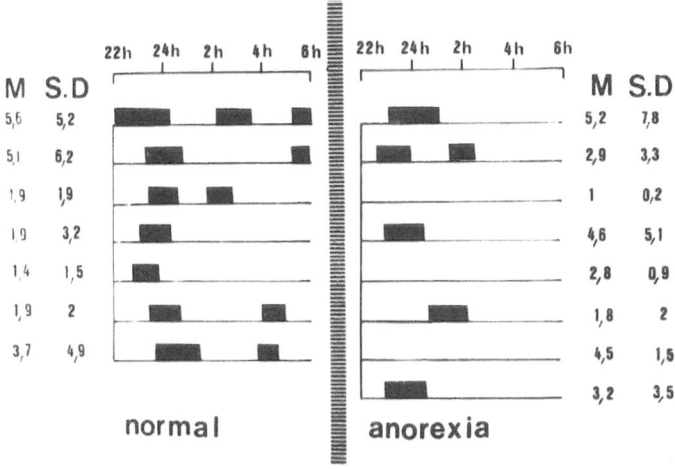

Figure 2 : Nocturnal burst of GH (ng/ml) (for definition see text) observed in normal subjects (left part) and in patients with anorexia nervosa (right part).

24 h mean PRL plasma levels did not differ significantly from normal values in all 8 cases. A significant PRL rise occurred during sleep (Fig. 3) in the 8 patients and the maximum PRL level was found between 24.00 h and 02.00 h in 7 cases and between 02.00 h and 04.00 h in the remaining patient.

PRL responsiveness to TRH was normal in the 8 patients.

3° Gonadotropins
Results of the study are shown in Table III.

The mean 24 h FSH plasma levels are similar to values in normal adults. An infantile plasma LH pattern (Fig. 4) was found in 3 patients (cases 1, 5, 7), a puberal pattern (Fig. 4b), in 3 patients (cases 2, 3, 8) and an adult pattern (Fig. 4c) was evidenced in the 2 remaining patients (Fig. 5). No correlation was found between LH pattern type and any one of the following parameters : body weight, duration of amenorrhea, age.

In all 8 patients FSH responded normally to LHRH. On the

Table III. Results of gonadotropin study in 8 cases of anorexia nervosa : mean diurnal and nocturnal levels and response to LHRH injection (100 µg I.V.). Patients are classified according to LH pattern (see text).

	CASE NB	% Ideal body weight	FSH (mIU/ml)				LH (mIU/ml)				LHRH test (cumulative response)	
			SLEEP		AWAKE		SLEEP		AWAKE		FSH (IU/ml/2 H)	LH (IU/ml/2H)
			Mean	SEM	Mean	SEM	Mean	SEM	Mean	SEM		
INFANTILE	1	70	2.6	0.36	2.3	0.31	0.7	0.10	0.4	0.12	0.83	0.08
	5	94	6.1	0.23	4.9	0.20	0.5	0.11	< 0.2	–	0.71	0.10
	7	76	6.4	0.20	5.5	0.17	< 0.2	–	< 0.2	–	0.79	0.03
PUBERAL	2	80	12.5	1.42	9.7	1.81	2.3	0.22	1.2	0.23	0.74	0.44
	3	83	3.15	0.15	3.5	0.14	2.1	0.33	< 0.2	–	1.43	0.16
	8	75	12.6	0.49	9.0	0.36	4.6	–	0.5	0.18	0.60	0.88
ADULT	4	78	8.9	0.22	9.8	0.35	6.1	0.25	5.7	0.29	0.38	2.10
	6	94	5.9	0.38	4.6	0.38	1.6	0.32	1	0.35	0.24	1.47

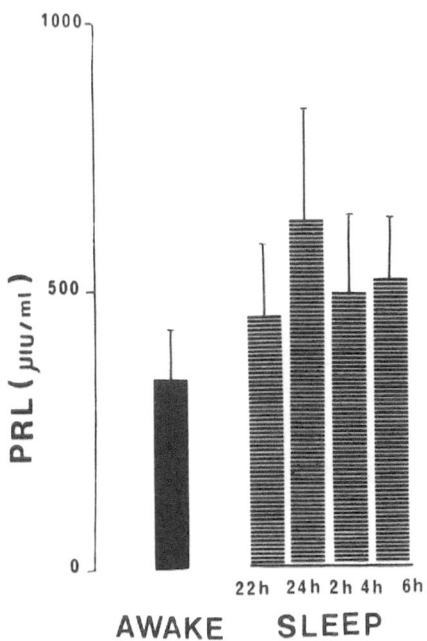

Figure 3 : *Mean prolactin levels observed in 8 cases of anorexia nervosa.*

other hand, LH responsiveness to LHRH varied according to cases : no or very weak response in 4 cases, a normal response in 4 cases. The absence of LH response to LHRH was observed in the patients with an infantile LH pattern (Fig. 6a) whereas the 2 patients with an adult pattern displayed normal LH responsiveness to the stimulation (Fig. 6c). Thus, the ratio of LH response to FSH response was practically zero in the infantile LH pattern group, normal (> 3) in the patients with an adult LH pattern, and ranged between these 2 values in the group with a puberal LH pattern (Fig. 6b).

DISCUSSION

Despite the many precautions taken during the sleep studies, reduction in total sleep time and especially in REM sleep occurred on the third night of testing (insertion of catheter) in normal subjects as well as in patients with anorexia

318

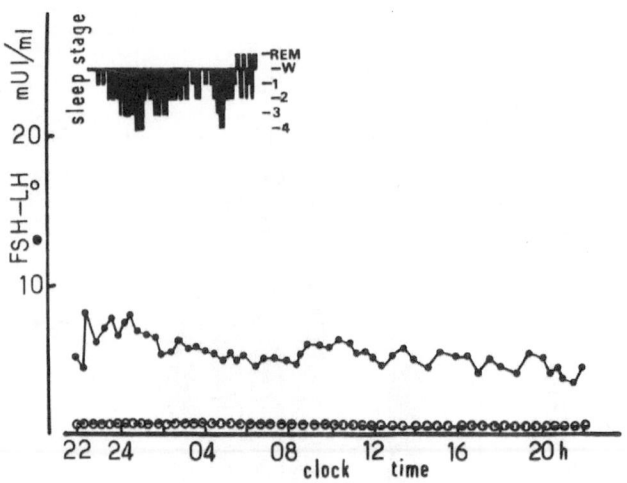

Figure 4a

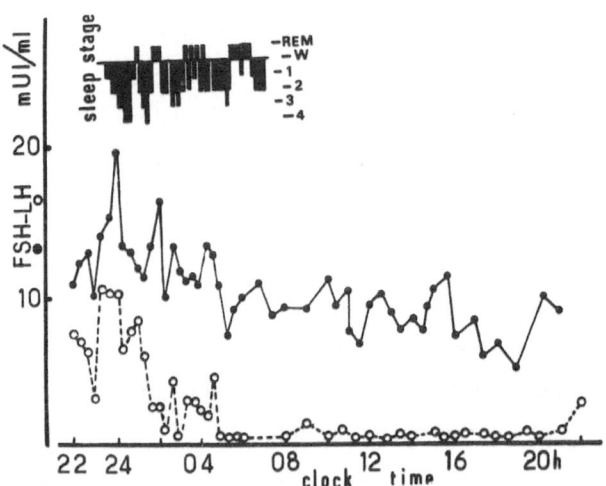

Figure 4b

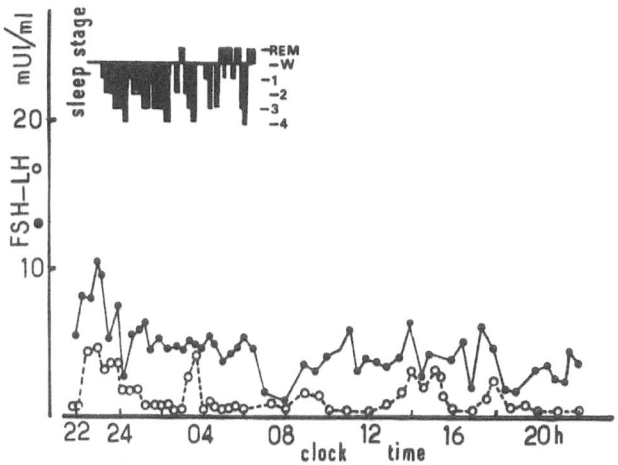

Figure 4c
Figure 4 : Typical infantile (4a), puberal (4b) and adult (4c) 24 - hour LH pattern observed in individual cases of anorexia nervosa.

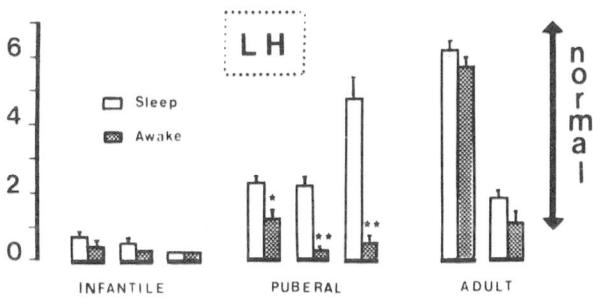

Figure 5 : 24-hour LH pattern in 8 cases of anorexia nervosa. Patients are classified according to LH pattern (see text).

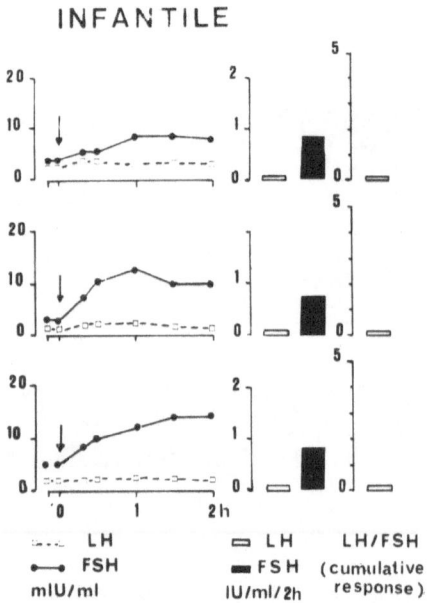

Figure 6a

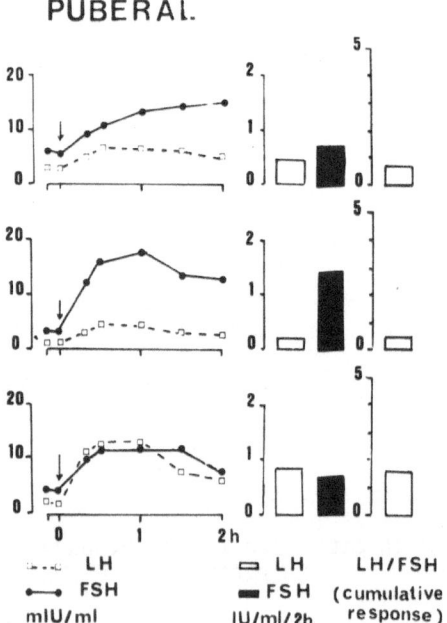

Figure 6b

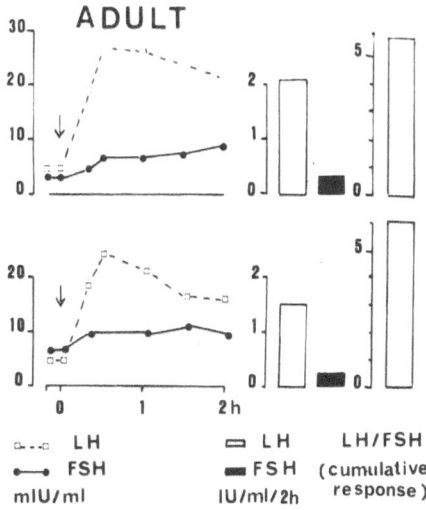

Figure 6c
Figure 6 : Results of LHRH test in anorexia nervosa with infantile
(3 cases : Fig. 6a), puberal (3 cases : Fig. 6b) and adult (2 cases :
Fig. 6c), 24-hour LH pattern.

nervosa. Conversely sleep was not modified on the 3 tests
nights in group A normal subjects (without catheter). Ins-
talling an indwelling catheter seems to be a stress producing procedure disturbing sleep which should be taken into
account when interpreting results of such studies.

In 3/8 patients with anorexia nervosa no GH rise occurred
at the onset of sleep. The five remaining patients who
displayed a nocturnal rise in plasma GH values did not differ from the 3 preceding cases when compared on the basis
of body weight and EEG sleep data. These abnormalities of
GH secretion can be linked to results obtained by other
workers studying GH responsiveness to dynamic tests. Such
results include a decreased GH response to insulin induced
hypoglycemia (9), lack of response to L-dopa (10) and a
paradoxical GH rise after I.V. TRH (11) which is not abo-

lished after administration of oral bromocriptine (12).
These results combined with those of the present study are
in favour of disturbed secretory regulation of GH in some
cases of anorexia nervosa. Certain authors (13) suggest
that the abnormality lies in disrupted dopaminergic control
of GH secretion. However, regulation of GH secretion in
normal subjects is complex and the precise role of biogenic
amines in the regulation of this hormone is not clear.

As shown by studies of 24-h PRL variations and responses to
TRH, PRI regulation was normal in all our cases of anorexia
nervosa. These findings confirm a previous study (2) in
which a normal PRL response to TRH persisted during follow-
up of weight in 23 cases of anorexia nervosa. Our results
are in agreement with other studies (14, 15) which showed a
normal baseline PRL level and response to TRH in this
disease. However, in certain studies (16, 17), frankly elevated baseline PRL values have been reported. The latter
finding could be related to an accompanying disease state
or the use of certain drugs (neuroleptic) able to affect
PRL secretion.

Three types of 24-h sleep-wake LH patterns (infantile,
puberal, adult) were found in our patients. Similar 24 h
patterns of infantile and puberal LH levels have been described previously (18). On the other hand, our finding of
an adult type pattern in 2 cases is in disagreement with
the study of Boyar and Katz (19) who consistently observed
a prepuberal or puberal profile despite a return to normal
weight. Conversely in a recent study Pirke et al. (20) observed an adult type LH pattern in many cases of anorexia
nervosa when body weight exceeds 80 % of ideal weight.

Gonadotropin responsiveness to rapid I.V. LHRH also leads
to defining an infantile (no LH response), puberal (weak LH
response) and adult group (early pronounced LH response).
Since FSH reactivity is constant in the 3 groups, the ratio
LH response/FSH response increases from the infantile to
adult state (reaching > 3) (21). These 3 types of responsiveness to LHRH were found in our patients group. Furthermore each response type correlated to the 24 h pattern in

each patient. Discording results have been reported by Katz et al. (22) who found an adult type of response to LHRH (100 µg I.V.) in 6 cases studied despite the presence of prepuberal 24 h LH pattern.

Abnormal responses to LHRH in anorexia nervosa have been described by Warren et al. (23) and Beumont et al. (24) and Sherman et al. (25) who showed that the LH response is absent when weight is less than 70 % of ideal body weight whereas normal LH responsiveness occurs at more than 90 % of ideal body weight. In a previous study (26) based on changes in reactivity to LHRH during weight gain in 23 patients we observed similar results when patients groups were compared on the basis of weight. Nevertheless, this study showed that marked variations exist among patients with the same percent of ideal body weight. However, the most striking finding in these cases was an increase in the ratio of LH response/FSH response during weight gain in all cases (Fig. 7). Furthermore, the rate of increase in this ratio varied among the patients. These data of variable alteration of gonadotropin function and variable resumption have been confirmed by Pirke et al. (20). These authors, studying 24 h LH patterns, suggest that a return to normal gonadotropin function is more rapid in young patients and in cases where amenorrhea is of short duration.

Whether gonadtropin regulation is estimated by 24 h LH patterns or reactivity to LHRH test (ratio of LH response/FSH response) the following conclusions emerge in typical cases: an infantile pattern is found when weight is very low, a puberal profile exists during weight gain and adult pattern arises when weight is practically normal.

However, there are 2 exceptions to this conclusion :
1. a puberal pattern occurs in some very low weight patients. However, weight improvement is accompanied by the progression of this pattern towards the adult type;
2. infantile patterns can persist despite weight gain. This notion points out that a definition of clinical improvement based only on weight gain may be insufficient to fully assess these patients.

324

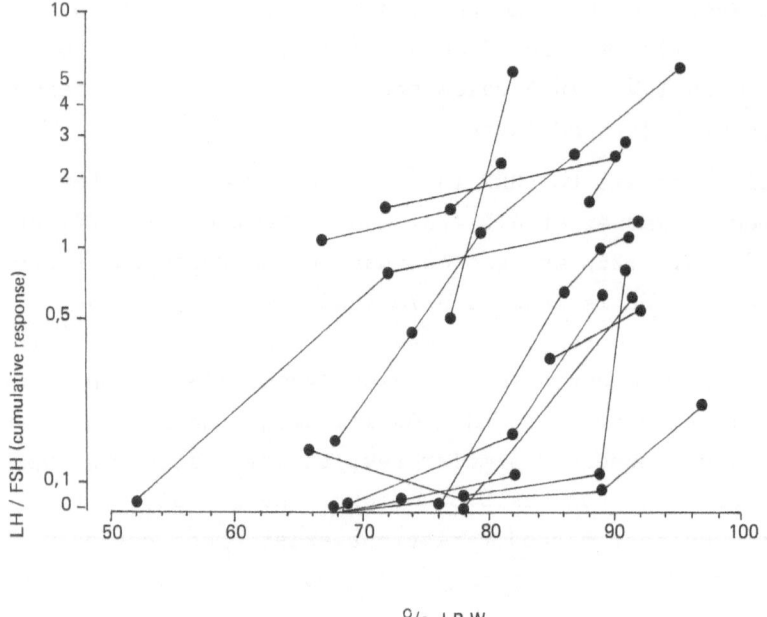

Figure 7 : Evolution of LH response/FSH response ratio in individual cases of anorexia nervosa during weight gain.

ACKNOWLEDGMENTS

To Claudie Andonian for her expert technical assistance.

REFERENCES

1. Halmi, KA, Anorexia nervosa : recent investigations. Ann Rev Med 29:137-48, 1978

2. Codaccioni, JL, R Roulier, B Conte-Devolx, A Berliner, Le status endocrinien dans l'anorexie mentale. Congrès de Psycho-neuroendocrinologie, Liège, 1979 (in press)

3. Feighner, JP, E Robins, SB Guze, RA Jr Woodruff, G Winokur, and R Munoz, Diagnostic criteria for use in psychiatric research. Arch Gen Psychiatry 26: 57-63, 1972

4. Geigy, JR, Stat Bull Metrop Life Insurance Company, 40, Bale Edit, 1959

5. Rechtsaffen, A, and A Kales (eds.). A manual for standardized terminology, techniques and scoring system for sleep stages of human subjects. National Institute of Neurological Disease and Blindness. Neurological Information Network, Bethesda, 1968 (NIH Publication n° 204)

6. Reuter, AM, F Kennes, Y Gevaert, and P Franchimont, A radioimmunoassay for human prolactin. J Nucl Med Biol 3:21-28, 1976

7. Armitage, P, Statistical methods in medical research. Blackwell, Oxford, p 217, 1971

8. Boyar, RM, JW Finkelstein, H Roffwarg, S Kapen, and ED Weitzman, Twenty-four hour luteinizing hormone and follicle-stimulating hormone secretory patterns in gonadal dysgenesis. J Clin Endocrin Metab 37: 521-525, 1973

9. Brauman, H, and F Gregoire, The growth hormone response to insulin induced hypoglycemia in anorexia nervosa and control underweight of normal subjects. Eur J Clin Invest 5:289-295, 1975

10. Sherman, BM, and KA Halmi, Effect of nutritional rehabilitation on hypothalamic pituitary function in anorexia nervosa. In: Anorexia Nervosa, Vigersky, RA (ed.), New York, Raven Press, 211-223, 1977

326

11. Maeda, K, N Yamaguchi, K Chihara, S Ohga, Y Iwasaki, Y
    Yoshimoto, K Moridera, S Kuromaru, and H Imura,
    Growth hormone release following thyrotropin-relea-
    sing hormone injection into patients with anorexia
    nervosa. Acta Endocrinol 81:1-8, 1976

12. Harrower, ADB, PL Yap, IM Nairn and JA Strong, Bromo-
    criptine and TRH induced growth hormone release in
    anorexia nervosa. Br Med J 2:264, 1977

13. Barry, VC, and HL Klawans, On the role of dopamine in
    the pathophysiology of anorexia nervosa. Journal
    of Neural Transmission 38:107-122, 1976

14. Beumont, PJV, HG Friesen, MG Gelder and T Kolakowska,
    Plasma prolactin and luteinizing hormone levels in
    anorexia nervosa. Psychol Med 4:219-221, 1974

15. Manciet, G, P Roger, L Mauriac, C Lataste, D Ducassou,
    B Schmitt, and J Rivière, Exploration endocrinienne
    dans l'anorexie nerveuse. Bordeaux Médical 10:1647,
    1977

16. Travaglini, P, P Beck-Peccoz, C Ferrari, B Ambrose,
    A Paracchi, A Severgnini, A Spada and G Faglia,
    Some aspects of hypothalamic pituitary function in
    patients with anorexia nervosa. Acta Endocrinol
    81:252-262, 1976

17. Mecklenburg, RS, DL Loriaux, RH Thompson, AE Andersen,
    and MB Lipsett, Hypothalamic dysfunction in
    patients with anorexia nervosa. Medicine 53:147-
    159, 1974

18. Boyar, RM, J Katz, JW Finkelstein, S Kapen, H Weiner,
    ED Weitzman and L Hellman, Anorexia nervosa : im-
    maturity of the 24-hour luteinizing hormone secre-
    tion pattern. N Engl J Med 291:861-865, 1974

19. Boyar, RM and J Katz, Twenty-four hour gonadotropin
    secretory patterns in anorexia nervosa. Anorexia
    Nervosa, Vigersky, RA (ed.). New York, 177-187,
    1977

20. Pirke, KM, MM Fichter, R Lund and P Doerr, Twenty-four
    hour sleep-wake pattern of plasma LH in patients
    with anorexia nervosa. Acta Endocrinol 92:193-204,
    1979

21. Franchimont, P, A Demoulin and JP Bourguignon,
    Clinical use of LHRH test as a diagnostic tool.
    Horm Res 6:177-191, 1975

22. Katz, JL, RM Boyar, H Roffwarg, L Hellman and H Weiner,
    LH-RH responsiveness in anorexia nervosa : intact-
    ness despite prepuberal circadian LH pattern.
    Psychosom Med 39:241-251, 1977

23. Warren, MP, R Jewelewicz, F Dyrenfurth, R Ans, S
    Khalaf and RL Vande Wiele, The significance of
    weight loss in the elevation of pituitary response
    to LH-RH in women with secondary amenorrhea. J
    Clin Endocrinol Metab 40:601-611, 1975

24. Beumont, PJV, GCW George, BL Pimstone and AI Vinik,
    Body weight and the pituitary response to hypotha-
    lamic releasing hormones in patients with anorexia
    nervosa. J Clin Endocrinol Metab 43:487-596, 1976

25. Sherman, BM, KA Halmi and R Zamudio, LH and FSH res-
    ponse to gonadotropin releasing hormone in anorexia
    nervosa. J Clin Endocrinol Metab 41:135-142, 1975

26. Roulier, R, R Djian, Reprise pondérale et fonction
    gonadotrope chez les femmes atteintes de maigreur
    nerveuse. Rev Franç Endocrinol Clin 1:58-62, 1976

DISCUSSION

L'HERMITE: Regarding PRL secretion in patients with
anorexia nervosa, you have shown that no change in PRL
levels was associated with weight gain. We have a similar
observation. In fact, there is a relation between œstra-
diol secretion and PRL levels. At puberty, PRL levels
increase a little later than estrogen secretion. There is
thus an apparent paradox between the well-known decrease
of estrogenic secretion in anorexia nervosa and loss of
body weight and the absence of change of PRL secretion in
such states. Do you think that the levels of sex hormone
binding globulin or changes in the half-life of PRL might
be involved?

ROULIER: We did not study these parameters. In our
studies, oestradiol levels did not increase significantly
with weight gain except in patients with weight over 190%
of the ideal body weight.

L'HERMITE: But, in contrast, oestradiol levels significantly decrease with weight loss. It is possible that
the absence of clear correlation between the type of gonadotrophin secretory pattern and body weight reflects differences in psychological states.

ROULIER: It is well possible.

L'HERMITE: Moreover, considering the ideal body
weight is certainly artificial. Would there be a better
correlation if the actual absolute weight losses and gains
were considered?

ROULIER: In our studies, we did not find a better
correlation with these parameters. Pirke and others showed
a good correlation between the duration of amenorrhea and
age of the patients. Increase of LH response was more
rapid with young patients and amenorrhea of short duration.

CAUFRIEZ: We studied a group of patients with anorexia nervosa and subdivided them into patients with primary amenorrhea and patients with secondary amenorrhea.
We then studied the TRH stimulation test. In patients
with secondary amenorrhea and a very important loss of
body weight, the peak of PRL was delayed. Did you observe the same phenomenon?

ROULIER: We do not have comparable data.

L'HERMITE: In our study with Dr. Caufriez, some
patients with anorexia nervosa and primary amenorrhea
experienced puberty onset and growth arrest.

GENERAL DISCUSSION

*The general discussion consisted of two parts. First, specific
points which were raised in the course of the Workshop were further
debated (methodology of statistical analysis, relationship between
sleep and hormonal secretion, hormonal profiles in pathologies and
after drug administration). Second, proposals aiming at organizing
international collaboration in the field of endocrine rhythms were
discussed.*

METHODOLOGY OF STATISTICAL ANALYSIS

VAN CAUTER: The methodology that we have developed
has been considered as rather complicated and generating
more parameters than needed to describe the data. Does
anyone want to comment on this criticism?

REINBERG: I think that there is no general recipe
for the analysis of chronobiological data. One has to
look at the data and at the methodology used to collect
them and then look for the best available procedure to
solve the problem of analyzing these specific data. It
is not valid to comment on a method of analysis without
considering its field of application. Van Cauter's
method is perfectly adequate for the data she has in
hand and provides a good statistical analysis of this
type of data. There is no need to try to generalize and
to propose a recipe for the statistical analysis of
chronobiological data.

VAN CAUTER: I totally agree with you. My method
aims specifically at analyzing 24-hour hormonal profiles,
taking into account the simultaneous presence of circadian
and episodic variations and the limitations of the sampling procedure.

KRIEGER: We all have to realize that the correct
choice of statistical approach depends on the particular type of curve one has to deal with. For example,
one should avoid attempting to fit a cosine function onto
data which don't have a cosine configuration. Another
determinant of the choice of a statistical method is the
type of question that is asked. Some approaches may be
too detailed if the only information required concerns
the presence or the absence of a predominant 24-hour
rhythm but may be adequate if other frequencies or episodic fluctuations are to be investigated. We all agree
that there are some minimal parameters that we want to
extract from the data, including period and amplitude.
After that, further analysis depends on the variables
measured. It may be appropriate to determine a design of
statistical analysis before starting the experiment in
order to obtain meaningful results. A number of experiments have been performed with such a timing that no matter how the data are analyzed, on the basis of what we
know of the hormone kinetics or of the assay procedure,
no meaningful information can be obtained.

VAN CAUTER: So far, our methodology has been used
over the last 2 years to analyze about 500 hormonal profiles and has generally provided a useful description of
the data. The procedure has been fully described and
published and the program is available to everyone. I am
willing to assist in its implementation without participating in any other aspect of the study. There are some
other approaches which may be more suitable in certain
types of chronobiological data collected in endocrinology.
At some point, it may be interesting to review all the
statistical approaches which have been proposed to analyze
endocrine rhythms.

ROSSMAN: Except for the way of performing the procedure, the cosinor is a least square fit. The type of analy-

sis provided by Van Cauter's method is not the only way to describe a time series. I believe that the steps of her method involving the Fourier transform and the Rao test on the acrophases are legitimate. The further definition of parameters deduced from the significant best-fit curve is, in my opinion, an interpretative process. If the outputs of the significant Fourier components were used as statistical variables, the procedure would be sounder.

VAN CAUTER: I disagree. If the parameters characterizing each of the Fourier components, namely, the phase and the amplitude, were to be taken into account instead of equivalent parameters deduced from the curve obtained by addition of these significant components, a larger number of parameters would have to be dealt with and the interpretation would be more difficult. Adding up the significant components does not generate any new parameter, it instead summarizes the information.

ROSSMAN: I think that the detection of the significant components ought to be the end point of your analysis.

REINBERG: Coming back to the standard parameters used in chronobiological analysis, I would like to know whether it is possible to determine the exact period of a circadian rhythm when sampling occurs only over one 24-hour span. It is a critical question. For example, as we discussed earlier, in patients with manic depression and in comatose subjects, it would be interesting to know whether their circadian period differs from 24 hours. Professor Halberg has been using the cosinor to study this problem. Do you know of any other procedure?

VAN CAUTER: It is probably impossible to determine the exact length of a circadian period from chronobiological observations collected over one 24-hour cycle. One

needs at least two or three consecutive cycles. If, in a
homogeneous set of 24-hour profiles, every individual best-
fit pattern includes a circadian component of period shorter than 24-hours, it is tempting to conclude that the
actual period is indeed shorter than 24 hours. However,
in our experience, the confidence interval for the acrophase of a hormonal profile sampled every 15 minutes over
a 24-hour span, is usually of about one hour and almost
never shorter than 50 minutes. Therefore, it is dangerous
to conclude that the circadian period is shorter or longer
than 24 hours on the basis of observations over one 24-hour
span.

COPINSCHI: It appears from all data which were presented and discussed that we should try to analyze individual data and no more transverse means. Does everybody
agree?

REINBERG: It depends on the aim of your study. If
you want to study a group phenomenon such as a given
physiological parameter in a group of so-called healthy
subjects, a transverse profile is adequate. If you want
to investigate a given subject, a longitudinal study is
necessary.

COPINSCHI: The point is that, even if you study a
group, the analysis of transverse means may mask some
phenomena and result in artefactual conclusions.

REINBERG: This is true. However, in a problem such
as aging, investigators study several groups of subjects
of comparable age and this is not valid since they are
studying several groups of ages instead of aging. It is
difficult to obtain a longitudinal study of aging in a
human. It is an important problem of data gathering which
is also encountered in chronobiology.

VAN CAUTER: The calculation of a transverse mean

profile for a group of individuals is perfectly legitimate
if it has been previously established that each of the individual profiles presents the same reproducible characteristics. For example, if 10 individual 24-hour profiles
of prolactin all exhibit a significant nocturnal increase
which can be quantitated and reported in a table, the presentation of a transverse mean to illustrate this property
is adequate. However, what has often been published is a
transverse mean profile incorporating individual profiles
where the characteristic looked after was absent. Then,
the transverse mean shows characteristics for the group of
subjects which were really only present in a certain percentage of the individuals.

ROSSMAN: Are you recommending that the neurologists
stop doing evoked potentials?

VAN CAUTER: I do not see the relevance of the question.

ROSSMAN: The relevance is that an evoked potential
is a transverse mean of about 1,000 to 2,000 samplings
which is used to test the neural function of an individual.

VAN CAUTER: There are not many similarities between
summing up electrical impulses from different parts of the
brain of a given individual and averaging hormonal profiles obtained in different individuals. In the first
case, one looks at a global response whereas in the other,
one investigates the reproducibility of a given characteristic in a series of individuals.

ROSSMAN: The transverse mean is a very useful way of
gathering information. If an investigator looks at your
slide showing the fictive data on six individuals and tries
to draw a general conclusion from these data, he should
not be doing research.

BARDIN: By and large, statistics are a way of pooling data. When one uses statistics, one should know what one is doing. It is often not the case in biology because many biologists don't know statistics well enough. One cannot make a universal statement that transverse means should not be used in biology. Sometimes they are very useful. For example, the pooling of hormonal data collected during the menstrual cycle can give a good summary of the information and no more can be learned from looking at the individual patterns. However, only ovulatory cycles should be considered. The procedure would be inadequate if anovulatory cycles were included.

ROBYN: Statistical analyses can be applied only if specific criteria are fulfilled. Unfortunately, it is not always the case in biology. In some papers, one really wonders whether the application of the statistical procedure was valid. What is difficult with the data we have to deal with here is the fairly large interindividual variability. Pooling the data often masks individual characteristics. Maybe one way to deal with this problem would be to define a reference point in the 24-hour cycle and to align the data.

KRIEGER: Dr. Aschoff has proposed and applied successfully to some hormonal patterns the use of mid-sleep or sleep onset as reference point. That smoothes out some of the inter-individual variability. Taking such types of reference points may make some rhythms apparent whereas otherwise they would seem to be out of phase with each other. Regarding the use of transverse versus individual data, it is not always possible, especially in animal studies, to investigate the same subject sequentially. A number of animal studies have attempted to demonstrate or to deny the presence of a periodicity on the basis of sacrifices of groups of animals at different time points. If such a procedure is used when constant conditions are perturbed or an additional variable is introduced, individual variations may be completely missed especially if some animals are free-running or phase-shifted.

ROBYN: During the menstrual cycle, one tries to define relationships between different hormonal patterns and this is facilitated by using the LH surge as a reference point. To look for such relationships between 24-hour profiles is much more difficult because of the complexity of the data. In a transverse mean of PRL patterns, the episodic fluctuations will be smoothed out because they do not occur at the same time in each individual. However, significant secretory episodes during daytime are apparent on individual profiles.

VAN CAUTER: The lack of inter-individual synchronization in human studies is indeed one of the major problems encountered in analyzing pooled data. Animals can be synchronized before the investigation by being maintained on a fixed L-D cycle for a certain period of time. It is much more difficult to synchronize human subjects.

QUABBE: How do you deal with missing data in a series of consecutive hormonal values? In our experiments, blood sampling was performed at 30 minute intervals, and when a data was missing, we interpolated it linearly. Is this procedure valid?

VAN CAUTER: It depends on the type of variation you are considering. If you study a circadian variation using 24-hour profiles obtained at 30-minute intervals, to interpolate linearly one or two missing data will not affect much your estimation of the circadian rhythm since the interpolation will not add any new fluctuation but instead smooth the variation. If you look at episodic secretion, then interpolating missing data in a series obtained at 30-minute intervals will bias the estimation and the section where the data are missing should be left out from the analysis.

QUABBE: We were looking for a 4-hour periodicity in a profile sampled every 15 minutes.

VAN CAUTER: I would discard the section of the profile where data were missing unless only one sample was missing.

RELATION BETWEEN SLEEP AND HORMONAL SECRETION

COPINSCHI: In the course of this Workshop, discrepancies between the results obtained by different groups were apparent. At least, two explanations are possible. First, it could be that the different groups were not measuring exactly the same hormonal compound because they used different assays. Second, the analysis of sleep and of the relation between sleep stages and hormonal peaks was not performed in the same way in different centers and this could also lead to discrepancies.

DESIR: Dr. Rossman agrees with us that we need a more accurate procedure to assign hormonal data to the concomitant event in the sleep record. I am however surprised by Dr. Rossman's statement that investigators who include in the calculation of transverse means profiles or sections of profiles where the characteristic under study is absent should quit research. In my opinion, the transverse means of REM - non-REM cycles which formed the basis for the claim that PRL elevations were concomitant with non-REM stages did indeed include individual cycles where no such relation was seen. The authors referred to this by writing that "most but not all" PRL increases were concomitant with SW sleep. In our hands, this relationship was also present in a certain percentage, maybe 25 or 30%, of all

the cycles studied but certainly not in the majority of
them. Thus, in my opinion, the transverse mean of all
cycles shows a characteristic which is not systematically
found in individual patterns. We have however to complete
all our calculations to reach a final conclusion.

COPINSCHI: Do you think that it would be useful to
put all the raw data regarding the PRL-sleep relationship
of Dr. Parker and of our group in the hands of one team of
neurologists in order to get an independent analysis using
standardized procedures?

DESIR: I do not believe that the discrepancy results
from the neurological part of our studies, namely, the
scoring of sleep stages. The problem really arise when
hormonal data, collected at 15- or 20-minute intervals,
have to be assigned to neurological events, scored at 20-
second intervals. Maybe we have to use a different method
of sleep analysis than the scoring standardized by Rechtstaffen and Kales over 15 years ago.

ROSSMAN: I do not disagree with anything Dr. Desir
said. I am not claiming that variations in PRL secretion
are dominated by the REM - non-REM cyclicity. Not every
REM is associated with a nadir and not every non-REM is
associated with an elevation. The transverse mean indeed
is not describing every individual pattern. An analysis
of variance of the data across time might give further
support to our results.

ROBYN: Again, we have here a problem of reference
point in the REM - non-REM cycle. Maybe there is a way to
perform a transverse mean which would show the individual
characteristics by defining an adequate zero point in the
REM - non-REM cycle.

DESIR: I do not believe that the discrepancy in our results is entirely related to the choice of a reference point in the REM - non-REM cycle although this is of course a procedure needing further standardization.

ROBYN: It could also be that the structure of sleep was different in Brussels and in Southern California. The quality of sleep may be very important regarding the type of relationship that can be observed. Others however have also had troubles confirming this relationship between PRL bursts and REM - non-REM cyclicity.

KRIEGER: To those of us who have been trying to correlate changes in sleep EEG with hormonal fluctuations, I would like to ask whether we have enough information concerning which events are meaningful in the various stages of sleep and in the hormonal variations to justify the expenditure of a detailed analysis of their possible correlations. Past studies trying to correlate standardized sleep records with hormonal variations have resulted in a relative paucity of positive findings. Before extending such correlative studies, is it possible to define what we should look for and what type of information we should try to extract?

ROSSMAN: REM is certainly the event which is easiest to identify in the sleep EEG. We have difficulties trying to make associations for the other stages of sleep. Start and end of stage II or slow wave sleep are often difficult to define. I personally don't believe that the sleep stage is a predominant control of nocturnal hormonal secretion. The relationship between REM - non-REM cycles and PRL episodes is a result which reflects the neural pathways involved in controlling PRL secretion.

KRIEGER: Little is known at the present time about the substrates underlying the various sleep stages. We try to use the sleep stages as an intermediate to reach the level of neural controls. I believe that the state of the art is not good enough yet to rely on it.

ROSSMAN: I agree with that.

QUABBE: There is, at the present time, no proof for the hypothesis that the relationship between hormonal secretion and sleep is neuronal. Therefore, we do not know what is the delay between the occurrence of a certain sleep stage or whatever generates it and the secretion by the pituitary. We assume that the relation is neural, that neural pathways are fast and that therefore the delay is short, probably a few seconds. Actually, the delay involved in the transmission from the locus coerulens, if this would be involved in controlling REM sleep, to the hypothalamus, then to the releasing hormone, then to the pituitary and then to peripheral hormonal levels is unknown. Even the description I just gave makes several assumptions for which there is no proof at the present time. The problem is thus not at the level of the reading of the EEG and the determination of REM, even if one or two minutes are misinterpreted, but is at the level of the blood sampling which we perform at intervals much longer than the 20-second epochs of the sleep record. We try to correlate EEG events recorded at 20-second intervals and hormonal values obtained at 15-minute intervals. We have also developed a computer approach, similar to that of Dr. Van Cauter, but we do not have results yet.

DESIR: Our purpose in obtaining sleep records in the jet lag study was primarily to control the amount and quality of sleep of our volunteers before and after travel. The study of possible correlations between hormonal events and REM - non-REM cycles was a secondary output. Our aim was not to demonstrate that hormonal secretion was con-

trolled by sleep stages but to assess the sleep-activity
cycle of our subjects.

KRIEGER: It is perfectly valid to assess the quality
of sleep to find out to which category the subjects belong.
For instance, there has been a number of studies on hormonal changes in aging, a process during which sleep is
modified, and to use sleep records to monitor this variable
is adequate. Trying to use the sleep stages to relate
hormonal secretion to certain control mechanisms is probably premature, considering the present state of knowledge.

DESIR: In addition, our language is not the same as
the one used by sleep neurologists who, for instance, define different types of REM stages.

QUABBE: We have deprived animals of either REM sleep
or slow wave sleep. This may be a better way to investigate possible effects on hormonal secretion than to calculate statistical correlations. However, we found that it
was relatively easy to deprive the animal of slow wave
sleep and still maintain a normal pattern of REM sleep but
the converse was impossible. I assume the same difficulty
would be encountered in humans.

VIGNERI: We must be cautious in considering the
plasma levels we measure as direct indicators of hormonal
secretion. For example, if at a certain point, we have a
very elevated hormone concentration in blood, a further
increase in hormonal secretion will result only in a small
change in plasma level which we would not even consider
as a peak. Such artefactual interpretations occur often.

HORMONAL PROFILES IN PATHOLOGIES AND AFTER DRUG ADMINISTRATION

JAQUET: I would like to ask a question regarding the
modifications of the PRL nyctohemeral pattern induced by

neuroleptics. The Belgian group and Boyar and Finkelstein
have shown persistence of the normal pattern of PRL in
estrogen stimulated states, such as pregnancy. Only at the
end of pregnancy or when the estrogen levels were in a high
range were there alterations. What happens during a
chronical treatment with phenothiazine or similar drugs?
Besides a report on one case by Dr. Meltzer, little data
seem to be available in the literature. Is anyone aware
of other studies?

ROBYN: As far as I know, there are no such data.
Moreover, the type of pattern present after the treatment
has been interrupted is not known either. Investigators
have a tendency to study the effect of drugs after they
are administered but not after withdrawal.

JAQUET: We have some preliminary data. The decrease
in PRL level depends on the type of drug but is generally
very rapid whereas the effect on the 24-hour pattern of
PRL is slow. Meltzer showed that 72 hours after withdrawal, the PRL levels had returned to normal values.

ROBYN: Were these studies based on single doses?

JAQUET: No, they were based on long-term treatment.

REINBERG: I would like to make a general comment.
Last year, in Paris, we had as part of the Congress of
Pharmacology a section on chronoendocrinology where times
of administration of the drug were discussed. There was
a general agreement that, not only the time of the day,
but also the time of the year, has to be taken into account, whether it is a single dose treatment or chronic
administration. This seems to be a critical data in
gathering information regarding drug effects. In the case
of corticosteroids, there is an abundant literature to
support this concept. We also showed that the effects of

HCG depend on the time of the day and on the time of the
year. I am ready to bet that, for many other variables,
these temporal factors are critical. Attention has to
be called upon controlling these factors in pharmacological studies.

COPINSCHI: Regarding rhythms in patients with pituitary tumors, I was very impressed by Dr. Jaquet's data.
Such data are very important as far as the patho-physio-
logy of the disease is concerned. I would hypothesize
that diseases such as acromegaly, prolactin adenoma and
Cushing's disease are of pituitary origin.

KRIEGER: At the moment, it is not possible to make
an all-or-none statement. The data available, even the
data on recovery unless there is a very long time course,
do not allow to rule out the possibility that there was
a primary inciting effect to produce the adenoma and that
there is a delay before the appearance of other adenomas.
The fact that the remaining pituitary function is suppressed is however an argument against this view. It may
be an over-simplification to consider a single etiology for
all adenomas. The 24-hour periodicity may be restored in
some patients with Cushing's disease but not in all of
them. Some, but not all, acromegalics respond to treatment. There may be at least two etiologies of these
diseases.

COPINSCHI: If after surgery, there is no return to
normal, you wonder whether surgery was complete. Also,
the fact that some patients are sensitive to drug administration is not a strong argument against the hypothesis
of pituitary origin because pituitary tumor cells have
been shown to be sensitive to a number of drugs in vitro.
How many years of cure would you consider as necessary to
prove the pituitary origin?

KRIEGER: This is purely arbitrary. There have been cases of adenomectomy where there has been a cure and then a recurrence. You may say that the surgery missed micro-adenomas but this is not sure. Also, both for PRL adenomas and for Cushing's disease, there has been a pathological demonstration of changes such as hyperplasia in the absence of adenomas. As far as drug action on pituitary is concerned, certain drugs indeed have been shown to have some effect on pituitary function in vitro. However, some of the drugs that are used for treatment have not yet been shown to have any in vitro effect on the pituitary. Moreover, two cases of acromegaly with pituitary adenoma have demonstrated circulating GH releasing factor of ectopic origin. Therefore, I don't think we can make a final statement regarding the origin of pituitary adenoma.

DESIR: A few years ago, Dr. Krieger reported abnormalities in the 24-hour profile of PRL in a few patients with Cushing's disease. Has this study been confirmed in larger series of patients? Are abnormalities in the PRL pattern a potential diagnosis tool for Cushing's disease?

KRIEGER: Our observation was that the 24-hour pattern of PRL was different in patients with adrenal adenoma and hyperproduction of cortisol and in patients with pituitary-dependent Cushing's disease. In the adrenal adenoma case, the PRL periodicity was normal whereas the nocturnal rise was absent in patients with Cushing's disease. We have not studied patients before and after microadenomectomy to see if the periodicity was restored after surgery. Patients with Cushing's disease who were brought into remission by pituitary irradiation and became thus eucortisolemic had no resumption of a normal periodicity. This could mean that the therapy was just decreasing the disease state without curing the condition. An interesting question is: "What is the basis for hyperprolactinemia in patients with

Cushing's disease?" If one assumes the presence of a pituitary adenoma, is it a multi-hormonal tumor with two types of hypersecreting cells which might then explain the differences between findings in adrenal adenomas and findings in pituitary adenomas? There are animal models of tumors which secrete both ACTH and PRL and may thus be responding to a common stimulus. If you make the assumption of neurotransmitter involvement, serotoninergic stimulation of PRL cells and ACTH cells could be hypothesized.

JAQUET: A theoretical possibility regarding the ACTH-PRL interaction in Cushing's disease would be that the endorphins secreted by the corticotroph cells compete with the dopaminergic control of PRL cells. We actually know that endorphin competes with dopamine, either at the hypothalamic level, or directly at the interface between dopamine and the pituitary receptors for dopamine. There is thus the possibility that the hypersecretion of endorphin could compete with the dopamine system and block it, either at the hypothalamic level or at the pituitary level. It is possible to test this hypothesis in vivo by using naloxone to block endorphin production in hyperprolactinemic states. We have some preliminary data showing no effect on the basal level of PRL but some effects on dynamic tests of PRL secretion. This could be a working hypothesis. Regarding the origin of the disease, we have a situation which we would describe in French as "un serpent qui se mord la queue" (the snake which is biting its tail). We should not forget that the first investigators who provoked the growth of a tumor did it by injecting oestradiol. Then, when these tumors were transferred in vitro, their secretory output shifted spontaneously. The GH_3 clones secreted GH and PRL and then sub-clones only GH. It is thus impossible to discuss the point of the localization of the initial disturbance.

KRIEGER: The hypothesis regarding the endorphin-
PRL interaction is interesting. However, one has to
determine whether naloxone is not affecting ACTH secretion. We and others have performed such studies. Whereas, in normal controls, we have no effect of naloxone on
ACTH levels, in Cushing's disease and Nelson's syndrome,
ACTH levels are markedly lowered by naloxone.

ROBYN: Recently, Dr. Pasteels showed that ACTH and
PRL were present in the same neurones and neuronal termi-
nals inside the hypothalamus.

FRAMEWORK FOR POSSIBLE INTERNATIONAL COLLABORATION

VAN CAUTER: We would like to propose a framework
of international collaboration in the field of hormonal
circadian rhythms in man. It often happens that, when
studying hormonal periodicities in pathologies or after
drug administration, control patterns, though extensively
described in the literature, are not available to the
investigators, who have then, in order to be able to make
quantitative comparisons, to repeat long, tedious and
expensive control studies. At the present time, it seems
that largely enough information on rhythms of pituitary
hormones and cortisol in control subjects has been collected and reported in the literature. Pooling the data
collected in the different centers around the world would
probably show that over a hundred control profiles are
available for each pituitary hormone, except for β-LPH.
One of the aims of an Euratom Workshop as this one is to
foster international collaboration. We would like to submit to your consideration a proposal consisting of creating
a data bank of 24-hour hormonal profiles in control subjects
in order to permit exchange of data. The data bank could
be extended in a further step by including information on

pathological subjects. This proposal should now be discussed in order to see if a general agreement on the
principle of this collaboration can be reached.

KRIEGER: It might be valuable to have a central
facility where the nature of the study, the characteristics of the subjects, the methods of analysis and of
collection and the data could be codified according to
certain criteria and a retrieval system would be available. This would allow the investigator or the person
who would like to use this information for statistical
analysis to have access to the data. Also, providing
access to computer programs for data analysis might also
be a meaningful way of collaborating. Simply listing
available data, with a careful description of how they
were obtained would already be useful.

WEEKE: I think that it is a good idea if a full
description of the methods is provided.

ROSSMAN: Will you calculate transverse means?

VAN CAUTER: I do not propose to analyze the data
which would be made available. I propose to make their
exchange possible.

QUABBE: We have performed a prospective study on
acromegalic patients in West Germany. We gathered about
250 - 300 patients. All the 9 participating clinics were
enthusiastic about the idea. The return of data from a
very strict protocol varied between 40 and 60%. Your
proposal consists instead of a retrospective sampling of
data, at least the way it is presented now. I would not
be surprised if the return would not surpass what we obtained. The variability of the conditions under which the
data were collected may invalid comparisons. I would be
ready myself to give access to all my data but I would be
hesitant to rely on other data unless I would know exactly

what was the methodology. For instance, when we do a
study on humans, we submit them to two preparatory
nights for adaptation. Some investigators perform only
one preparatory night and some not at all.

COPINSCHI: Of course, if we implement such a pro-
ject, we have to make a very careful and strict protocol
and try to ensure its application. Personally, I don't
find that 40 - 50% of responses is a bad result.

VAN CAUTER: Maybe we should keep this discussion
focused on the principle of such a collaboration, which
is: enough control data seem to have been collected and
described to allow investigators to have access to data
on adequate controls through a central facility. The
participants to this Workshop have collected approximately 80% of data on rhythms of pituitary hormones
published in the literature. This Workshop offers an
opportunity to develop an actual collaboration.

ROBYN: The principle is excellent. I don't know
however if we know enough on the physiology of rhythms
to be able to apply it realistically. The data have
been collected on presumably normal and healthy subjects.
But what are our criteria of normality? Maybe we should
look for relationships between the characteristics of
the subjects and the type of profiles recorded. The amount
of data available would allow such investigations which
would help us to define what is a "normal" profile. The
inter-individual heterogeneity is often large in controls and even more in pathologies.

VAN CAUTER: If a standard methodology of analysis
would be applied to all available control profiles of a
given hormone, confidence intervals could be defined and
used to determine the "normality" of a profile. This type

of research program goes well beyond our proposal of collaboration. It is an excellent suggestion, probably difficult to implement. I personally believe that it is the right approach to define group statistics from 200 rather than, as usually in the literature, 10 to 20 profiles.

ROSSMAN: With the discrepancies between different investigators that have appeared during this Workshop, grouping data to define normality may not be the proper thing to do. I certainly don't want to define my normal population from a group including disparate results. I would be willing to give access to our data for further analysis using your methodology but everyone may not accept that this is a standardized methodology which will define normality.

VAN CAUTER: The standardized methodology should not include only one procedure.

KRIEGER: The methodology of analysis to be used depends on the parameters considered and on what one wants to describe. Dr. Van Cauter made reference to some of the diagrams on endocrine periodicites in the chapter by Aschoff and myself in "Endocrinology", edited by DeGroot. In this chapter, Dr. Aschoff pooled the results of a number of studies reporting periodicities using a common reference time point and the concordance between results from different centers became amazing. This type of approach is adequate for circadian variations but probably not for episodic secretion. No one can accept someone else's data unless he or she knows how they have been obtained. Then, a decision can be made as to whether they constitute controls for valid comparisons.

COPINSCHI: How does Dr. Van Cauter plan to implement such a proposal from the practical point of view?

VAN CAUTER: A report on this Workshop has to be pre-
pared for Euratom. This report could include tentative
protocols of international collaboration which could be
forwarded to all participants. In return, they would
indicate their willingness to participate in one or
other of the protocols.

LIST OF PARTICIPANTS

ASCHOFF, J., Max-Planck-Institut für Verhaltensphysiologie, D-8131 Erling-Andechs, F.R.G.

BARDIN, C.W., The Population Council, The Rockefeller University, York Avenue and 66th Street, New York, New York 10021, U.S.A.

CAUFRIEZ, A., Clinique de Gynécologie et d'Obstétrique et Laboratoire de Gynécologie et de Recherches sur la Reproduction Humaine, Université Libre de Bruxelles, Hôpital Universitaire Saint-Pierre, Rue Haute 322, B-1000 Bruxelles, Belgium.

CERESA, F., Clinica Medica Generale e Terapia Medica B, Università di Torino, Via Genova 3, I-10126 Torino, Italy.

CONTE-DEVOLX, B., Service d'Endocrinologie et des Maladies du Métabolisme, Hôpital de la Conception, F-13385 Marseille Cedex 4, France.

COPINSCHI, G., Département d'Endocrinologie, Hôpital Universitaire Saint-Pierre et Laboratoire de Médecine Expérimentale, Université Libre de Bruxelles, Rue Evers 2, B-1000 Bruxelles, Belgium.

DESIR, D., Département d'Endocrinologie, Hôpital Universitaire Saint-Pierre et Laboratoire de Médecine Expérimentale, Université Libre de Bruxelles, Rue Evers 2, B-1000 Bruxelles, Belgium.

DUMONT, J.E., Institut de Recherche Interdisciplinaire, Faculté de Médecine, Université Libre de Bruxelles, Rue Evers 2, B-1000 Bruxelles, Belgium.

FEVRE-MONTANGE, M., Laboratoire d'Endocrinologie, Hôpital de l'Antiquaille, Rue de l'Antiquaille 1, F-69321 Lyon Cedex 1, France.

GOLSTEIN, J., Institut de Recherche Interdisciplinaire, Faculté de Médecine, Université Libre de Bruxelles, Rue Evers 2, B-1000 Bruxelles, Belgium.

HANSEN, A.P., 1st and 2nd University Clinic of Internal Medicine, Kommunehospitalet, DK-8000 Aarhus C, Denmark.

JAQUET, P., Clinique Endocrinologique, CHU Timone, Boulevard Jean Moulin, F-13385 Marseille Cedex 4, France.

KRIEGER, D.T., Department of Medicine, Division of Endocrinology, Mount Sinai School of Medicine of the City University of New York, Fifth Avenue and 100th Street, New York, New York 10029, U.S.A.

LAGOGUEY, M., Laboratoire de Physiologie, Equipe de
Recherches de Chronobiologie Humaine, Fondation A. de
Rothschild, Rue Manin 29, F-75019 Paris, France.

L'HERMITE, M., Service de Gynécologie-Obstétrique, Hôpital
Universitaire Brugmann, Place A. Van Gehuchten 4,
B-1020 Bruxelles, Belgium.

MENDLEWICZ, J., Service de Psychiatrie Clinique, Cliniques
Universitaires de Bruxelles, Hôpital Erasme,
Université Libre de Bruxelles, Route de Lennick 808,
B-1070 Bruxelles, Belgium.

MINORS, D.S., Department of Physiology, Stopford Building,
University of Manchester, Manchester M13 9PT, United
Kingdom.

QUABBE, H.J., Endokrinologische Abteilung, Medizinische
Klinik und Poliklinik (WE 1), Klinikum Steglitz (FB2),
Freie Universität Berlin, Hindenburgdamm 30, D-1000
Berlin 45, F.R.G.

REINBERG, A., Laboratoire de Physiologie, Equipe de
Recherches de Chronobiologie Humaine, Fondation A. de
Rothschild, Rue Manin 29, F-75019 Paris, France.

ROBYN, C., Clinique de Gynécologie et d'Obstétrique et
Laboratoire de Gynécologie et de Recherches sur la
Reproduction Humaine, Université Libre de Bruxelles,
Hôpital Universitaire Saint-Pierre, Rue Haute 322,
B-1000 Bruxelles, Belgium.

ROSSMAN, L.G., Endocrine Section, Veterans Administration
Hospital, 3350 La Jolla Village Drive, San Diego,
California 92161, U.S.A.

ROULIER, R., Service d'Endocrinologie et des Maladies du
Métabolisme, Hôpital de la Conception, F-13385
Marseille Cedex 4, France.

VAN CAUTER, E., Institut de Recherche Interdisciplinaire,
Faculté de Médecine, Université Libre de Bruxelles,
Rue Evers 2, B-1000 Bruxelles, Belgium and Thyroid
Study Unit, Department of Medicine, Box 138, The
University of Chicago, 950 E. 59th Street, Chicago,
Illinois 60637, U.S.A.

VANHAELST, L., Dienst Endocrinologie, Academisch Ziekenhuis,
Vrije Universiteit Brussel, B-1090 Brussel, Belgium.

VIGNERI, R., Istituto di Endocrinologia, Via Ofelia 35,
I-95124 Catania, Italy.

WEEKE, J., 2nd University Clinic of Internal Medicine,
Kommunehospitalet, DK-8000 Aarhus C, Denmark.